AF323128

Non-Umbilical Laparoscopic Entry Ports

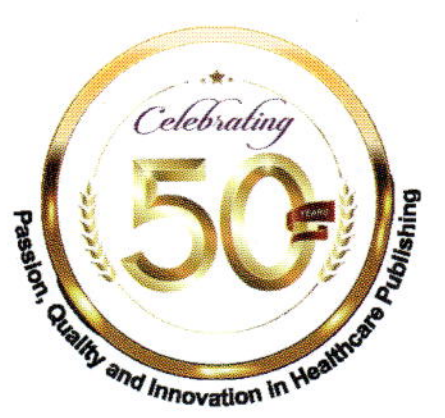

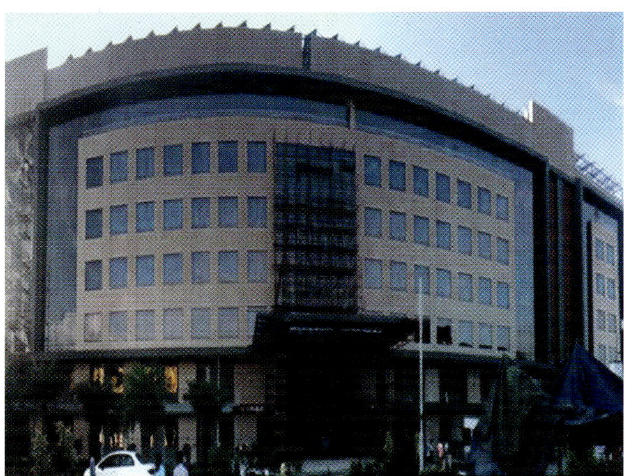

Vardhman Super Specialty Hospital, Muzaffarnagar, Uttar Pradesh, India

Non-Umbilical Laparoscopic Entry Ports

Nutan Jain MS
Director
Department of Obstetrics and Gynecology
Vardhman Super Specialty Hospital
Muzaffarnagar, Uttar Pradesh, India

Forewords
Harry Reich
Ceana Nezhat
Pawanindra Lal
Parveen Bhatia
Sven Becker

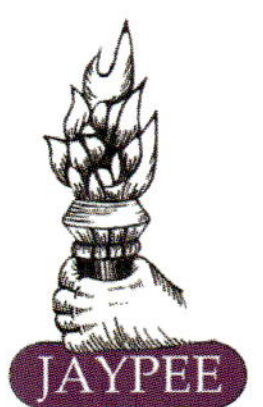

JAYPEE BROTHERS MEDICAL PUBLISHERS
The Health Sciences Publisher
New Delhi | London

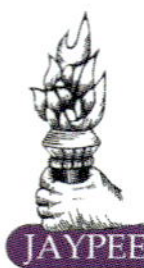 **Jaypee Brothers Medical Publishers (P) Ltd**

Headquarters

Jaypee Brothers Medical Publishers (P) Ltd
4838/24, Ansari Road, Daryaganj
New Delhi 110 002, India
Phone: +91-11-43574357
Fax: +91-11-43574314
E-mail: jaypee@jaypeebrothers.com

Overseas Office

JP Medical Ltd
83 Victoria Street, London
SW1H 0HW (UK)
Phone: +44 20 3170 8910
Fax: +44 (0)20 3008 6180
E-mail: info@jpmedpub.com

Website: www.jaypeebrothers.com
Website: www.jaypeedigital.com

Non-Umbilical Laparoscopic Entry Ports

First Edition: **2020**

ISBN 978-93-89776-45-4

Printed at: Samrat Offset Pvt. Ltd.

Dedication

This book is dedicated to all my worthy endoscopy fellows and trainees who contributed by trying and learning the "Jain point" entry in different types of challenging situations and thereby giving us insights to further improving and improvising the technique and bringing it up to its present methodology of almost flawless insertion of the first blind nonumbilicalentry port.

Contributors

Anadeep Chandi MS(Obs & Gyne) DNB
Fellow in Gynecology-Endoscopy at
Vardhman Super Specialty Hospital
Muzaffarnagar, Uttar Pradesh, India

Anshu Gupta MS(Obs & Gyne)
Senior Resident
Department of Obstetrics and
Gynecology
All India Institute of Medical Sciences
Rishikesh, Uttarakhand, India

Artin Ternamian MD FRCSC
Associate Professor
Department of Obstetrics and
Gynecology
Faculty of Medicine
University of Toronto
St Joseph's Health Centre, Toronto
Division of Gynecological Endoscopy
Toronto, Ontario, Canada

Aruna Arya MBBS MD
Assistant Professor
Department of Anatomy
Muzaffarnagar Medical College
Muzaffarnagar, Uttar Pradesh, India

Aruna Tantia MBBS MS DGO
Diploma in Gynecology-Endoscopic
Surgery(Germany) FMAS
ILS Hospitals
Kolkata, Howrah, Dum Dum, Agartala

Barıs Mulayim MD
Saglık Bilimleri University
Antalya Education and Research Hospital
Associate Professor
Department of Obstetrics and Gynecology
Supervisory Board Member of Turkish
Society for Gynecological Endoscopy
Vice-President of Antalya Branch Office
of Turkish Gynecology and
Obstetrics Society
Antalya, Turkey

Bhumika Bansal MS(Obs & Gyne)
Research Fellow in Gynecology-
Endoscopy at
Vardhman Super Specialty Hospital
Muzaffarnagar, Uttar Pradesh, India

Chetna Agarwal MS(Obs & Gyne)
Research Fellow in Gynecology-
Endoscopy at
Vardhman Super Specialty Hospital
Muzaffarnagar, Uttar Pradesh, India

CS Ramesh Babu MSc(Biology)
Associate Professor
Department of Anatomy
Muzaffarnagar Medical College
Muzaffarnagar, Uttar Pradesh, India

Gunjan Saxena MS(Obs & Gyne)
Head, Department of Reproductive
Medicine and Fertility
Apollo Spectra
Amritsar, Punjab, India

Harry Reich
Retired
Honorary Member, AAGL
Past President, ISGE, SLS
Southern Ocean Medical
Center, Hackensack—Meridian Health
Center, New Jersey, USA

Jonathan M Reich MD
Chairman
Department of Surgery
Southern Ocean Medical
Center, Hackensack—
Meridian Health Center
New Jersey, USA

Kaustubh Srivastava MS(Obs & Gyne)
Research Fellow in Gynecology-
Endoscopy at
Vardhman Super Specialty Hospital
Muzaffarnagar, Uttar Pradesh, India

Kiran Kumari Mandal
MS(Obs and Gyne)
Fellow in Gynecology-Endoscopy at
Vardhman Super Specialty Hospital
Muzaffarnagar, Uttar Pradesh, India

Medhavi Tomar MS(Gen Surg)
General and Laparoscopic Surgeon
Star Hospital and Laparoscopic Surgical
Center
Meerut, Uttar Pradesh, India

Monika Ranwa MS(Obs & Gyne)
Research Fellow in Gynecology-
Endoscopy at
Vardhman Super Specialty Hospital
Muzaffarnagar, Uttar Pradesh, India

Nutan Jain MS
Director
Department of Obstetrics and
Gynecology
Vardhman Super Specialty Hospital
Muzaffarnagar, Uttar Pradesh, India

Parima Jain MBBS MS(Obs & Gyne)
Research Fellow in Gynecology-
Endoscopy at
Vardhman Super Specialty Hospital
Muzaffarnagar, Uttar Pradesh, India

Prateek Gupta MBBS MS(Gen Surg)
MAMC(Delhi) MCH(Urology)
Department of Urology
All India Institute of Medical Sciences
Jodhpur, Rajasthan, India

Praveen Bhatia
MBBS MS(Gen Surg)
Consultant Surgeon and Medical
Director
Bhatia Global Hospital and
Endosurgery Institute
New Delhi, India

Priyanka Bansal
MS(Obs & Gyne) FICOG
Associate Professor
FH Medical College
Agra, Uttar Pradesh, India

Rhythm Bhalla MS(Obs & Gyne)
Research Fellow in Gynecology-
Endoscopy at
Vardhman Super Specialty Hospital
Muzaffarnagar, Uttar Pradesh, India

Rooma Sinha MD DNB MNAMS
Hon. Professor (AHERF)
Senior Consultant Gynecologist
Minimal Access and Robotic Surgeon
Apollo Health City
Hyderabad, Telangana, India

Rupa B MS
Consultant
Apollo Health City
Hyderabad, Telangana, India

Shivam Vatsal ASI ISO IASO
Senior Consultant
Department of Surgical Oncology
Sarvodaya Hospital and Research Center
Faridabad, Haryana, India

Siddharth Gupta
DNB(Gen Surg) FMAS FIAGES
Lifetime Member of ASI, SELSI and IHS
Fellow (Pursuing) in Advanced
Laparoscopy and Robotics
Gastroenterology Medical Centre and
Hospital
Coimbatore, Tamil Nadu, India

Sonam Singh MS(Obs & Gyne)
Research Fellow in Gynecology-
Endoscopy at
Vardhman Super Specialty Hospital
Muzaffarnagar, Uttar Pradesh, India

Sonika Mann MS(Obs & Gyne)
Research Fellow in Gynecology-
Endoscopy at
Vardhman Super Specialty Hospital
Muzaffarnagar, Uttar Pradesh, India

Sonil Srivastava MS(Obs & Gyne)
Consultant Laparoscopic Surgeon
Lake City Hospital
Bhopal, Madhya Pradesh, India

Sunil Gupta MS(Gen Surg)
Director
Jyoti Nursing Home
Muzaffarnagar, Uttar Pradesh, India

Swati Dubey MS(Obs & Gyne)
Research Fellow in Gynecology-
Endoscopy at
Vardhman Super Specialty Hospital
Muzaffarnagar, Uttar Pradesh, India

Swati Kanawa MS
Laparoscopic Surgeon, Infertility
Specialist and Gynecologist
Research Fellow in Gynecology-
Endoscopy at
Vardhman Super Specialty Hospital
Muzaffarnagar, Uttar Pradesh, India

Swati Varshney
MS(Obs & Gyne)
Research Fellow in Gynecology-
Endoscopy at
Vardhman Super Specialty Hospital
Muzaffarnagar, Uttar Pradesh, India

Vandana Jain MS
Consultant
Department of Obstetrics and
Gynecology
Vardhman Super Specialty Hospital
Muzaffarnagar, Uttar Pradesh, India

Foreword

Being asked to write a forward is always an honor but to do so for Dr Nutan Jain who I have greatly admired for many years is surely a pleasure. This book describes the rationale for Jain's point and explains it very well. I agree that perforation of large vessels would be extremely rare at this point. Usually I am more concerned about perforation of intestine in adhesion cases and thus I go higher, in the ninth intercostal space, as this area has served me well since 1990. But I must commend Dr Jain for presenting a technique much easier and safer for the average laparoscopic surgeon. I never liked Palmer's point as I never knew what I could get into there. I like the concept that I can 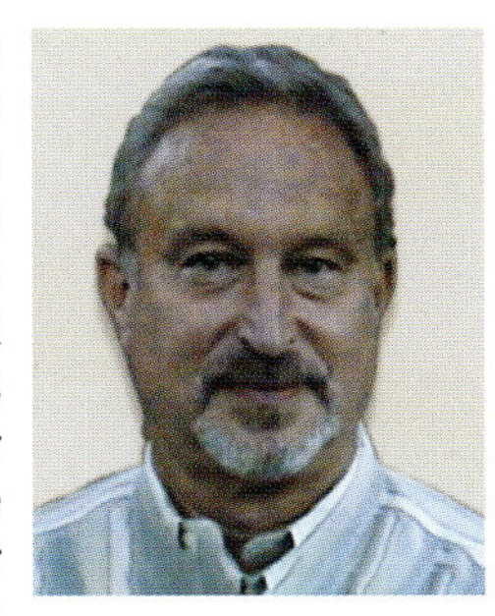 feel the ribs for my point and that the anterior-superior iliac spine is readily available for Dr Jain's point. Actually it seems that Dr Jain's point is the lowest of the three points and may be best for routine use.

Harry Reich
Retired
Honorary Member, AAGL
Past President, ISGE, SLS
Southern Ocean Medical Center, Hackensack—Meridian Health Center
New Jersey, USA

Foreword

Dr Nutan Jain has taken on the role of international educator and is revered as one of the most distinguished surgeons in the minimally invasive arena. Her focus on teaching is admirable. This book provides another opportunity for Dr Jain to share her innovative expertise on laparoscopic surgery with colleagues.

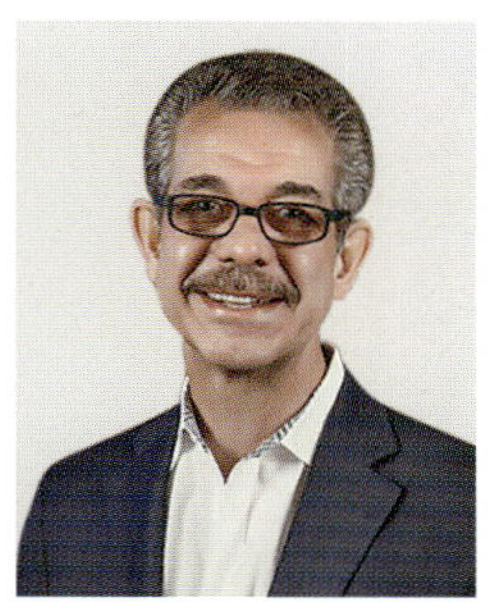

Video Assisted Laparoscopic Surgery, with and without robotic assistance, has become the most innovative and effective technique for performing intra-abdominal procedures. As advancements in technology and operative technique continue to develop, the basic principles of laparoscopic surgery remain pivotal when considering patient safety and outcomes. While instrument choice, energy source, and knowledge of pelvic anatomy are of utmost importance, abdominal entry remains the most critical step in laparoscopic surgery. To date, a single, ideal method of entry for all patients has yet to be described. The best approach is truly individualized, and must consider the patient's risk of prior adhesion formation, the possibility of distorted anatomy, size and contour of the pelvic organs, the patient's body habitus, and the planned surgical approach.

Umbilical port placement is the conventional method used to gain access to the abdominal cavity, and approaches include direct entry, the Veress needle technique, the open "Hassan" technique, or visual entry using an optical trocar. Complications include failed entry, bowel injury, inadequate exposure, vascular injury, and extraperitoneal insufflation. Several alternatives to blind port placement have been used when umbilical entry is deemed hazardous. These include Palmer's point, Left ninth intercostal space, and vaginal or uterine entry by way of natural orifice transluminal endoscopic surgery (NOTES). Perioperative ultrasonography has also been utilized to map out safe entry sites using periumbilical ultrasound-guided saline infusion (PUGSI). I agree "as the prevalence of surgical management increases, alternative entry sites will be necessary". Jain point is a novel entry site that has not been previously reported.

This book provides a brief overview of relevant abdominal anatomy and previously described abdominal entry techniques, while focusing more on the utility and application of new trocar entry sites. This detailed composition is a must-read for both aspiring laparoscopists, and master surgeons, alike.

Ceana Nezhat MD FACS FACOG
Fellowship Director, Nezhat Medical Center
Medical Director of Training & Education and
Director of Minimally Invasive Surgery & Robotics,
Northside Hospital, Atlanta Georgia
Adjunct Professor of Gynecology and Obstetrics, Emory University
Past President, Society of Reproductive Surgeons
Past President, American Association of Gynecologic Laparoscopists
Editor-in-Chief, Atlanta Medicine

Foreword

It gives me a great pleasure to write the foreword to the book entitled "Non-Umbilical Laparoscopic Entry Ports" by a pioneer laparoscopic gynecologist Dr Nutan Jain. In this book, which is itself, a rarity, as there are very limited books on port access in laparoscopic surgery, Dr Jain has taken the readers through the surgical anatomy of the abdominal wall and then discussed the existing alternate entry points that are already established. She then takes the readers through the challenges posed in entry especially in a previously scarred abdomen. The highlight of the book is the description of the "Jain point" which she has described after thousands of cases done using 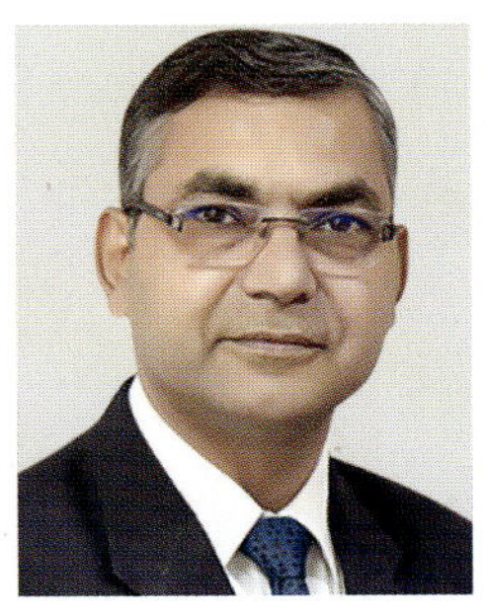 the same and the chapters related to these are authored by herself with detailed description of the evolution, rationale and the ergonomics of this point. This point was described her in her publication of 2016 in the Journal of Human Reproductive Sciences as an original article where Dr Jain described the point in 624 patients operated from 2010 to 2014. The Jain point has been described to be located in the left paraumbilical region, in a straight line drawn vertically upward from a point 2.5 cm medial and 10 cm above the anterior superior iliac spine.

Having described the safe technique for open trocar placement in laparoscopic surgery using the umbilical cicatrix tube which was published in Surgical Endoscopy in 2002 and later on the follow-up original article in 2012 on 6000 cases using the same technique, I am very happy to say that an Indian gynecologist has used her vast experience to help the surgical community by describing the Jain point for closed entry and reported it to be as safe as the Palmer's point. The advantage being that while placing it in the lower abdomen and laterally, this point becomes one of the ports for surgical procedure as well.

I am sure this publication will find favor with all practicing gynecologist and surgeons and will form a reference for all those who wish to acquire knowledge about open and closed access techniques. I congratulate, Dr Nutan Jain for a publication that has the potential to bring Indian surgery to an international pedestal.

Pawanindra Lal
MS DNB FIMSA FCLS FRCSEd FRCSGlasg FRCSEng FACS FAMS
Consultant Laparoscopic Gastrointestinal, Oncology and Bariatric Surgeon
Chairman, Division of Minimal Access Surgery
Head of Clinical Skills Centre
Editor-in-Chief, MAMC Journal of Medical Sciences
Vice-President, International College of Laparoscopic Surgeons
EC Member, Association of Surgeons of India
President, ASI Delhi Chapter
President Elect, Indian Hernia Society
Director Professor and Head
Department of Surgery
Maulana Azad Medical College (University of Delhi) and
Associated Lok Nayak Hospital
New Delhi, India

Foreword

"It is puncture itself that causes risk" was the bold statement by Dr Hans Jacobaeus (1879–1937), Inventor of Laparoscopy and Thoracoscopy in 1910. This century has made the surgeons, gynecologist, urologist, cardiac, ENT surgeon, etc. minimal access surgeons—the cerebral laborers rather than the manual laborers. Still, we have not reached "Zero harm goal" level surgeons.

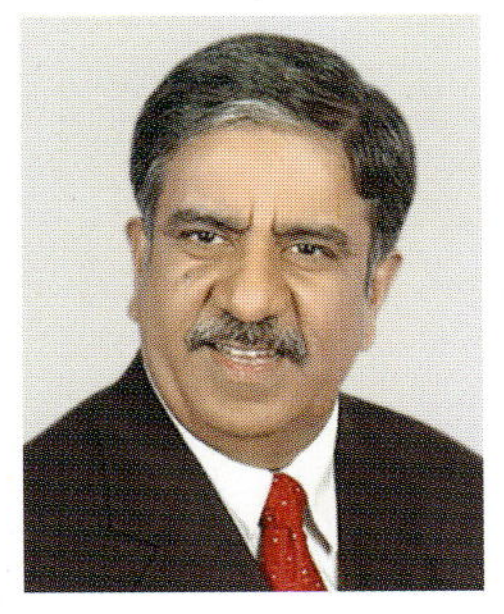

In specific situations like battered abdomen with previous abdominal surgeries scars, morbid obesity, complex ventral hernias, organomegaly, etc, the surgeon has to pray before entering into the pandora box to be safe. We strongly believe on "There is safety in more safety." Safety is the avoidance of a negative outcome; quality is the achievement of a positive outcome. To enter into the abdomen, umbilicus and nonumbilicus points have been described by both nonoptical and optical entries.

I must compliment, Dr Nutan Jain, the thinking surgeon (gynecologist), to write this book on a single theme-safety in abdominal wall access. 'Jain point' re-emphasizes the importance of relatively avascular horizontal line of umbilicus and the fixed bony landmark (anterior-superior iliac spine). Surgeon is always advised to think of all the three muscle layers of abdominal wall, i.e. external oblique, internal oblique and transversus abdominis at the time of blind Veress needle entry. The chances of injury to the viscera and vessels (including inferior epigastric vessels) are further reduced by this point entry.

Happy to note that one chapter has been dedicated to the complications of entry and exits. To be safe, "all entries and all exits must be shown by the camera person."

Dr Nutan Jain's immense experience, innovative thoughts and sharing of the knowledge in this color atlas is highly commendable. "Knowledge shared is Knowledge gained."

Parveen Bhatia
MS FRCS(Eng) FICS FIAGES(Hon) FMAS FIMSA FAIS FALS FCLS
Senior Consultant Laparoscopic, Bariatric and Robotic Surgeon
Institute of Minimal Access, Metabolic and Bariatric Surgery (IMAS)
Institute of Robotic Surgery (IRS)
Sir Ganga Ram Hospital, New Delhi, India
Medical Director
Bhatia Global Hospital and Endosurgery Institute, New Delhi
Editorial Board, Journal of Minimal Access Surgery
Author of 3 books: Laparoscopic Hernia Repair: A Step-by-Step Approach; Art of
Endosuturing: A Step-by-Step Approach; Comprehensive Laparoscopic Surgery

Foreword

Laparoscopy has become the most common approach to gynecologic surgery.

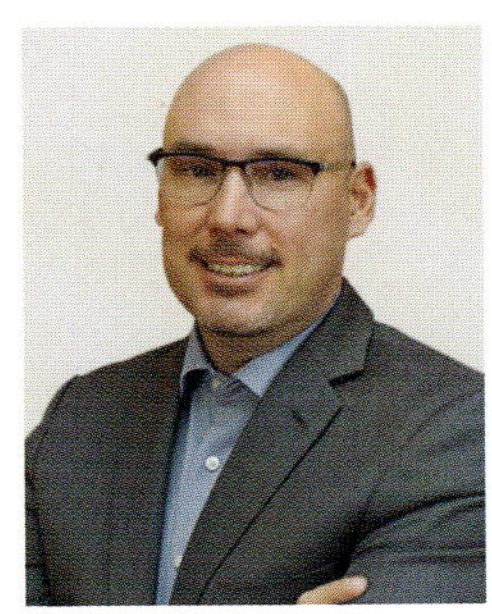

Hysterectomy, myomectomy, treatment of ovarian cysts, management of ectopic pregnancies, surgery for endometriosis, adhesiolysis, fertility-surgery and management of oncologic disease have all become standardized as minimally invasive surgeries.

While the command of the actual surgery is central to the art and science of laparoscopy, obtaining safe access to the abdominal cavity remains the first step of this surgery and is particularly for the less experiences surgeon—the most dangerous and complicated part of the procedure.

In this wonderful book, the focus is exactly on different laparoscopic entry-techniques. Dr Nutan Jain has to be commended for her efforts to thoroughly explain the different approaches, their histories, advantages and disadvantages. And also to introduce a new safe portal for laparoscopic entry, the Jain point, which could be feasible in many challenging situations.

This book is an excellent reference for those eager to learn about this basic part of everyday laparoscopy but also for the experienced surgeons as a review of the available options of entry in difficult situations.

Sven Becker MD PhD
Director, Frankfurt University Women's Hospital
Goethe University
Frankfurt, Germany

Preface

Laparoscopic entry has always been a daunting task, and, even, the most experienced laparoscopists would admit they still feel a relief after seeing safe entry in the face of a challenging case. Previous surgery is the first situation which alarms the surgeon to the possibility of periumbilical adhesions, rendering umbilicus a hazardous site to make entry. Palmer's point has been the trusted site by general surgeons, urologists and gynecologists for several decades, since the inception of operative laparoscopy. It has all the merits and few contraindications. But the contraindications such as, upper abdominal large gastropancreatic masses, upper abdominal 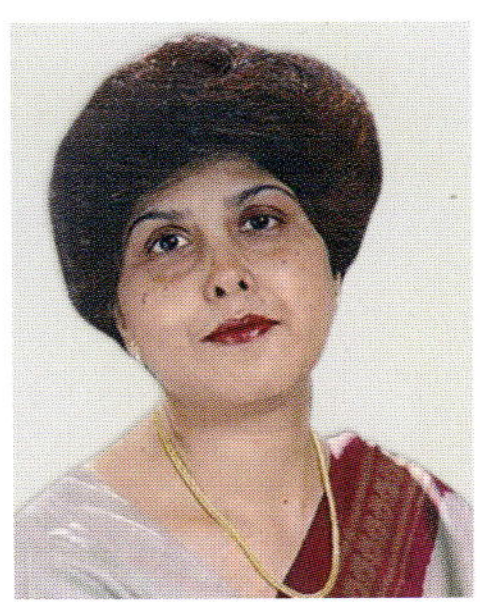 previous surgery scars as the open Kocher's incision, Chevron incision, enlarged spleen due to portal hypertension and bloated stomach, are formidable situations where there is a glaring need of an alternate nonumbilical entry port. Jain point offers a fresh thought, fresh perspective to laparoscopic entry in challenging situations. It is located in left paraumbilical position on a line drawn vertically upwards, 2.5 cm medial to ASIS. It is most versatile as can be used in all types of previous surgery scars. It is applicable in all body types for obesity, extremely thin and extreme lax abdomen patients.

By the medium of this book, we bring forth a new concept, a new approach which can make laparoscopic entry much safer. It can be used as a universal first blind entry port to avoid the major, retroperitoneal vessels beneath the umbilicus, a lurking fear at least in, the minds of novice endoscopist. Many a careers are nipped in the bud by the occurrence of catastrophic bleeding by major retroperitoneal vessels that lie beneath the umbilicus. By making first blind entry from Jain point this can be avoided.

This book has been presented as an atlas to clearly demonstrate a new technique. We have explained all existing entry points and their indications and contraindications, if any. We have elaborated a special section detailing the concept of Jain point entry, its evolution, rationale and ergonomics. The reader will go through the entire process by which this new safe entry port was tried, evolved and improvised over passage of time by the contributions of several endoscopy fellows and trainees over a decade. And now in its present technique, it is, almost infallible with very low complication rate, and very easy to learn and master in different clinical situations.

A separate section deals with all possible clinical situations such as in obese and very thin patients, extraordinary lax abdominal wall, large masses, previous surgeries and previous infectious pathologies. Jain point has favorable applications in general surgery also, hence, chapters defining its role in various general surgeries have been described. Ventral hernia and previous mesh hernia repair are one indication where compared to any entry point, Jain point is most suitable. Lastly a chapter on entry related complications. A chapter by endoscopy fellows on their experience of usage of Jain point entry summarizes the ease of learning.

I feel this book offers rich content with a very practical Cook Book such as steps with surgical snapshots feasible for both gynecologist and general surgeons, to help them tide over the challenging situations. It is a practical guide for budding as well as expert endoscopists.

Finding reference to Jain point in the Evidence-Based Clinical Decision Support the—UpToDate was an honor. With our several international presentations and peer-reviewed publications on Jain point, we present this book to "All Lovers and Learners of Innovations in Endoscopy".

Nutan Jain

Acknowledgments

As I sit to write this draft, I have immense feelings of gratitude for my fellows, trainees and junior consultants who tried Jain point, first blind port entry in laparoscopy. According to their level of expertise they kept on trying it in different clinical situations. Most of them conversant only with umbilical entry as a routine, found Jain point entry, a big relief to the lurking fear they have regarding first blind entry with sharp trocars. After having understood the anatomical rationale and methodology of Jain point they found it very easy and safe and none of them wanted to go back to umbilical entry. As their expertise grew they kept on making laparoscopic entries in previous surgery cases and other complex situations. Over last ten years the fellows and trainees kept changing but our perseverance to develop this entry point persisted. We finally managed to make the endoscopy world believe the new entry port. And this was accepted by surgeons and gynecologists alike. In situations of limitations to Palmer's point, the general surgeons also appreciated this new approach. And I keep getting positive feedbacks from endoscopy colleagues from every corner of the world. So, I sincerely express gratitude to all my colleagues, within gynecologist, urologists and general surgeon fraternity who have used Jain point entry and have instilled in us the confidence to move ahead.

My sincere thanks to many good friends who are illustrious members of AAGL, SLS, ISGE, ESGE, MESGE, APAGE, AMASI, SELSI, IAGES, USI and ICS. Technical discussions with them, suggestions and constructive criticism have kept us motivated all through and improvised the Jain point technique.

I thank the publisher M/s Jaypee Brothers Medical Publishers (P) Ltd, Mr JP Vij (Group Chairman) has steered this company through his dynamic leadership as one of the largest medical publisher in Asia. He is duly assisted by Ms Chetna Malhotra Vohra (Associate Director—Content Strategy) and Ms Kritika Dua (Senior Development Editor). My books have been translated in Chinese, Spanish and available worldwide due to their efforts. I feel happy that rightful dissemination of medical knowledge has become a virtual reality by their efforts.

I would like to acknowledge my hospital staff especially the Gyne-Endoscopy unit who have taken pride in latest developments in the department. The Junior Doctors, Fellows and Residents and other consultants working with me have been greatly helpful and enthusiastic about the project. I would especially mention Dr Sunil Gupta, Dr Vandana Jain, Dr Aruna Arya, Dr Anadeep Chandi, Dr Kiran Kumari Mandal and Dr Parima Jain who have worked day and night to fulfill this dream project. The general surgeons and urologist Dr Siddharth Gupta, Dr Prateek Gupta and Dr Shivam Vatsal an oncosurgeon have contributed immensely in shaping up this project.

My technical staff headed by Mr Pranay, Ms Nimisha Jain and Mr Vishram Singh duly assisted by Mr Saurabh, Ms Asha, Mr Bhopal Singh have given their best in giving high quality pictures, videos and data from OT records.

In the end, I would like to raise a toast to my family for their unique help and mental support during the compilation of this book. My husband, Dr Mukesh Jain and my son Dr Anubhav Jain, both Orthopedic Surgeons, have been my pillar of strength.

Dr Vandana Jain my daughter-in-law has been most enthusiastic about the usage of Jain point and this project.

Lastly, I would like to thank my teachers and mentors who enabled me to reach this point in my career. Nonetheless, I profusely thank my patients who posed faith in my skills.

Above all, I am indebted to my late parents Mrs Vimla Gupta and Shri Ramesh Chandra Gupta who inculcated in me the spirit of, "To aim as high as possible, then, let nothing deter your faith!!."

Contents

Section 5: Application of Jain Point

Section 6: Jain Point in the Practice of General Surgery

Section 7: Complications

Videos Title*

- What is Jain point
- Direct trocar entry through Jain point
- Jain point entry in a case of previous cesarean section
- Jain point entry in flabby abdomen
- Jain point entry in obese patient with previous cesarean sections
- Jain point entry in thin patients
- Jain point entry in a very thin patient with large broad ligament myoma
- Jain point entry in very large myomas
- Jain point entry in a large dermoid cyst
- Laparoscopic management of endometriotic rectovaginal nodule
- Laparoscopic management of extensive endometriosis
- Jain point usage in Burch colposuspension
- Jain point entry in case for paravaginal defect repair
- Laparoscopic pectopexy
- Laparoscopic management of cesarean scar ectopic
- Laparoscopic isthmocele repair
- Tubo-tubal reanastomosis
- TLH with extensive endometriosis
- TLH with extensive adhesions
- TLH with large broad ligament myoma.

The videos are available on www.emedicine360.com.

General

Surgical Anatomy of Anterior Abdominal Wall

CS Ramesh Babu, Aruna Arya

INTRODUCTION

Anterior abdominal wall (AAW) is a hexagonal area bounded superiorly by the xiphoid process and costal margins (formed by 7th to 10th costal cartilages), inferiorly by upper border of pubic symphysis, pubic crest, pubic tubercle, inguinal ligament and iliac crest and laterally by midaxillary lines. It consists of skin, superficial fascia, deep fascia, muscles and their aponeuroses, fascia transversalis, extraperitoneal (preperitoneal) fat, and parietal peritoneum. A thorough knowledge of anatomy of this region is most essential to surgeons and understanding of its neurovascular anatomy became imperative especially after the advent of laparoscopic surgery. In this chapter surgical anatomy of blood vessels of AAW, relevant to laparoscopic portals is discussed.

UMBILICUS

The fibrous cicatrix umbilicus represents the site of attachment of the umbilical cord. Its position is highly variable especially in multiparous obese women. It is one of the commonly used sites of laparoscopic entry because at this site skin and linea alba are in close contact with parietal peritoneum with little intervening fat. Attached to the umbilical scar are four remnants of fetal structures (1) ligamentum teres hepatis (remnant of left umbilical vein) running along the free margin of falciform ligament attached at 12 o'clock position, (2 and 3) right and left medial umbilical ligaments (remnants of umbilical arteries) attached at 4 o'clock and 8 o'clock positions, (4) median umbilical ligament (remnant of urachus) attached at 6 o'clock position.[1] During embryonic period midgut loop as physiological umbilical hernia and vitellointestinal duct extend into umbilical cord. Meckel's diverticulum which is a remnant of vitellointestinal duct, if remains patent, opens at the umbilicus. The urachus connected to apex of urinary bladder sometimes remains patent and opens at umbilicus.

SUPERFICIAL FASCIA

Many text books of anatomy customarily describe the superficial fascia as a single fatty layer in the supraumbilical region and as a bilaminar structure in the infraumbilical region made up of superficial fatty layer (Camper's fascia) and a deep membranous layer (Scarpa's fascia). A trilaminar arrangement of superficial fascia as superficial fatty layer, middle membranous layer, and a deep fatty layer with adipose tissue metabolically different from that of the superficial fatty layer has recently been suggested.[2,3] Computerized tomographic analysis has revealed that the membranous layer was observable in whole of AAW and the superficial fascia was a three layered structure.[4]

ARTERIAL SUPPLY

Arteries supplying the AAW include superficial and deep set of arteries which are branches of external iliac, femoral, subclavian, and descending aorta. The superficial set supplies the skin and subcutaneous tissues and is located between the superficial fatty layer and Scarpa's fascia. Three superficial branches of the femoral artery supply the infraumbilical region and small arteries accompanying the cutaneous nerves and cutaneous perforating branches from deep set of arteries supply the supraumbilical region. The deep set supplies the muscles and deeper tissues and lie between the muscles.

It is convenient to divide the AAW into three zones based on the arterial supply.[5] Zone I is the midcentral portion of supraumbilical AAW supplied by vertically oriented deep superior epigastric and inferior epigastric arteries. Zone II is the entire infraumbilical region supplied by femoral and external iliac artery branches generally oriented vertically. Zone III is the lateral parts (flank) of supraumbilical region supplied by musculophrenic, posterior intercostal, lumbar, and deep circumflex iliac arteries **(Fig. 1)**.

- *Superficial inferior epigastric artery (SIEA)* or simply superficial epigastric artery is a branch of common femoral artery present nearly in 85–94% cases[6] and arises 1.0–1.5 cm below the midinguinal point **(Fig. 2)**. Enters AAW just lateral to midinguinal point and ascends up to umbilicus to supply infraumbilical region lying 2 cm lateral to linea semilunaris. The diameter ranges from 0.6 mm to 1.5 mm.[7]
- *Superficial circumflex iliac artery (SCIA)* arises from common femoral artery and passes obliquely parallel to inguinal ligament to reach the anterior superior iliac spine (ASIS) to supply superficial tissues anterosuperior to ASIS up to the level of umbilicus. The diameter ranges from 0.9 mm to 2 mm.[8]
- *Superficial external pudendal artery (SEPA)* a small branch from common femoral passes medially towards pubic symphysis to supply labium majus and infraumbilical AAW.

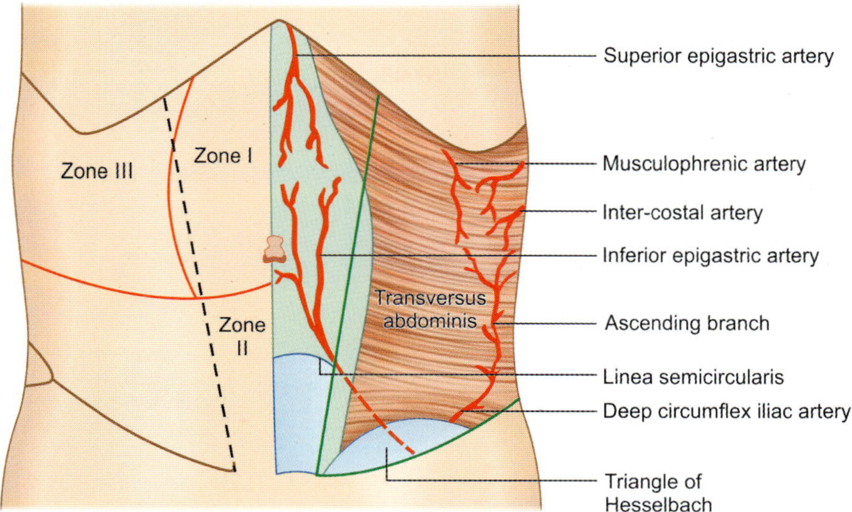

Fig. 1: Vascular zones of anterior abdominal wall. Deep arteries are shown on the left side.

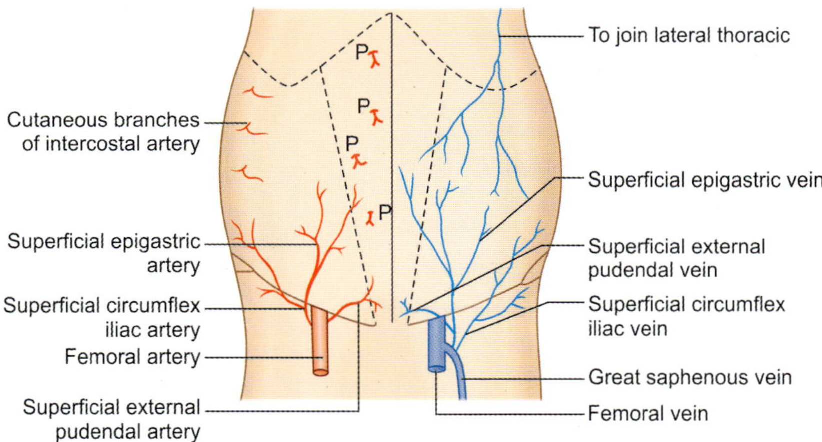

Fig. 2: Cutaneous vessels of anterior abdominal wall. Superficial arteries on the right and veins on the left. (P: perforator).

- *Deep circumflex iliac artery (DCIA)* is a branch arising from lateral aspect of external iliac above the inguinal ligament in 72–91% cases and in rest of the 9–28% cases from common femoral artery below the inguinal ligament.[8,9] Its diameter ranges from 1.1–3.2 mm. It passes upwards and laterally towards ASIS and gives branches to iliacus muscle and ilium. Curving posterolaterally along the iliac crest it gives off a large ascending branch which runs between internal oblique and transversus abdominis muscles to supply them and anastomose with posterior intercostal and musculophrenic arteries **(Figs. 1 and 3)**. Ascending branch of DCIA runs more laterally in the flank region to supply zone III.

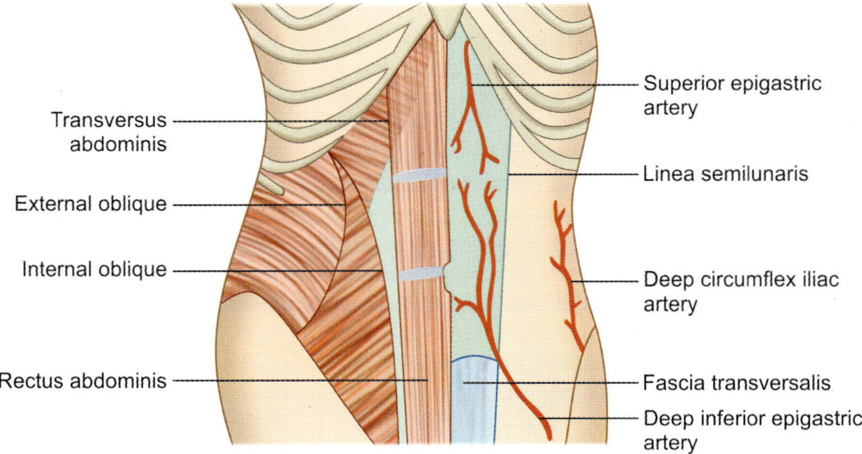

Fig. 3: Deep arteries are shown on the left. On the right the anterior extent of three flat abdominal muscles are shown, beyond which their aponeuroses contribute to formation of rectus sheath.

- *Superior epigastric artery (SEA)* is one of the terminal branches of internal mammary branch of subclavian artery arising in 6th intercostal space. It enters the rectus sheath to descend between the muscle and posterior rectus sheath. Generally it divides into branches to anastomose with inferior epigastric artery midway between umbilicus and xiphoid process **(Figs. 1 and 3)**. Mean diameter of SEA at its origin is 1.6 mm.[10] At the level of xiphoid process it lies at a distance of 4.0–4.5 cm and midway between umbilicus and xiphoid process at a distance of 5.3–5.5 cm from the midline.[11]

- *Deep inferior epigastric artery (DIEA)* or simply inferior epigastric artery is the most widely studied vessel of the AAW because of its susceptibility to injury during laparoscopic and other interventional procedures (0.3–2.5% cases). Since it is the dominant artery supplying the AAW, perforator based cutaneous and myocutaneous flaps [deep inferior epigastric artery perforator (DIEAP) flap and transverse rectus abdominis myocutaneous (TRAM) flap] are frequently used for breast reconstruction. It arises from anteromedial aspect of external iliac just above the inguinal ligament and passes superomedially along the medial margin of deep inguinal ring towards lateral border of rectus abdominis **(Figs. 1 and 3)**. It is estimated that it arises from the external iliac in 83.6% cases but may also arise from femoral below the inguinal ligament, from obturator artery or in common with obturator from the external iliac.[12] Its origin from external iliac was above inguinal ligament in 76% cases, behind the inguinal ligament in 12% and from femoral below the ligament in 8% cases.[13] Its origin above the inguinal ligament ranges from 0.5 cm to 2.0 cm.[14] Initially it lies in the extraperitoneal tissue in the posterior wall of inguinal canal forming the

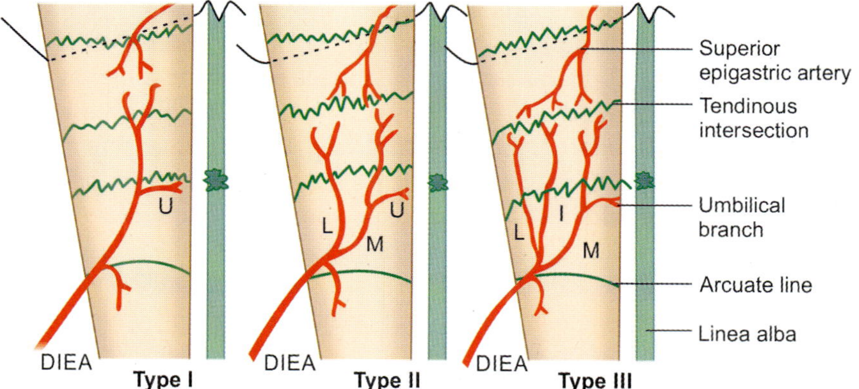

Fig. 4: Three types of deep inferior epigastric artery. (DIEA: deep inferior epigastric artery; M: medial branch; L: lateral branch; I: intermediate branch; U: umbilical branch).

lateral boundary of inguinal triangle of Hesselbach and raises a peritoneal fold named as lateral umbilical fold. Piercing the transversalis fascia it enters the rectus sheath generally at the level of arcuate line (linea semicircularis of Douglas). Length of the DIEA measured from its origin to entry into the rectus sheath was as short as 1.2 cm on the left and 3.5 cm on the right side and as long as 6.8 cm on the right side and 6.9 cm on the left.[15] It ascends with in the rectus sheath posterior to the muscle and anastomoses with SEA midway between umbilicus and xiphoid process. In about 28% cases the DIEA did not reach the umbilicus.[15,16] It gives a pubic branch which anastomoses with a similar branch from obturator artery on the pelvic surface of pubis forming arteria corona mortis. Branching pattern of DIEA within the rectus sheath was classified according to number of branches into three types: Type I single artery found in 29%, Type II bifurcation into two branches in 57%, and Type III trifurcation in 14% cases **(Fig. 4)**.[10] An umbilical branch from DIEA supplies the umbilicus. It also gives muscular branches to supply rectus abdominis and perforator branches to the overlying skin. It was noted that more branches arose from the lateral aspect and were contained within the rectus sheath.[16]

Many cadaveric and radiological studies focused their attention to map a safety zone of entry by measuring the distance of deep epigastric arteries from midline at certain levels to avoid vascular injuries.[17-21] To minimize the risk of vascular injury, Hurd et al. (1994) suggested that the lateral trocars should be placed 8 cm lateral to midline and 5 cm above the pubic symphysis.[17] Sriprasad et al. (2006) indicated that the ideal primary port entry is in the midline and the ideal lateral port entry is more than 6 cm from the midline both at the level of ASIS.[22] Kulkarni et al. (2013) suggested that a zone of safety for access in the midline is 2 cm (1 cm on each side of midline) at the level of xiphoid process, 4 cm at umbilicus (2 cm on either side of midline) and 5 cm at ASIS.[23] They also suggested that more laterally the safe area of access is >8 cm from the midline at the level of umbilicus. It was observed that the position of deep epigastric vessels shifted more laterally after insufflation ranging from 0.6 cm to 1.1 cm.[24]

VENOUS DRAINAGE

Veins draining the AAW accompany the corresponding arteries and are grouped into superficial and deep veins. Superficial veins drain the skin and subcutaneous tissues whereas the deep veins drain the muscles. Infraumbilical AAW is drained by three superficial veins; the superficial inferior epigastric, superficial circumflex iliac, and superficial external pudendal, which are tributaries of the great saphenous vein whereas the supraumbilical region is drained by small veins which unite to form the thoracoepigastric vein which joins the lateral thoracic vein, a tributary of the axillary vein **(Fig. 2)**. The superficial inferior epigastric and superficial circumflex iliac veins anastomose with the thoracoepigastric vein. Thus this longitudinally arranged superficial venous system can act as a collateral channel connecting the superior vena cava with inferior vena cava. The deeper veins include deep circumflex iliac and deep inferior epigastric veins draining into external iliac vein, superior epigastric vein draining into internal mammary vein, subcostal, lower posterior intercostal, and lumbar veins draining into azygos venous system. At the umbilicus the veins of the AAW establish an important anastomosis with paraumbilical vein and smaller veins in the falciform ligament which drain into portal vein. Thus umbilicus is one of the sites of portocaval anastomosis and in cases of portal hypertension enlarged tortuous radiating veins appear around umbilicus, a condition called as "caput medusae".

MUSCLES

There are three flat abdominal wall muscles in the flank region, the external oblique, internal oblique, and transversus abdominis which are arranged in a plane similar to that of the three intercostal muscles in the thoracic region. These muscles end in aponeuroses more medially at variable distances from the linea semilunaris and contribute to the formation of rectus sheath enclosing vertically oriented paramedian rectus abdominis and pyramidalis muscles. The aponeuroses of muscles of both sides interlace with each other at linea alba resulting in a digastric arrangement of the muscles with linea alba acting as the intermediate tendon.

- *Linea alba*: It is a median fibrous raphe formed by the interlacement and decussation of aponeuroses of three anterolateral muscles forming the anterior and posterior rectus sheath. It extends from tip of xiphoid process to upper border of pubic symphysis. It is wider above the umbilicus than below and widest at the level of umbilicus.[25] The width of the linea alba indicates the inter-recti distance. A recent sonographic study in nulliparous women suggested that the linea alba can be considered normal up to a width of 22 mm at a point 3 cm above the umbilicus, 16 mm at a point 2 cm below the umbilicus, and 15 mm at the xiphoid process.[26] Linea alba is not a simple merging line of the aponeuroses of both sides forming the rectus sheath. Fibers from each layer decussate to the opposite side forming a continuous aponeurosis with the contralateral muscles. Thus linea alba acts as a central tendon for the digastric arrangement of the three flat muscles. Moreover, fibers also decussate anteroposteriorly passing from anterior sheath to the posterior sheath. Linea alba is relatively avascular and is a preferable site for various surgical approaches.

TRANSVERSALIS FASCIA

It is a thin fascial layer lining the AAW on the deep surface of the transversus abdominis and is a part of endoabdominal fascia. It is separated from the parietal peritoneum by the extraperitoneal fat. Superiorly it is continuous with the fascia on the abdominal surface of diaphragm. Posteriorly it is continuous with thoracolumbar fascia. Posteroinferiorly it is attached to iliac crest where it is continuous with the iliac and parietal layer of endopelvic fascia. Anteroinferiorly it is attached to inguinal ligament and shows a thickening called as iliopubic tract (deep crural arch), an important structure during inguinal hernia surgery. Opposite to midinguinal point it presents the deep inguinal ring through which vas deferens in male and round ligament of uterus in female enter the inguinal canal surrounded by a prolongation of the transversalis fascia named as internal spermatic fascia. Along the medial margin the deep inguinal ring it is thickened to form interfoveolar ligament. It is also prolonged around femoral vessels forming anterior wall of femoral sheath. Above the pubic symphysis and below the arcuate line the rectus abdominis muscle rests on it.

EXTRAPERITONEAL FAT

It is a loose connective tissue layer with fat separating the parietal peritoneum from the abdominal wall. Along the medial margin of the deep inguinal ring it is traversed by the deep inferior epigastric vessels. A considerable accumulation of subperitoneal fat named as "yellow island" is present at the lateral third of a line joining the ASIS with umbilicus. The "yellow island" is well developed especially in obese women and it is suggested that this site is suitable for safe introduction of ancillary trocars since vascular injury is avoided. The DIEA and other major vessels are never present in this area.[27,28]

CONCLUSION

This article is not an exhaustive description of anatomy of the AAW. Its main focus is to discuss about the surgical anatomy of the AAW more relevant to laparoscopic gynecological surgery. Therefore the detailed anatomy of the muscles, nerves, inguinal canal, and associated structures are not discussed. In an attempt to identify a safety zone of entry, though lot of morphometric data on deep epigastric vessels was generated, there was no uniformity because different authors have used different anatomical landmarks. It will be more fruitful if both cadaveric/surgical and radiological studies employ same bony landmarks for measuring the distance of the epigastric vessels from midline. More studies on the positional anatomy of DCIA and its ascending branch are required. Similarly morphometric data on vascular anatomy in nulliparous and multiparous women and women with normal body mass index (BMI) and increased BMI are necessary. Similarly positional anatomy of the vessels in resting and insufflated abdomen is needed.

REFERENCES

1. Skandalakis PN, Skandalakis JE, Colborn GL, et al. Abdominal wall and hernias. In: Skandalakis JE (Ed). Surgical Anatomy: The Embryologic and Anatomic Basis of Modern Surgery. Athens: Paschalidis Medical Publications; 2004. pp. 393-492.
2. Rosen MJ, Petro CC, Stringer MD. Anterior abdominal wall. In: Standring S (Ed) Gray's Anatomy: The Anatomical Basis of Clinical Practice, 41st edition. Amsterdam, Netherlands: Elsevier; 2016. pp. 1069-82.
3. Lancerotto I, Stecco C, Macchi V, et al. Layers of the abdominal wall: anatomical investigation of subcutaneous tissue and superficial fascia. Surg Radiol Anat. 2011;33:835-42.
4. Chopra J, Rani A, Rani A, et al. Re-evaluation of superficial fascia of anterior abdominal wall: a computed tomographic study. Surg Radiol Anat. 2011;33:843-9.
5. Huger WE Jr. The anatomic rationale for abdominal lipectomy. Am Surg. 1979;45:612-7.
6. Rozen WM, Chubb D, Grinsell O, et al. The variability of the superficial inferior epigastric artery (SIEA) and its angiosome: A clinical anatomical study. Microsurgery. 2010;30(5):386-91.
7. Fathi M, Hatamipour E, Fathi HR, et al. The anatomy of superficial inferior epigastric artery flap. Acta Cirurgica Brasileira. 2008;23(5):429-34.
8. Penteado CV. Anatomosurgical study of the superficial and deep circumflex iliac arteries. Anat Clin. 1983;5:125-7.
9. Vasanthakumar T, Priyadarisini SE. A study on the variations in the origin of deep circumflex iliac artery. Int J Anat Res. 2017;5:4451-3.
10. Taylor GI. The angiosomes of the body and their supply to perforator flaps. Clin Plast Surg. 2003;30:331-42.
11. Saber AA, Meslemani AM, Davis R, et al. Safety zone for anterior abdominal wall entry during laparoscopy. Ann Surg. 2004;239:182-5.
12. Al-Talalwah W. The inferior epigastric artery: Anatomical study and clinical significance. Int J Morphol. 2017;35(1):7-11.
13. Jakubowicz M, Czarniawska-Grzesinska M. Variability in origin and topography of the inferior epigastric and obturator arteries. Folia Morphol (Warsz). 1996;55:121-6.
14. Anandhi V, Rajeshwari K, Jebakani CF. A study of the origin and course of the inferior epigastric artery and its significance in laparoscopic surgery. Int J Anat Res. 2016;4(3):2692-7.

15. Rao MP, Swamy V, Arole V, et al. Study of the course of inferior epigastric artery with reference to laparoscopic portal. J Min Access Surg. 2013;9:154-8.
16. Joy P, Pritishkumar IJ, Isaac B. Clinical anatomy of the inferior epigastric artery with special relevance to invasive procedures of the anterior abdominal wall. J Min Access Surg. 2017;13:18-21.
17. Hurd WW, Bude RO, De Lancey JO, et al. The location of abdominal wall blood vessels in relationship to abdominal landmarks apparent at laparoscopy. Am J Obstet Gynecol. 1994;171(3):642-6.
18. Joy P, Simon B, Pritishkumar IJ, et al. Topography of inferior epigastric artery relevant to laparoscopy: a CT angiographic study. Surg Radol Anat. 2016;38(3):279-83.
19. Andrade D, Abranches D, Souza N, et al. An analysis of the anatomical trajectory of the inferior epigastric arteries in the era of videolaparoscopic surgery: Is there in fact a 'safety zone' for the prevention of iatrogenic lesions? Eur J Anat. 2012;16(1):43-8.
20. Rahn DD, Phelan JN, Roshanravan SM, et al Anterior abdominal wall nerve and vessel anatomy: clinical implications for gynaecologic surgery. Am J Obstet Gynecol. 2010;202:234-6.
21. Epstein J, Arora A, Ellis H. Surface anatomy of inferior epigastric artery in relation to laparoscopic injury. Clin Anat. 2004;17:400-8.
22. Sriprasad S, Yu DF, Muir GH, et al. Positional anatomy of the vessels that may be damaged at laparoscopy: new access critera based on CT and ultrasonography to avoid vascular injury. J Endourol. 2006;20(7):498-503.
23. Kulkarni M, Ambiye M. Positional anatomy of deep epigastric arteries. Int J Biol Med Res. 2013;4(3):3350-4.
24. Burnett TL, Garza-Cavazos A, Groesch K, et al. Location of the deep epigastric vessels in the resting and insufflated abdomen. J Minim Invasive Gynecol. 2016;23(5):798-803.
25. Rath AM, Attali P, Dumas JL, et al. The abdominal linea alba: an anatomo-radiological and biomechanical study. Surg Radiol Anat. 1996;18:281-8.
26. Beer GM, Schuster A, Seifert B, et al. The normal width of the linea alba in nulliparous women. Clin Anat. 2009;22:706-11.
27. Tinelli A, Gasbarro N, Lupo P, et al. Safe introduction of ancillary trocars. JSLS. 2012;16:276-9.
28. Vitale SG, Gasbarro N, Lagana AS, et al. Safe introduction of ancillary trocars in gynaecological surgery: the yellow island anatomical landmark. Ann Ital Chir. 2016;87:608-11.

Overview of Laparoscopic Entry

Artin Ternamian

■ INTRODUCTION

Endoscopy allows optically guided procedures to be performed within the body, through surgically created temporary ports (laparoscopy, thoracoscopy, and arthroscopy) or through natural conduits, without requiring an entry wound (hysteroscopy, bronchoscopy, natural orifice transluminal endoscopic surgery—NOTES).

These minimally invasive measures are practiced in most specialties and have become a preferred method for diagnosis and treatment of several surgical conditions. Endoscopy is a technology driven dynamic discipline that challenges conventional open surgery and introduces innovative advances that renders robotic surgery, telesurgery, remote telepresence, high-resolution imaging, and surgical macrorobots and makes frameless stereotactic surgery possible.

Principal difference between open and laparoscopic surgery is size of surgical wound. The most important and potentially hazardous first step in laparoscopy is safe and successful insertion of a primary port. As more surgical specialties practice laparoscopy, conventional methods of blind umbilical peritoneal entry may not be uniformly acceptable.

Recently, the US Food and Drug Administration (FDA) in a Laparoscopic Trocar Injuries report recommended surgeons performing sophisticated endoscopic operations to be well-versed in alternate laparoscopic access methods and instruments to address evolving patient expectations and societal safety requirements.[1]

Publication of the USA Institute of Medicine Committee Report on Patient Safety suggests that over 90% of unintended medical mishaps are human error related. Accordingly, surgeons and industry now recognize the need for less hazardous laparoscopic access options especially in high-risk situations.[2]

Moreover, entry methods that can anticipate, avoid, or at the very least recognize error are advocated, where error recovery is possible, before permanent patient harm occurs.[3] Ultimately, surgeons must use those access methods and instruments that they are schooled in, feel comfortable using and are safest in their hands. In this chapter, several access instruments and their safe deployment techniques will be reviewed.

ACCESS INSTRUMENTS

Laparoscopic ports perform several important functions, including administration of distending gas, maintenance of operative envelope, placement of optical and operating instruments, safe retrieval of tissue, and preservation of port competence.

Conventional first generation laparoscopic access instruments generally consist of two parts—(1) a removable central trocar and (2) an encasing outer sheath or cannula **(Fig. 1)**. Once placed inside a body cavity, the central trocar is removed to accommodate a laparoscope or various operating instruments. Trocars have a proximal end to accommodate the surgeons' dominant palm and transmit penetration force (PF) generated to the instrument-tissue interface. The distal end is traditionally designed to have a pointed sharp conical, beveled pyramidal, or cutting bladed tip.

Cutting pyramidal or bladed trocars are the most commonly employed devices; as extremely sharp bladed tips render trajectory propulsion, require less PF. These trocars, with the outer casing cannula mounted, transect different myofascial abdominal tissue layers, en route to the intended body cavity.[4]

Extremely sharp disposable access instruments make insertion less forceful and more controlled. However, risk of inadvertent bowel or vessel injury because of extreme sharpness and blind insertion cannot be denied. In some

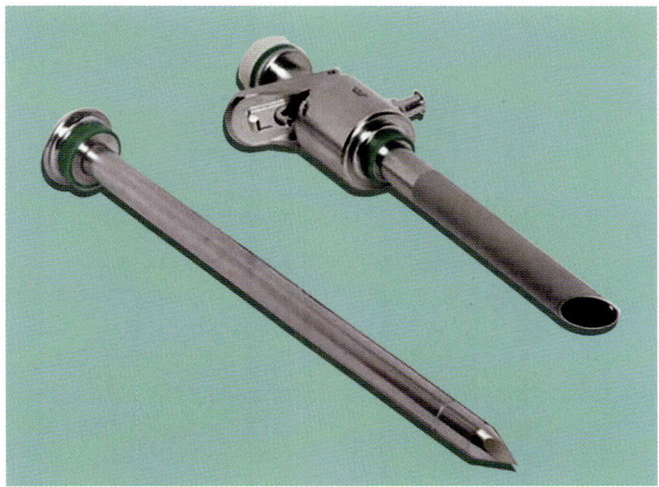

Fig. 1: Conventional first-generation laparoscopic access instrument with a central trocar and encasing outer sheath or cannula.

series, risk of bowel injury with disposable access trocars is three times that previously reported for reusable trocars while blunt-tipped trocars present less access risk to vascular or tissue injury.

Disposable bladed access trocars with automatic extending shields were designed to decrease the risk of inadvertent injury. However, as injuries continued to occur, the FDA ordered all device manufacturers and distributors of shielded access trocars to remove all claims of added "safety".

Leibl showed that incisional hernia risk is 10 times greater when disposable cutting pyramidal trocars are used instead of reusable conical trocars (1.83 versus 0.17%).[5]

Conical trocars have pointed nonbladed sharp tips with no cutting edges; these recruit considerably more PF as tissue layers are not transected, but radially parted to accommodate cannulas' outer diameter.[6]

These would have to inflict a "direct hit" on vessels to cause injury as only the tip is sharp, whereas a same sized cutting pyramidal or bladed trocar can do exact significant injury to any vessel along its path.[7] Clearly, trocar tip design is very important when evaluating entry accident causation and port competence **(Figs. 2A to D)**.

The cannula portion of access devices has a proximal valve section to allow insertion and removal of optics or laparoscopic instruments without losing insufflated gas. They may also have a CO_2 insufflation stopcock, particularly those used at primary port site.

The shaft's outer surface is usually smooth or serrated and ends either horizontally or in an oblique slant with a small venting window at their distal end. Recently, threaded shafts have gained popularity as they anchor cannulas at entry site and discourage unintended intraoperative displacement.

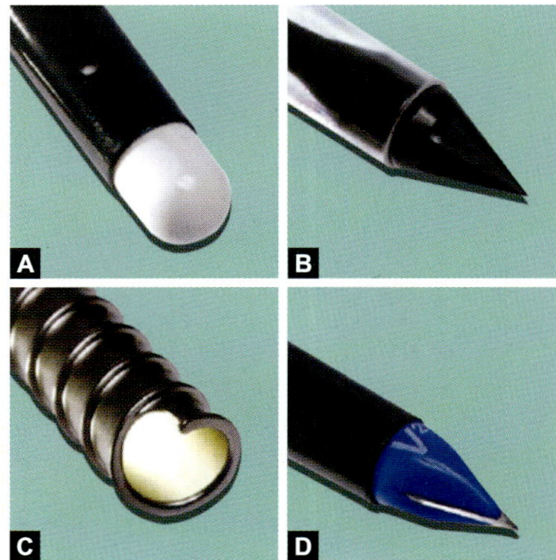

Figs. 2A to D: Different trocar and cannula tips.

Laparoscopic access instruments are either intended for single or multiple use. Environmental and societal concerns in addition to mounting healthcare costs generally encourage use of reusable instruments.[8]

Moreover, multiple use of single-use designated instrument, especially trocars and cannulas are generally not recommended.[9] Unfortunately, surgeons world over, have less say in operating room purchasing decisions and are called upon to defend outcomes only when mishaps are publicized.

Since exposure of a primary port is not possible unless when using visual access systems, it is always advisable to inspect the parietal peritoneal aspect of primary ports, through an ancillary port, at the end of each laparoscopy.[10] Most gynecologists use a Veress needle to preinsufflate the peritoneal cavity with a noncombustible and easily absorbable gas, usually CO_2, prior to insertion of the primary laparoscopic port. This is intended to further minimize inadvertent access injury during placement of sharp blind trocars; though complications related to their use are rare and well-documented.[11]

Concern regarding their safety, especially at primary port has been expressed as considerable axial PF is applied blindly to thrust a sharp trajectory into the abdomen, resulting in inevitable overshoot. Despite significant advances in endoscopic techniques and instrumentation; potentially avoidable access injuries continue to occur. Several publications indicate that inadvertent trauma to major vessels and bowel remains underreported.[12]

Many of these serious injuries are related to closed laparoscopy, where insertion of the Veress needle during preinsufflation or a sharp trocar and cannula are generally blind steps.

Alternatively, during open laparoscopy, peritoneal entry through a mini cutdown is first secured, followed by insertion of the Hasson trocar and finally the peritoneal cavity is insufflated **(Fig. 3)**. This method is intended to avoid major vessel and bowel injury; however, inadvertent large vessel or bowel injury is not entirely eliminated.[13-16]

Given continued incidence of serious access complications, "visual access" trocars were introduced in 1994 to mitigate access injury by allowing visually guided layered entry.

Two disposable "optical access" trocars are available—one has a conical crystal tip at the distal end of a hollowed trocar that accommodates a sheathed 0° laparoscope to display entry images on the monitor (OptiView XCEL; Ethicon Endo-Surgery, Cincinnati, OH) **(Fig. 4)**; while the other trocar has a spherical crystal tip at the end of a hollowed trocar with an embedded wire blade at the equator that transects anterior abdominal tissue layers at the strike of a trigger. The optical trocar with a 0° laparoscope mounted, is pushed down toward the CO_2 distended peritoneum to display access sequences on the monitor (VisiPort; COVIDIEN, TYCO, Norwalk, CT) **(Fig. 5)**.

Despite their ability to optically display entry tissue layers on the monitor, these instruments retain a conventional trocar and cannula insertion

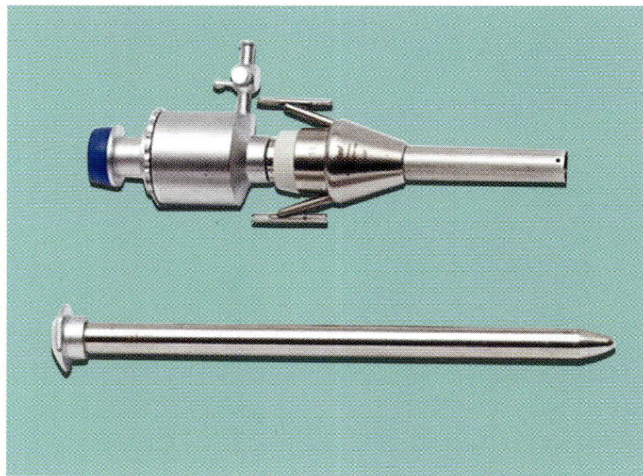

Fig. 3: Hassons' open entry trocar and cannula with cone.

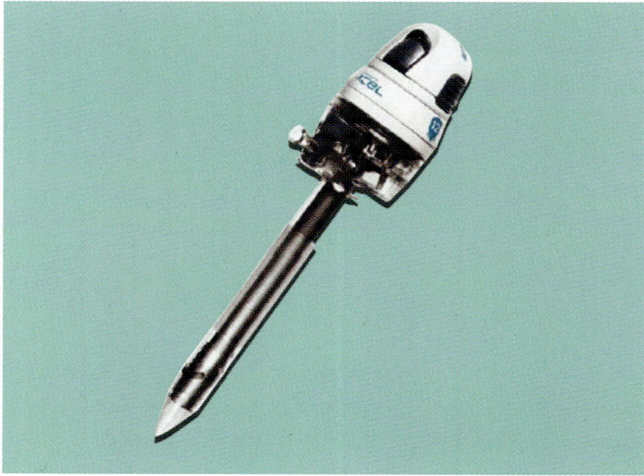

Fig. 4: OptiView XCEL, Ethicon, Endo-Surgery. Disposable visual trocar and cannula.

dynamics where entry is achieved by palming the access device and applying considerable perpendicular PF to propel the trajectory into the peritoneal cavity, with no means to control overshoot. Although the degree of risk or serious complications compared to conventional blind sharp trocar and cannula systems remains uncertain, serious access injury can still occur with their use. Moreover, extreme caution has to be exercised, especially when surgeons fail to interpret or recognize displayed entry images.

Some endoscopists advocate gasless laparoscopy where visualization is achieved by suspending the anterior abdominal wall by a mechanical lifting device instead of CO_2 insufflation. Specialized valveless threaded ports with a scored side are used to accommodate conventional open surgical instruments.

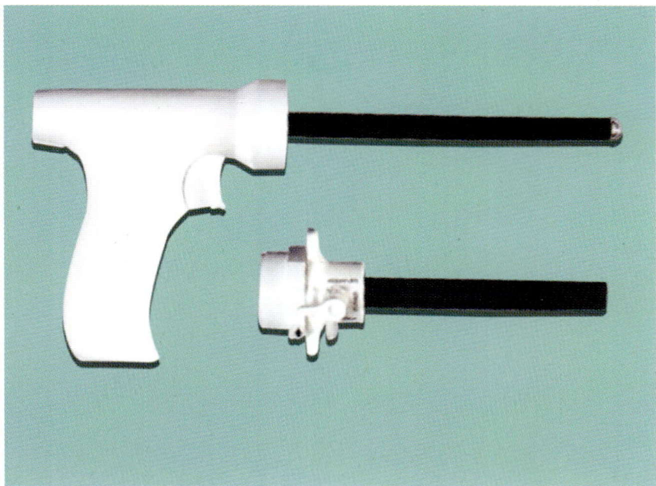

Fig. 5: VisiPort, COVIDIEN, TYCO. Disposable visual trocar and cannula.

The primary access site is dissected down to peritoneum through a mini cutdown and then a lifting device is suspended through the umbilical primary port site to create a tented operating compartment. This method has limited clinical application but may be of value especially in patients who have cardiovascular compromise.[17]

More recently, a radially expanding trocar system has been introduced to decrease the incidence of unintended access injury by sharp trocars (VersaStep trocar; COVIDIEN, TYCO, Norwalk, CT). This disposable instrument retains a conventional trocar design and method of application. It comprises an expandable polymeric outer sleeve that covers a Veress like needle. Following insertion of the sleeve a dilating trocar is deployed for the sleeve to accommodate a laparoscope **(Fig. 6)**.[18]

Better optics, miniaturization and advances in instrument design allowed improvements in rigid and flexible narrow caliber microlaparoscopes that require very small diameter access ports with potential advantages. Some have introduced a visual access system that requires a 1.2 mm semirigid 0° microlaparoscope that fits into a modified Veress type needle (Optical Veress Entry System; Karl Storz Endoscopes GMBH, Tuttlingen, Germany).

This reusable system offers excellent optics. However, it is expensive, has a very short focal point, is very delicate, and can easily fracture given its narrow diameter and heavy top end camera. They can be used through the left upper quadrant in high-risk cases, during diagnostic conscious pain mapping and in critical care or outpatient diagnostic units **(Fig. 7)**.[19]

Second generation laparoscopic access instruments are a more recent addition and consist of only a cannula, where no trocar is required and access is visually monitored in real-time. The reusable bladeless cannula has a

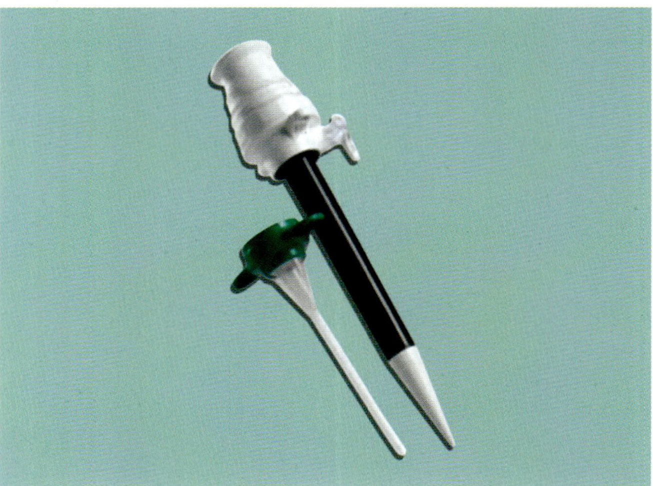

Fig. 6: VersaStep, COVIDIEN, TYCO. Disposable radially dilating trocar and cannula.

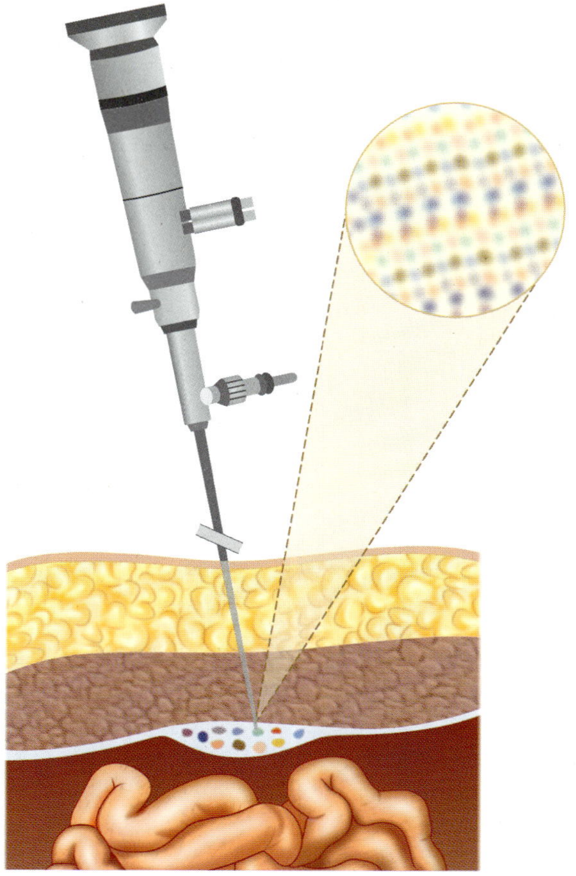

Fig. 7: Microlaparoscopy optical Veress access system.

conventional valve section at one end to allow insertion and removal of optics or laparoscopic instruments without losing insufflated gas and may house a CO_2 insufflation stopcock. The shaft's outer surface has a single diagonal thread that ends distally in a blunt notched tip **(Fig. 8)**.

During deployment, a 0° laparoscope is sheathed into the cannula and held 1 cm short of the cannulas' distal end by a telescope stopper (TS). Cannulas' rotation engages the myofascial tissue with the notched tip to lift successive anterior abdominal wall layers using the Archimedes' principle **(Fig. 9)**.

As the cannula has no cutting or sharp end, tissue planes are not transected, instead are parted. This preserves port competence as it is shown to result in a smaller fascial entry wound area with less muscle damage compared to pyramidal trocar wounds.[20]

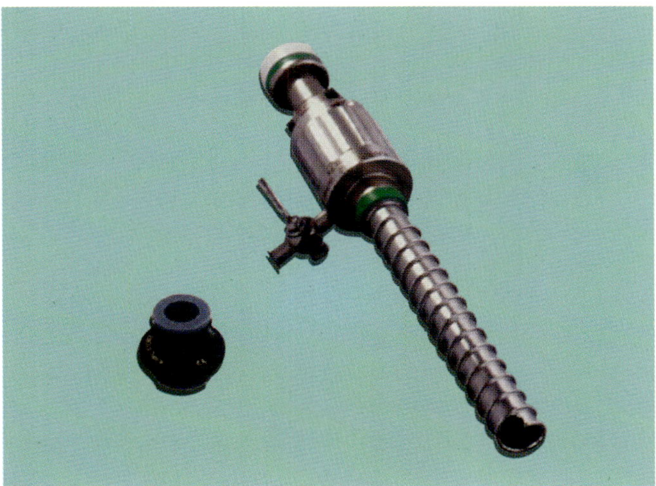

Fig. 8: Endoscopic threaded imaging port (EndoTIP) reusable visual access cannula with telescope stopper.

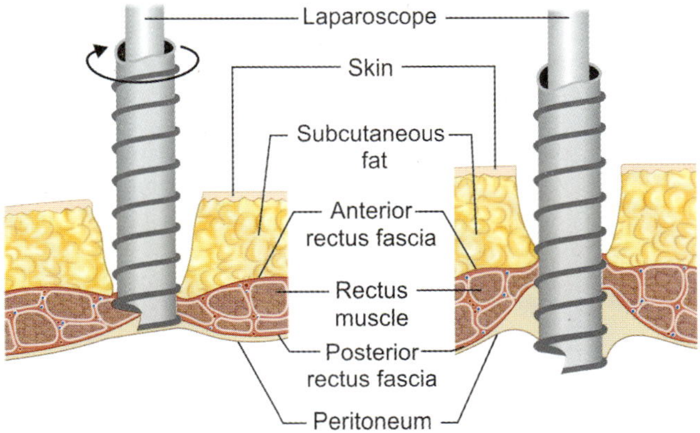

Fig. 9: Layered access with EndoTIP.

This bladeless visual access cannula system (Endoscopic Threaded Imaging Port, EndoTIP; Karl Storz Endoscopy GMBH, Tuttlingen, Germany) has no crystal tip compressing and distorting monitor images at tissue—cannula interface. Therefore, interpretations of monitor images are easier and layered entry more interactive.

Endoscopists agree that visual and controlled access systems, that deploy less axial PF, require no sharp trocars and allow real-time error analysis, recognition and recovery are preferred. Intuitively, these systems are less dangerous, infer added safety, improve understanding of entry complications, and reduce recurrent inadvertent error.[21,22]

Port Dynamics during Laparoscopy

Like all surgical methods, laparoscopy is associated with some inadvertent patient risk. Serious peritoneal entry complications, such as bowel and vascular injury, continue to occur despite innovative port creation techniques and well-trained surgeons.

Laparoscopic access injury is best understood when tissue dynamics at port site is studied in real-time. Careful error analysis is essential to unravel interaction between surgeon, instrument and tissue. It is known that a minimum of 25% of practicing gynecologists have experienced Veress needle or cannula injuries.[23,24]

Two primary access methods are available in laparoscopy—(1) first-generation conventional access method where a push-through spike principle is applied and (2) second-generation access method where an Archimedean spin principle is employed **(Table 1)**.

Irrespective of instrument make or model, conventional access requires two components, a central trocar with a sharp, cutting, or pointed distal end and an encasing cannula. Surgeons palm the access instrument by their dominant hand and apply PF, generated through the upper arm muscles, axially at port site. This propels the spike across different tissue layers toward the intended

TABLE 1: Laparoscopic access techniques.

First generation spike principle	Trocar and cannula design
Insufflated access	Closed conventional T and C high-pressure T and C radially expanding T and C visual T and C
Noninsufflated	Visual Veress mini-laparoscope open Hassons' T and C access direct T and C access gasless laparoscopy
Second generation spin principle	*Visual cannula design*
Endoscopic threaded	Imaging port
EndoTIP	Closed preinsufflated access Open direct access Extraretroperitoneal access

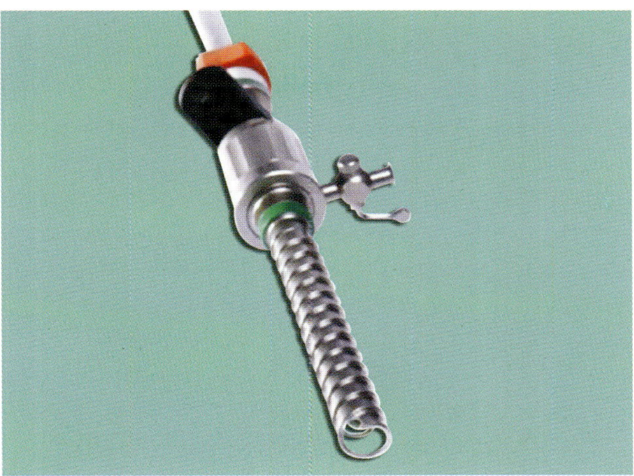

Fig. 10: EndoTIP with laparoscope mounted and held in position with telescope stopper.

body cavity. Several versions, modifications, and models have attempted to render this access system less perilous while maintaining the spike and cannula design principle intact.

A more contemporary second generation access method uses the spin principle where the entry instrument comprises a reusable bladeless threaded cannula that ends in a notched, blunt tip. No central trocar is required; instead a zero degree laparoscope is mounted into the cannula during insertion and removal. No axial PF is deployed; tissue layers part radially and the visually guided cannula pulls tissue up along its outside thread **(Fig. 10)**.[25]

FIRST-GENERATION INSUFFLATED ACCESS METHODS

A primary port is the first access conduit through which a lens, camera, and light are introduced. Its insertion is a critical step during laparoscopy when most serious unintended injuries occur.

Veress or trocar placement is particularly perilous, as considerable uncontrolled axial PF is applied blindly to sharp instruments. Moreover, all practitioners agree that subsequent ancillary ports must be inserted under direct vision; consequently some endoscopists favor insertion of the primary port under visual control as well, since intuitively, this can further mitigate inadvertent access complications.[26]

Most gynecologists prefer insufflating the peritoneal cavity prior to primary port insertion. Available evidence demonstrates that vascular injuries are seven times more likely to be caused by either the primary or ancillary trocar placement than by the Veress needle.[10]

In a nationwide prospective multicenter Dutch study, Jansen reviewed 25,764 laparoscopies. Five complications were caused by Veress and 68 by trocar insertion.[27]

In another survey, Veress was implicated in only 2% of Medical Device Reports (MDR) to the US FDA primary access injury reports.[28,29] However, Veress injury was associated with 18% of reported cases in the Physician Insurers Association of America (PIAA) statistics.

Inspection of the supine nondraped abdomen, notation of previous surgical scars, careful abdominopelvic examination, and palpation of the bony landmarks must precede every laparoscopic insufflation and primary port insertion. Patients must remain horizontal until insufflation and primary access is successfully achieved.

The umbilical skin incision should be larger than the diameter of the primary cannula used, to avoid "skin dystocia" and obviate use of excessive PF. Clearly CO_2 leak around a cannula has very little to do with skin incision size and everything to do with the anterior rectus fascial incision size, relative to the cannula's diameter, and tissue recoil.

The Veress needle is then inserted to distend the peritoneal cavity with CO_2 gas. This gas cushion, interposed between an advancing sharp trocar and abdominal viscera compensates for inevitable trocar overshoot and may avert unintended injury.

The braced abdominal wall and distended peritoneum offer counter pressure against the considerable axial PF applied during accessing. In addition, a gas filled spacious cavity allows unobstructed visualization of pelvic-abdominal organs during surgery.

The Veress needle is first inspected, spring mechanism tested and CO_2 stopcock kept open to allow room air to stream into the sealed abdominal cavity as soon as the peritoneal membrane is penetrated. The needle held at the hub by the dominant hand, like a dart, is advanced toward the pelvic hollow in the midline sagittal plane, where there are no large vessels and nonadherent bowel generally moves out of harm's way.

Some advocate lifting the relaxed abdominal wall with the nondominant hand to offer counter pressure against the advancing Veress needle. Two distinct "pops" are usually felt, as it first punctures through anterior rectus fascia, followed by the posterior fascia and peritoneum. Once a second pop is felt, the needle insertion is stopped. When insertion is intraumbilical, only one pop will be felt.[30]

Determining correct placement prior to insufflation has always been a very important step, as failure to achieve and maintain adequate pneumoperitoneum is a common cause of procedural failure. Earlier, correct needle placement was verified with the saline drop and other confirmatory tests; only then the insufflator was connected, set to 15 mm Hg and total instilled CO_2 volumes measured.

It is now accepted that by far the most reliable indicator of correct peritoneal placement is an intraperitoneal pressure reading less than 10 mm Hg (range 4–10 mm Hg). More recently, investigators described a Veress needle insertion technique where the Veress tubing is connected and insufflator flow rate set to deliver 1 L/minute during needle insertion.

Only when intraperitoneal needle placement is secure and the pressure reading is less than 10 mm Hg, the insufflation flow rate is safely cranked to high flow and target pressure is raised to 25 mm Hg.[31-33]

More importantly, as soon as the desired intraperitoneal pressure is achieved, the Veress is retrieved, primary and ancillary ports inserted and insufflation pressure dropped to 15 mm Hg. Remember that inadvertent improper Veress needle placement and a high-flow rate may lead to serious complications. The accepted intraperitoneal pressure during laparoscopic surgery is about 15 mm Hg.

When high initial peritoneal insertion pressures are encountered, needles' position may be carefully changed by drawing out or moving it gently sideways, to dislodge the tip that may be resting against a viscus. Alternatively, the abdominal wall can be manually elevated with similar results. Injecting a few milliliters of saline could also be tried.

It is important to make sure that the patient is well-anesthetized with relaxed anterior abdominal muscles, as bucking could record similar elevated readings. When all fails, it is better to remove, inspect for malfunction and then reinsert the Veress anew. If Veress insertion fails on three consecutive attempts for whatever reason, it is recommended to resort to open, visual, or left upper quadrant entry.

Manual abdominal palpation remains a preferred method of determining degree of distention, as measurement of total instilled gas volume is unreliable. Having attained adequate insufflation, the Veress needle is removed and conventional trocar and cannula is inserted toward the distended peritoneal cavity. This basic entry principal has not changed much, since its inception several decades ago and remains a common access method.

Higher intraperitoneal pressure CO_2 gas insufflation is a variation on the conventional closed insertion technique, where insufflation to an intraperitoneal pressure of 25–30 mm Hg is attained using a Veress needle. This splints the anterior abdominal wall and braces the parietal peritoneum against the axial PF of the advancing trocar.

The larger interposes CO_2 gas cushion reduces tenting of peritoneal membrane between the advancing trajectory and great vessels or abdominal viscera.[34-36]

Bowel adherent to parietal peritoneal wall remains susceptible to injury, as insertion is blind and sharp. Once a primary cannula is placed and correct insertion is verified, intraperitoneal pressure must be lowered to about 10–15 mm Hg.

It is recognized that obesity does not adversely affect insufflation volume for a given intra-abdominal pressure. The actual intra-abdominal volume is a finite value and 94% of this capacity is distended at an abdominal pressure of 15 mm Hg.[37]

Radially expanding disposable trocar system comprises an expandable polymeric outer sleeve that covers a modified Veress needle. The abdomen is first insufflated with the sleeve covered Veress, then the needle is withdrawn, leaving the hollow outer sleeve in the abdominal wound. A trocar is then rammed into the hollow polymeric sleeve, gradually expanding it to accommodate the trocars' larger diameter. Then the trocar is withdrawn and replaced with a laparoscope.[38]

Professor K Semm of the University of Kiel, was first to endorse benefits of visual access; his group used a beveled reusable cannula to insert primary ports under visual control. His teaching proscribed blind puncture of abdominal wall at all costs to improve access safety.[39]

To improve primary access safety, visual access trocar methods were introduced. Two methods are available, Optiview XCEL and VisiPort trocars. These instruments have traded blind sharp trocar for a hollow trocar with a transparent crystal tip at its distal end. With a 0° laparoscope sheathed in the hollowed central trocar, the distal crystal tip transects abdominal tissue layers and transmits entry images during insertion.

These visual entry instruments retain a push-through trocar and cannula design where the spike principle is employed to thrust a clear tipped trajectory across abdominal wall layers. Insertion requires considerably more PF applied axial to tissues that tent toward viscera and often tissue compression by the distal crystal tip, renders layer recognition off the monitor difficult.

Patients with previous midline laparotomy incisions are particularly at risk of developing umbilical adhesions. Consequently, alternate primary port entry sites and visually guided access techniques may have to be practiced. In high-risk situations, a visual Veress access technique may be preferred, where a 1.2 mm diameter semirigid fiberoptic microlaparoscope, sheathed into a 2.1 mm diameter modified visual Veress may be employed.[19]

They are inserted in the left upper quadrant, which is usually adhesion free, even in patients who have had previous lower abdominal surgery. Subsequent ancillary ports can then be safely inserted under direct visual control in an adhesion-free access site. Particular caution needs to be exercised in patient with portal hypertension, hepatosplenomegaly, gastric surgery, or previous left upper quadrant incisions. Small caliber microlaparoscopes are usually available to visually access peritoneum for conscious pain mapping, trauma units, and other diagnostic outpatient procedures.[40]

FIRST-GENERATION NONINSUFFLATED ACCESS METHODS

Hasson first introduced open laparoscopy as a primary port insertion method where a Veress needle with preinsufflation is not required. A generous umbilical skin incision is made and subcutaneous layer is dissected to expose the anterior rectus fascia using S-shaped retractors. Two Kocher clamps hold the fascia while stay sutures are applied at 3 and 9 o'clock. Anterior fascia is then incised between the two sutures using a curved long Mayo scissors and peritoneum is entered using a snap.[41]

The index finger is inserted into the peritoneal window to ensure absence of adhesions. The trocar and cannula is then introduced and cone-shaped obturator is secured to the fascia using stay sutures to discourage gas leakage around the cannulas' stem (*see* **Fig. 3**).

Several variations on this method have been described and a number of general surgeons practice this method, especially in patients who have had previous abdominal surgery or when parietal peritoneal adhesions are suspected. Moreover, possibility of access injury to adherent viscera at immediate entry site is not entirely eliminated; it is believed that fatal large vessel injuries are less likely. Although such vessel injuries can and has occurred, especially with thin patients.[42-44]

Open access is designed to avoid use of a Veress needle and sharp push-through trocars. Some endoscopists prefer direct primary port insertion using sharp or bladed blind trocars without preinsufflation. Although, a few small studies suggest direct primary trocar entry that may cause fewer minor access complications, it is clear that most of these studies involve low-risk patients.[45]

Direct trocar access advocates recommend elevation of the anterior abdominal wall with the nondominant hand while inserting the sharp primary trocar directly and blindly toward the peritoneal cavity with the other. CO_2 gas stopcock must be kept open, to relieve negative intra-abdominal pressure, as soon as the vented instrument tip enters the sealed peritoneal space. It is postulated that viscera falls off its parietal apposition prior to contact with advancing sharp trocar.[46]

Consequently, this laparoscopic primary port insertion method is not advised in those who have had previous abdominal surgery.

Published data generally do not support suggestion that direct entry is any safer than conventional closed access.

Studies recommending this entry method are too small and ambiguous to make reliable statistically valid observations. Many surgeons find insertion of sharp trocars blindly into a noninsufflated abdomen counter intuitive, potentially hazardous and sometimes indefensible. Bowel injury has been reported as a consequence of this direct entry technique, certainly larger trials are necessary to better understand limitations of this insertion method.[25,47,48]

Gasless laparoscopy is another method of endoscopy, where insufflation is not utilized during surgery. The primary port site is dissected down through peritoneum. Laparoscope is inserted to verify absence of adhesions and then, a special abdominal wall lifter is suspended, attached to the operating table.

The tented abdomen creates a peritoneal working compartment where additional ports are placed under direct vision.

Some believe that this method fails to offer a uniform and satisfactory displacement of viscera compared with the work envelope created by a pneumoperitoneum. Conventional laparotomy instruments are used to operate and it is suggested that laparoscopic learning curve becomes shorter. Several abdominal lifting instruments are available, some are intrusive and most surgeons prefer conventional insufflated laparoscopy.[49]

SECOND-GENERATION VISUAL ACCESS METHOD

Task performance studies have identified several important performance shaping factors (PSFs) that determine outcome **(Fig. 11)**.

It is believed that lack of redundancy in conventional access techniques and instrument design are responsible for most serious access accidents irrespective of the surgeons' competence and dexterity.

Conventional primary port insertion requires application of considerable axial PF to a sharp or bladed blind trocar. The anterior abdominal wall tents toward the viscera where entry is sudden and uncontrolled with inevitable overshoot. The compilation of these potentially dangerous PSFs during primary port insertion renders accessing less forgiving and sets the stage for inadvertent injury.

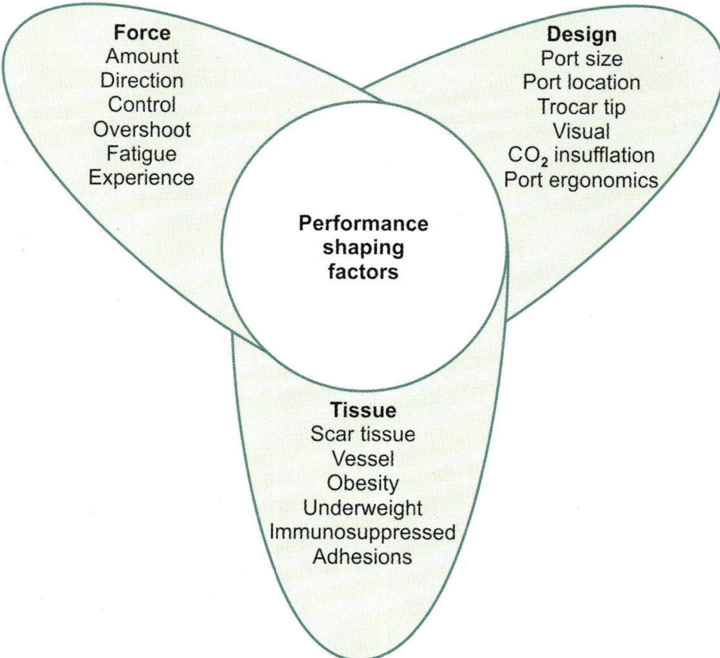

Fig. 11: Etiology of port complication-performance shaping factors.

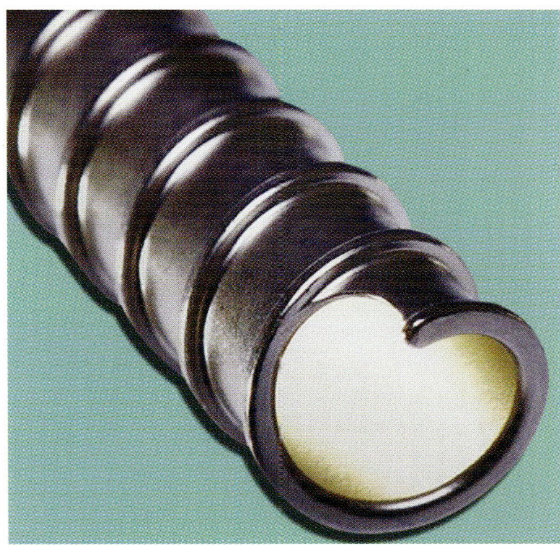

Fig. 12: EndoTIP cannula has a single thread that ends in a blunt tip.

Second-generation access systems buffer human error, through system redesign and elimination of identified PSF. When specific PSFs of conventional access are eliminated during primary entry, port insertion becomes less dangerous. Error recognition is likely when mishaps occur and recovery is possible before irreparable patient harm develops. Interactive and real-time visual access avoids application of axial force at port site, requires no sharp or pointed trocar to allow visual and controlled port placement without overshoot.[50]

The EndoTIP™ is a reusable visual access cannula system that may be used during closed or open laparoscopy. It can be applied as a primary or ancillary port and may be used to perform intra- or retroperitoneal operations.

It consists of a proximal valve and a stainless steel hollow distal cannula section. A single thread winds diagonally on its outer surface, which ends distally in a blunt notched tip **(Fig. 12)**. EndoTIP™ is available in several lengths and diameters for different surgical applications. The reusable retaining ring, TS is used to keep the sheathed 0° laparoscope from sliding out of focus during insertion (*see* **Fig. 10**).

Closed Laparoscopic Access with EndoTIP

As is recommended in the consensus document on laparoscopic entry, all port insertions should be performed when the patient is lying flat with no Trendelenburg tilt, since this position rotates the sacral promontory to bring the aortic bifurcation closer to the umbilicus, consequently increasing the likelihood of inadvertent vascular injury.[51]

A generous subumbilical skin incision is made using a 15-mm surgical blade to accommodate the cannulas' diameter and avoid skin dystocia. Ribbon retractors and "peanut sponges" are used to expose the white anterior rectus

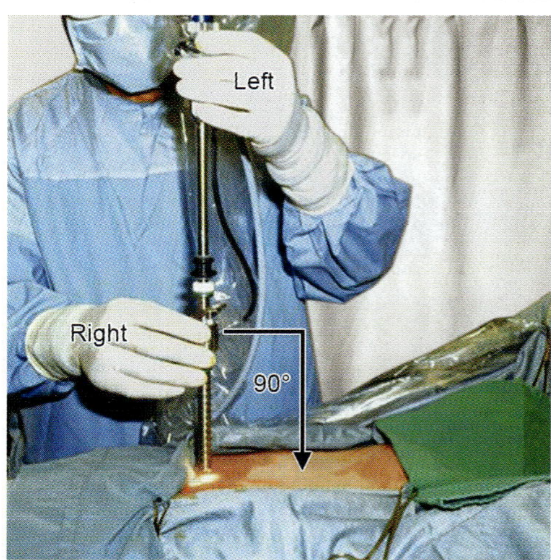

Fig. 13: Sheathed laparoscope is held perpendicular to supine abdomen with nondominant hand, while EndoTIP cannula is rotated clockwise with the dominant hand.

fascia, as insertion starts at fascial level. Then a Veress needle is inserted as described previously.

During insufflation, a 0° laparoscope is white balanced and defogged; then the TS followed by the visual cannula mounted. The TS is locked to hold the laparoscope 1 cm short of the cannulas' distal end and the camera is focused to the visual cannulas' tip.

When insufflation is complete, the Veress is removed. The cannula with mounted laparoscope is held vertical to the patient's supine abdomen, using the surgeons' nondominant hand and is lowered into the umbilical well with the CO_2 stopcock in the closed position **(Fig. 13)**. Using the surgeons' dominant hand wrist muscles, the cannula is rotated clockwise, while keeping the forearm horizontal and shoulders in a comfortable resting position facing the monitor.

The bladeless blunt cannulas' tip engages the anterior rectus fascia and lifts to transpose successive tissue layer sequentially onto the cannulas' outer thread. The white anterior rectus fascia red rectus muscle, pearly white posterior fascia, and yellowish preperitoneal fat are observed in sequence **(Figs. 14A to F)**.

The laparoscopes' intense light traverses the thin taut peritoneal membrane and the CO_2 filled peritoneal cavity appears gray-blue in color. Vessels, bowel or adhesions are recognized and inadvertent injury is avoided. Further clockwise rotation, parts the thin peritoneal membrane radially to advance the cannula intraperitoneally, under direct visual control, without requiring a sharp trocar, or applying axial PF. The visual cannula has to be kept perpendicular to tissues at all times to avoid tunneling.

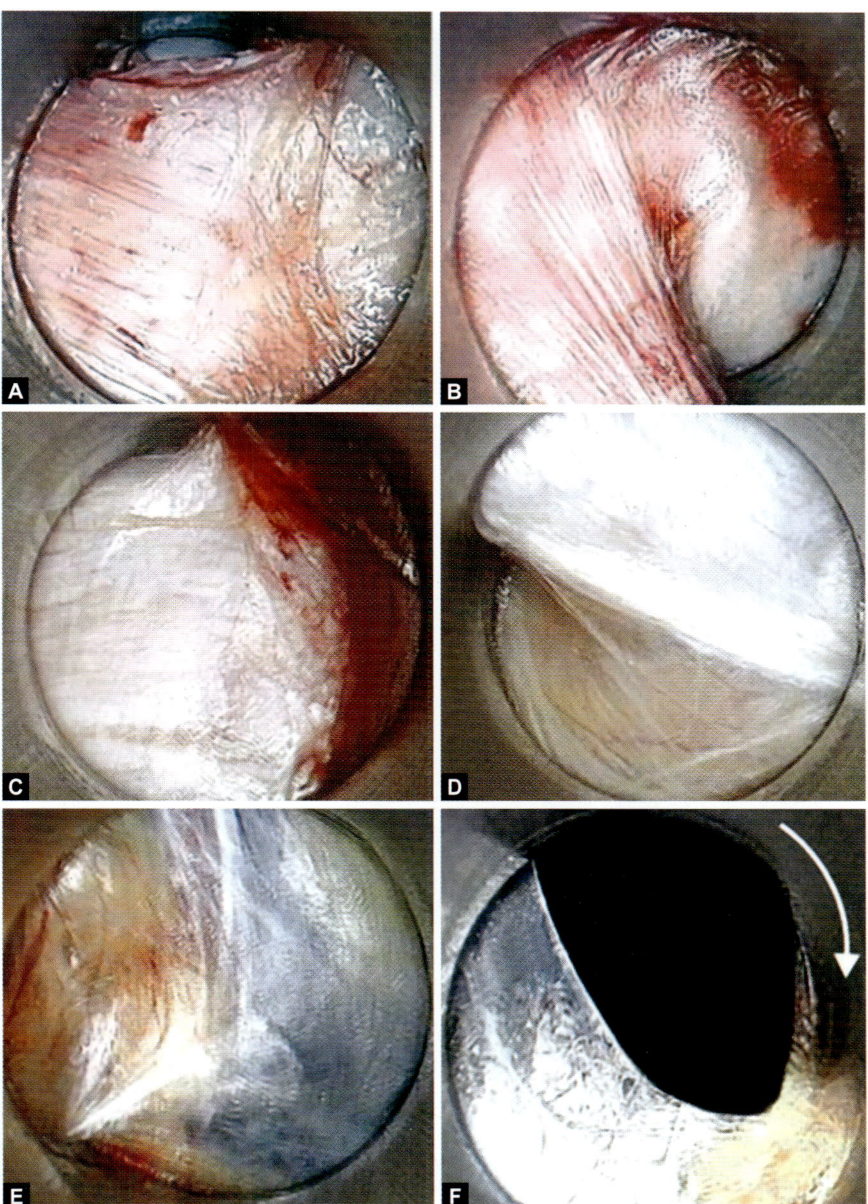

Figs. 14A to F: Abdominal wall layer sequencing during closed EndoTIP cannula application.

Open Laparoscopic Access with EndoTIP

Surgeons must be well-versed with closed EndoTIP™ insertion at primary port with preinsufflation before attempting application of the visual cannula without preinsufflation. It is essential for the operator to clearly recognize tissue plane transition off the monitor during entry and appreciate importance of not applying perpendicular PF during insertion.

A generous skin incision is made using a 15 mm surgical blade; ribbon retractors are used to expose the anterior rectus fascia, the laparoscope is defogged and camera white-balanced. Then the TS and cannula are mounted and stopper is locked to keep laparoscopes' end 1 cm short of the visual cannulas' distal tip (*see* **Fig. 10**). The camera is focused to cannulas' blunt end and laparoscope held vertical to the patients' supine abdomen using the surgeon's nondominant hand.

The EndoTIP^{TM} visual cannula, with the CO_2 stopcock in the open position, is lowered into the umbilical well and rotated clockwise, using the wrist muscles of the dominant hand while keeping the forearm horizontal and shoulders square in resting position, facing the monitor (*see* **Fig. 13**).

The cannulas' bladeless tip engages the anterior fascia, stretches it radially, and then lifts to transpose successive tissue layers on to the visual cannulas' outer thread. The white anterior rectus fascia, red rectus muscle, then pearly white posterior fascia, and yellowish preperitoneum are pulled up in sequence along outer pitch. It is very important for the surgeon to identify and recognize each layer to avoid unintended overshoot and visceral injury (**Figs. 15A to F**).

Given the intense light and magnification of laparoscope, bowel or omentum can be observed moving across a transparent peritoneal membrane with respiratory movements of patient. One may also observe bowel peristalsis across the peritoneal membrane.

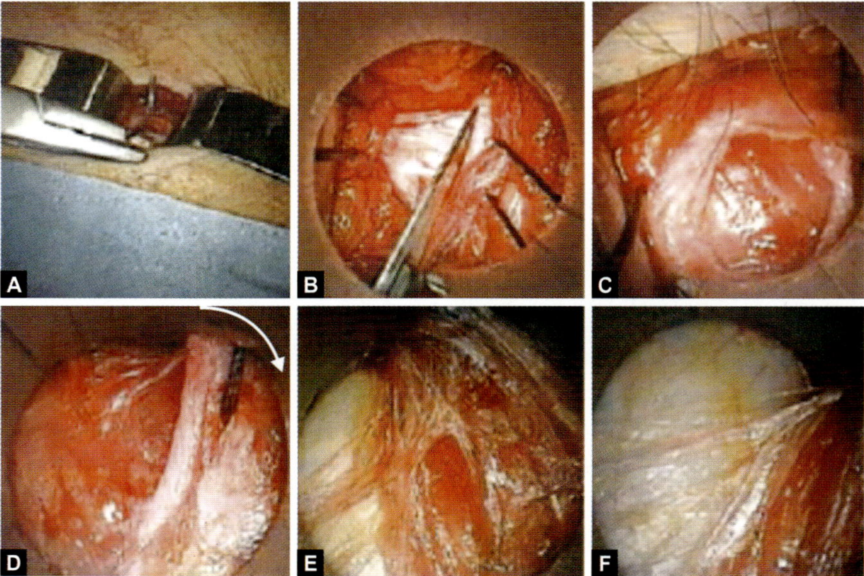

Figs. 15A to F: Abdominal wall layer sequencing during open application of EndoTIP cannula.

Upon peritoneal entry, room-air streams through the visual cannulas' open CO_2 stopcock into the virtual peritoneal cavity, interposed between presenting organ and cannula. At this point, clockwise rotation is stopped and CO_2 insufflation is initiated through a partially parted peritoneal membrane under visual control.

During closed preinsufflated laparoscopy, a CO_2 filled buffer zone is interposed between access device tip and intra-abdominal organs. Whereas, during open laparoscopy, the visual access cannula encounters abdominal contents directly upon peritoneal entry. It is, therefore, very important to identify location of the cannula at all times—situational awareness and distinguish access images at all times during port insertion. Surgeons must be familiar with normal anterior abdominal wall anatomy at entry site, learn when to stop rotation and know when to initiate insufflation.

Care must be exercised to minimize application of perpendicular PF as excessive axial force may cause unintended injury. Tissue sequencing at port site during open insertion of laparoscopic access instruments in general is different from closed laparoscopic access. Therefore, when applying the EndoTIP™ visual cannula in open laparoscopy, the surgeon must exercise extreme caution until well-versed in closed application of EndoTIP™ and fully familiar with anatomic image sequencing at access site.

Ancillary Access with EndoTIP

Ancillary port insertion is also a very important step during laparoscopic operations as through these strategically placed ports, various specialized instruments are introduced to perform complex operations.

The insertion site, number, and method of access depend on several important factors, including patient's anatomy, type of procedure performed, and surgeon's preference.

Given that the abdomen is already distended with CO_2 gas and laparoscope—camera inserted, it is essential that all ancillary ports be visually observed through the primary port during insertion, so as to minimize inadvertent injury.

Knowledge and careful attention to vascular anatomy are important, as injury to the deep epigastric vessels is the single most common vascular accident during operative laparoscopy.

The course of the epigastric vessel is identified through laparoscopic inspection (inferior epigastric—last branch of the external iliac vessels) and transillumination (superficial epigastric—first branch of the femoral vessels). Applying axial abdominal pressure with the advancing instrument-tip indents access-site. Direction and axis of entry can then be altered when vessels are suspected along a cannulas' path to avoid injury.

Sometimes the inferior epigastric vessels are difficult to identify by abdominal transillumination, especially in obese patients, those who have had

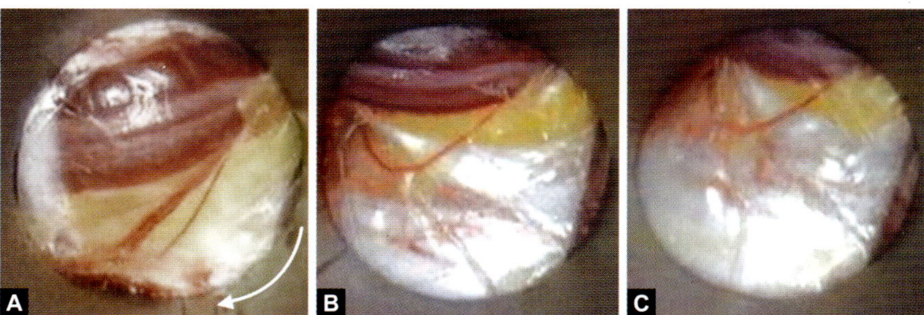

Figs. 16A to C: Vessels encountered along EndoTIP™ visual cannulas' entry path are not transected. They move laterally out of harm's way.

previous surgical scars and those with abdominal adhesions. As they invariably run lateral to the umbilical ligaments, they are easily identified laparoscopically on either side of the bladder, just medial to the internal inguinal ring.

In order to avoid vascular injury, ancillary ports must be inserted lateral to the internal inguinal ring or medial to the umbilical ligaments. The triangular area between these two lines should be avoided if possible. Vessels encountered along EndoTIP™ cannulas' path move radially out of harms' way and are not transected **(Figs. 16A to C)**.

When using EndoTIP™ at ancillary port, only a skin incision along Langer's lines and subcutaneous dissection is needed; an ancillary telescope is not necessary. As with all ancillary port insertions, ancillary EndoTIP cannulas must also be introduced under direct laparoscopic visual control.

To avoid peritoneal tenting or tunneling, EndoTIP™ cannula insertion must remain at right angle to skin surface until the abdominal cavity is entered **(Fig. 17)**.[50] The urinary bladder should always be emptied before suprapubic port insertion.

Alternate Access Sites

Alternate access sites are considered when umbilical placement of a Veress needle or primary trocar is deemed unsafe, such as in patients known to have umbilical adhesions. Palmers' point, located 3 cm below the left costal margin at mid clavicular line is a popular and safe alternative.[52]

A nasogastric tube is first inserted to prevent inadvertent gastric injury, as sometimes the stomach may get distended with anesthetic gases during intubation. Surgeons must be particularly careful in patients with portal hypertension, gastric or pancreatic masses, splenomegaly or when left upper abdominal pathology is suspected.[53]

In high-risk patients, a preliminary umbilical inspection is possible with the EndoTIP™ visual cannula, optical Veress microlaparoscope, or other visually guided cannulas. Peritoneal adhesions are mapped and additional ports inserted accordingly.

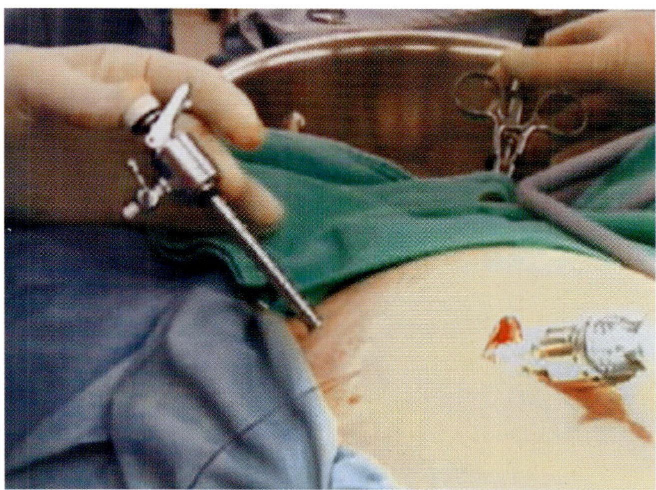

Fig. 17: Keep EndoTIP cannula at right angle to abdominal surface until safely in the peritoneal cavity.

Successful peritoneal access on first passage of a Veress needle through conventional sites does not exclude the possibility of umbilical adhesions or subsequent bowel injury upon insertion of conventional trocars.

The clinical burden of postoperative adhesions is well documented in the SCAR study and it is clear that 60–90% of women who have undergone major gynecologic surgery will have some adhesions.[54]

Some suggest that the incidence of umbilical adhesion is infrequent, <0.03%, however, in some instances it may be as high as 68% in those patients where the previous midline laparotomy surgical scar extends to the umbilical region.[55]

Patients with known peritoneal adhesions, more than one previous laparoscopy, morbid obesity, history of failed previous laparoscopy or insufflation, and others with special circumstances may be candidates for alternate access techniques, with specialized laparoscopic visual access instruments.

Importance of Port Removal

Increasingly, surgeons are appreciating the importance of safe cannula removal to maintain port competence and avoid implantation of malignant cells along port tract following oncological procedures. Introduction of the visual laparoscopic access systems allows surgeons to understand tissue dynamics at port-site during insertion and removal of cannulas. It helps to determine and maintain the integrity of different tissue planes that preserve port competence.

Without the ability to visually observe port tract during insertion and removal of cannulas, surgeons are unable to identify compromised access sites; consequently, appropriate pre-emptive measures are not taken.

The incidence of ventral hernia after laparotomy ranges between 11% and 20%, versus 0.02% incidence of port site herniation.[56,57] Published incidence of port herniation is about 0.3–1.3%.[58]

When inserting sharp pyramidal or cutting trocars, the bladed instrument transects tissue layers along its path, disrupting the shutter mechanism at port site. The fascial defect is significantly larger as compared to the noncutting bladeless visual cannula tip.[59] EndoTIP™ is designed to address port competence concerns, such that the radially displaced tissue layers regain their normal grid iron orientation and restore shutter mechanism at access site upon cannula removal.

In addition, entry point at the anterior rectus fascia, muscle, posterior fascia, and peritoneal membrane are not aligned along a straight vertical axis, instead they are scattered along the perimeter of the cannulas' path, thereby theoretically maintaining port competence.

In a randomized trial, Glass et al. demonstrated a smaller fascial wound area and less muscle damage, requiring less force when applying the EndoTIP™ visual cannula compared with the Ethicon Endopath TriStar Pyramidal Cutting Trocar of the same diameter **(Figs. 18A to F)**.[60]

When the operation is completed, the stopcock is closed, CO_2 tubing disconnected and laparoscopes' end retracted 1 cm into the cannula, TS locked and camera focused to the EndoTIP™ visual cannulas' tip.

All ancillary ports are removed under visual control, then peritoneal cavity dis-insufflated and finally the primary umbilical port is removed under visual control. The laparoscope is held perpendicular to the patients' abdomen with

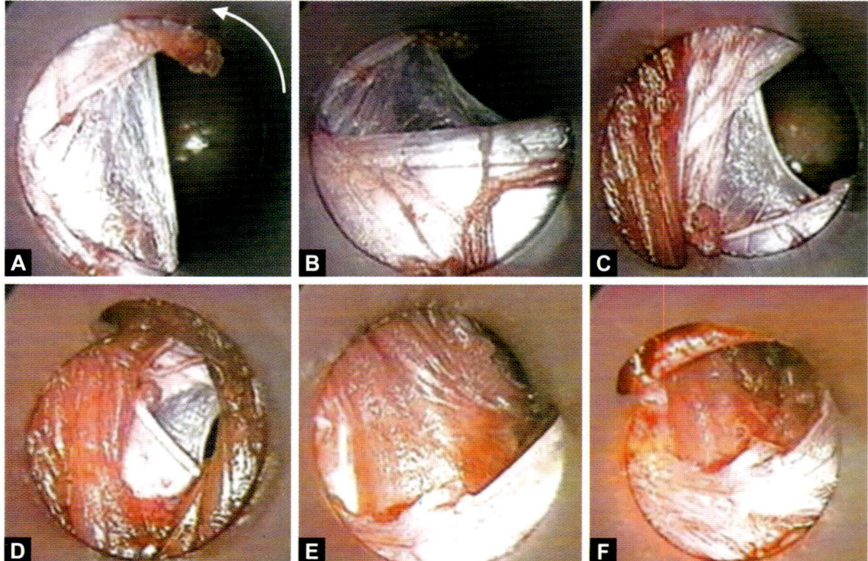

Figs. 18A to F: EndoTIP visual cannula removal.

the nondominant hand and cannula is rotated counterclockwise with the dominant hand.

As cannula removal is visual, incremental, and controlled, tissue injury or entrapment along the cannulas' tract is avoided. When fascia is extended to retrieve surgical specimens; fascial sutures are applied to that cannula entry site to further secure port competence.

Closure of fascial defects is particularly important in high-risk patients where predisposing factors may exist. Several direct port-site fascial closure instruments are available; however, it has been shown that fascial suturing of laparoscopic entry sites decreases but does not eliminate incidence of all hernias.[28]

CONCLUSION

Primary entry techniques have always been considered a critical first step in laparoscopy, as push-through conventional first generation trocar and cannula access systems apply considerable, uncontrolled axial PF at port- site to thrust the trajectory blindly toward the peritoneum, with no recourse for overshoot.

Second-generation access systems are redesigned to buffer inevitable surgical mishaps and render primary access and exit more error-tolerant. Application of perpendicular PF is avoided by realigning direction of entry from axial to spiral. Sharp or bladed trocars are not required and visual interactive port creation is possible.

Real-time recognition of mishaps, when accidents occur, allows timely error recovery and prevents access injury from progressing to patient harm. It is clear from the literature that delayed recognition of bowel injury is associated with very-high mortality, especially in patients over 60 years of age.[25]

Visual access systems can improve our understanding of laparoscopic entry complications and reduce recurring error. Surgeons can visualize tissue dynamics at port site; appreciate port toilette, and address port competence concerns. Controlled incremental access with a bladeless visual instrument that recruits less PF generated by weaker wrist muscles and dissipates force radially along horizontal tissue planes, offers unique instrument and method redundancy that renders access less hazardous.

Surgeons should not ascribe access complications to their colleagues' inexperience or carelessness; instead one must thrive to understand accident causation and always remember that such catastrophes lie in wait at every moment of an endoscopists' career.

It is important for surgeons to be versed in more than one safe laparoscopic access method and be knowledgeable in different entry techniques, as our patients have different medical needs. Careful access selection, meticulous attention to surgical technique during laparoscopic port entry and exit can significantly reduce inadvertent injury and improve patient safety.

REFERENCES

1. US Food and Drug Administration. Laparoscopic Trocar Injuries: A report from a US Food and Drug Administration (FDA) Center for Devices and Radiological Health (CDRH) Systematic Technology Assessment of Medical Products (STAMP) Committee. [online]. Available from http://www.fda.gov/cdrh/medicaldevicesafety/stamp/trocar.html [Last accessed December, 2019].
2. Institute of Medicine. To Err is Human. Building a Safer Health System. Washington, DC: National Academy Press. 1999.
3. Bogner MS. Medical Devices and Human Error in Human Performance. In: Mouloua M, Parasuraman R (Eds). Automated Systems: Current Research and Trends. Hillsdale, NJ: Lawrence Erlbaum; 1994. pp. 64-7.
4. Corson SL, Batzer FR, Gocial B, et al. Measurement of the force necessary for laparoscopy trocar entry. J Reprod Med. 1989;34:282-4.
5. Leibl BJ, Schmedt CG, Schwarz J, et al. Laparoscopic surgery complications associated with trocar tip design: review of literature and own results. J Laparosc Adv Surg Tech A. 1999;9:135-40.
6. Tarnay CM, Glass KB, Munro MG. Entry force and intra-abdominal pressure associated with six laparoscopic trocar-cannula systems: a randomized comparison. Obstet Gynecol. 1999;94:83-8.
7. Hurd WW, Wang L, Schemmel MT. A comparison of the relative risk of vessel injury with conical versus pyramidal laparoscopic trocars in a rabbit model. Am J Obstet Gynecol. 1995;173:1731-3.
8. Hurd WW, Diamond MP. There's a hole in my bucket, the cost of disposable instruments. Fertil Steril. 1997;67:13-5.
9. Chan AC, Ip M, Koehler A, et al. Is it safe to reuse disposable laparoscopic trocars? An in vitro testing. Surg Endosc. 2000;14:1042-4.
10. Soderstrom RM. Injuries to major blood vessels during endoscopy. J Am Assoc Gynecol Laparosc. 1997;4:395-8.
11. Hashizume M, Sugimachi K. Needle and trocar injury during laparoscopic surgery in Japan. Study group of endoscopic surgery in Kyushu, Japan. Surg Endosc. 1997;11:1198-201.
12. Yuzpe AA. Pneumoperitoneum needle and trocar injuries in laparoscopy. A survey on possible contributing factors and prevention. J Reprod Med. 1990;35:485-90.
13. Pring CM. Aortic injury using the Hasson trocar: a case report and review of the literature. Ann R Coll Surg Engl. 2007;89:W3-5.
14. Hasson HM, Rotman C, Rana N, et al. Open laparoscopy: 29-year experience. Obstet Gynecol. 2000;96:763-6.
15. Levy BS, Hulka JF, Peterson HB, et al. Operative laparoscopy: American Association of Gynecologic Laparoscopists, 1993 membership survey. J Am Assoc Gynecol Laparosc. 1994;1:301-5.
16. Wherry DC, Marohn MR, Malanoski MP, et al. An external audit of laparoscopic cholecystectomy in the steady state performed in a medical treatment facility of the Department of Defense. Ann Surg. 1996;224:145-54.
17. Uen YH, Liang AL, Lee HH. Randomized comparison of conventional carbon dioxide insufflation and abdominal wall lifting for laparoscopic cholecystectomy. J Laparoendosc Adv Surg Tech A. 2002;12:7-14.
18. Bhoyrul S, Payne J, Steffes B, et al. A randomized prospective study of radially expanding trocars in laparoscopic surgery. J Gastrointest Surg. 2000;4:392-7.
19. Audebert AJ. The role of micro-laparoscopy in the diagnosis of peritoneal and visceral adhesions and in the prevention of bowel injury associated with blind trocar insertion. Fertil Steril. 2000;73:631-5.

20. Munro MG. Laparoscopic access; complications, technologies, and techniques. Curr Opin Obstet Gynecol. 2002;14:365-74.
21. Ternamian A. Laparoscopy without trocars. Surg Endosc. 1997;11:815-8.
22. Levy BS. Litigation and laparoscopy. J Am Assoc Gynecol Laparosc. 2001;8:335-6.
23. Ahmed G, Duffy JM, Watson AJ. Laparoscopic entry techniques and complications. Int J Gynecol Obstet. 2007;99:52-5.
24. Rullo S, Ticconi C, Marchetti AA, et al. Common iliac artery injury during the abdominal entry phase of gynecologic laparoscopy. J Reprod Med. 2007;52:1052-5.
25. Corson SL, Chandler JG, Way LW. Survey of laparoscopic entry injuries provoking litigation. J Am Ass Gynecol Laparosc. 2001;8:341-7.
26. Marret H, Pierre F, Chapron C, et al. Complications of laparoscopy caused by trocars. Preliminary study from the national registry of the French Society of Gynecologic Endoscopy. J Gynecol Obstet Biol Reprod. 1997;26(4):405-12.
27. Jansen FW, Kapiteyn K, Trimbos-Kemper T, et al. Complications of laparoscopy: a prospective multicentre observational study. Br J Obstet Gynaecol. 1997;104: 595-600.
28. Leonard F, Lecuru F, Rizk E, et al. Perioperative morbidity of gynecological laparoscopy: a prospective monocenter observational study. Acta Obstet Gynecol Scand. 2000;79:129-34.
29. Harkki-Siren P. The incidence of entry-related laparoscopic injuries in Finland. Gynecol Endos. 1999;8:335-8.
30. Loffer FD. Endoscopy in high risk patients. In: Martin DC (Ed). Manual of Endoscopy. Santa Fe Springs, CA: J Am Assoc Gynecol Laparosc; 1990; p. 43.
31. Teoh B, Sen R, Abbott J. An evaluation of four tests used to ascertain Veress needle placement at closed laparoscopy. J Min Invas Gynecol. 2005;12:153-8.
32. Abu-Rafea B, Vilos GA, Vilos AG. High-pressure laparoscopic entry does not adversely affect cardiopulmonary function in healthy women. J Minim Invas Gynecol. 2005;12:475-9.
33. Vilos G, Ternamian A, Dempster J, et al. Laparoscopic Entry: A Review of Techniques, Technologies, and Complications. SOGC Clinical Practice Guidelines. J Obstet Gynecol Can. 2007;29:433-65.
34. Phillips G, Garry R, Kumar C, et al. How much gas is required for initial insufflation at laparoscopy? Gynaecol Endosc. 1999;8:369-74.
35. Garry R. Complications of laparoscopic entry. Gynae Endosc. 1997;6:319-29.
36. Sutton C. A practical approach to diagnostic laparoscopy. In: Sutton C, Diamond M (Eds). Endoscopic Surgery for Gynaecologists. London: WB Saunders; 1993. pp. 21-7.
37. McDougall E, Figenshau RS, Cdayman RV, et al. J Laparoscopic Surgery. United States: Mary Ann Liebert, Inc. Publishers; 1994.
38. Rothenberg SS, Georgeson K, Decou JM, et al. A clinical evaluation of the use of radially expandable laparoscopic access devices in the pediatric population. Pediatr Endosurg Innov Tech. 2000;4:7-11.
39. Semm K, Semm I. Safe insertion of trocars and the Veress needle using standard equipment and the 11 security steps. Gynae Endosc. 1997;6:319-29.
40. Okeahialam MG, O'Donovan PJ, Gupta JK. Microlaparoscopy using an optical Veress needle inserted at Palmer's point. Gynaecol Endosc. 1999;8:115-6.
41. Hasson HM. Open laparoscopy. A modified treatment and method of laparoscopy. Am J Obstet Gynecol. 1971;110:886-7.
42. Hanney RM, Carmalt HL, Merrett N, et al. Use of the Hasson cannula producing major vascular injury at laparoscopy. Surg Endosc. 1999;13:1238-40.

43. Voitk A, Rizoli S. Blunt Hasson trocar injury: long intra-abdominal trocar and lean patient—a dangerous combination. J Laparoendosc Adv Surg Tech A. 2001;11:259-62.
44. Pring CM. Aortic injury using the Hasson trocar: a case report and review of the literature. Ann R Coll Surg Engl. 2007;89(2):W3-5.
45. Nezhat FR, Silfen SL, Evans D, et al. Comparison of direct insertion of disposable and standard reusable laparoscopic trocars and previous pneumoperitoneum with Veress needle. Obstet Gynecol. 1991;78:148-9.
46. Byron JW, Markenson G, Miyazawa K. A randomized comparison of Veress needle and direct trocar insertion for laparoscopy. Surg Gynecol Obstet. 1993;177:259-62.
47. Vilos GA. Litigation of laparoscopic major vessels injuries in Canada. J Am Assoc Gynecol Laparosc. 2000;7:503-9.
48. Molloy D, Kalloo PD, Cooper M, et al. Laparoscopic entry: a literature review and analysis of techniques and complications of primary port entry. Aust NZJ Obstet Gynecol. 2002;42:246-54.
49. Smith RS, Fry WR, Tsoi EK. Gaseless laparoscopy and conventional instruments. The next phase of minimally invasive surgery. Arch Surg. 1993;128:1102-7.
50. Ternamian AM. A trocarless, reusable, visual-access cannula for safer laparoscopy; an update. J Am Assoc Gynecol Laparosc. 1998;5(2):197-201.
51. Garry R. A consensus document concerning laparoscopic entry: Middlesbrough. Gynaecol Endosc. 1999;8:403-6.
52. Palmer R. Safety in laparoscopy. J Repro Med. 1974;13:1-5.
53. Chapron C, Pierre F, Harchaoui Y, et al. Gastrointestinal injuries during gynaecological laparoscopy. Hum Repro. 1999;14:333-7.
54. Lower AM, Hawthorn RJ, Ellis H, et al. The impact of adhesions on hospital readmissions over ten years after 8849 open gynaecological procedures: an assessment from the Surgical and Clinical Adhesions Research Study. Brit J Obstet Gynecol. 2000;107:855-62.
55. Childers JM, Brzechffa PR, Surwit EA. Laparoscopy using the left upper quadrant as the primary trocar site. Gynaecol Oncol. 1993;50:221-5.
56. Luijendijk RW, Hop WC, van den Tol MP. A comparison of suture repair with mesh repair for incisional hernia. N Engl J Med. 2000;343:392-8.
57. Montz FJ, Holschneider CH, Munro MG. Incisional hernias following laparoscopy: a survey of the American Association of Gynecologic Laparoscopists. Obstet Gynecol. 1994;84:881-4.
58. Mayol J, Garcia-Aguilar J, Ortiz-Oshiro E, et al. Risks of the minimal access approach for laparoscopic surgery: multivariate analysis of morbidity related to umbilical trocar insertion. WJ Surg. 1997;21:529-33.
59. Tarnay CM, Glass BK, Munro MG. Incisions characteristics associated with six laparoscopic trocar-cannula systems; A randomized, observer-blinded comparison. Am J Obstet Gynecol. 1999;94:89-93.
60. Glass KB, Tarnay CM, Munro MG. Intra-abdominal pressure and incisional parameters associated with a pyramidal laparoscopic trocar-cannula system and the EndoTIP cannula. 2002;9:508-13.

3

Palmer's Point

Parima Jain, Prateek Gupta, Nutan Jain

■ INTRODUCTION

Minimally invasive surgery is a dynamic field that requires surgeons to be ambidextrous and acquire new sets of motor skills, with a long learning curve.[1,2] The most important and potentially dangerous is the first step in laparoscopy that is the insertion of a primary port, since half of complications with laparoscopy occur even before the start of the intended procedure.[3-5]

No single method has proven to be the safest approach to access peritoneal cavity for all patients. Body habitus of a patient, abdominal wall anatomy, underlying tissues, and underlying pathology are various factors that influence the best site for access. That is why a surgeon should be well versed with all alternative access sites. One of them is Palmer's point described by a French gynecologist, Raoul Palmer in 1974 in a paper titled 'Safety in Laparoscopy'.[6]

Raoul Palmer, well known in the field of laparoscopic surgery, in 1944, examined the pelvis of patients laparoscopically by placing the patients in Trendelenburg position so that air could fill the pelvis.[7] Importance of continuous intra-abdominal pressure monitoring during laparoscopy was also emphasized. In 1947, he advocated creation of pneumoperitoneum by Veress needle as a vital first step for blind entry.[8]

Then in 1974, he introduced this alternate primary port location in left upper quadrant for peritoneal entry—'Palmer's point'.[6] Thus Palmer changed laparoscopy from an occasionally performed technique to an absolutely indispensable means of obtaining invaluable diagnostic and therapeutic results.

Palmer's point, a point in the left upper quadrant is a safe and effective alternative approach compared to umbilicus in certain situations like.

- After three failed attempts at umbilical region[9] (two failed attempts according to some).[10]
- In morbidly obese patients, as subcutaneous adipose tissue is thicker at umbilical region than in left upper quadrant.[11] Palmer's point entry can

also be considered for obese and very thin individuals as in obese patients the umbilicus is shifted caudally to the aortic bifurcation and in very thin patients, especially those with a prominent sacral promontory and android pelvis, the great vessels lie 1–2 cm underneath the umbilicus.

- In case of suspected intra-abdominal adhesions (previous surgeries, Koch's abdomen).
- Previous midline incision.
- Umbilical hernia.

ANATOMICAL LANDMARK

Palmers point is situated in the left upper quadrant, 3 cm below the subcostal margin, in the midclavicular line (Fig. 1).[6]

Prerequisites before using Palmer's point:

- On the basis of prior history, physical examination and investigations, ruling out any splenomegaly, hepatomegaly, signs of portal hypertension, gastric or pancreatic masses or any left upper abdominal pathology.
- Proper marking of the landmark and positioning the needle.
- Nasogastric tube should be inserted prior to inserting Veress needle as distended stomach may come in the path, especially due to distension of stomach after bag and mask ventilation and use of certain anesthetic gases.

TECHNIQUE (FIGS. 2 TO 5)

Patient is first placed in supine position and surgeon preferably should stand on the left side of the patient with hand on left upper quadrant making skin taut between two fingers. Stab incision is given commonly using No. 11 blade. Veress needle inserted two fingers below the costal margin (3 cm) in midclavicular line in 15° cephalad direction.[6] Pneumoperitoneum created and after insufflation,

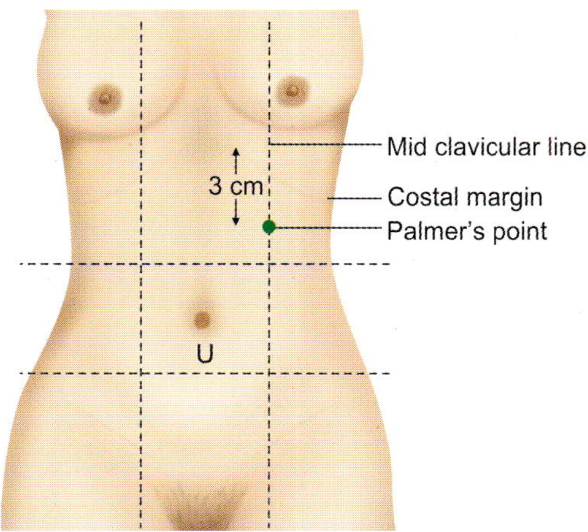

Fig. 1: Landmark of Palmer's point. (U: umbilicus).

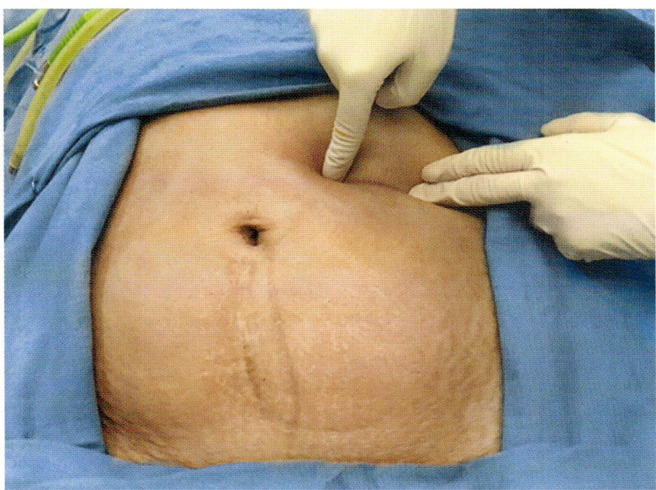

Fig. 2: Site for Palmer's point—left upper quadrant. Patient had a midline scar thereby suspected periumbilical adhesions.

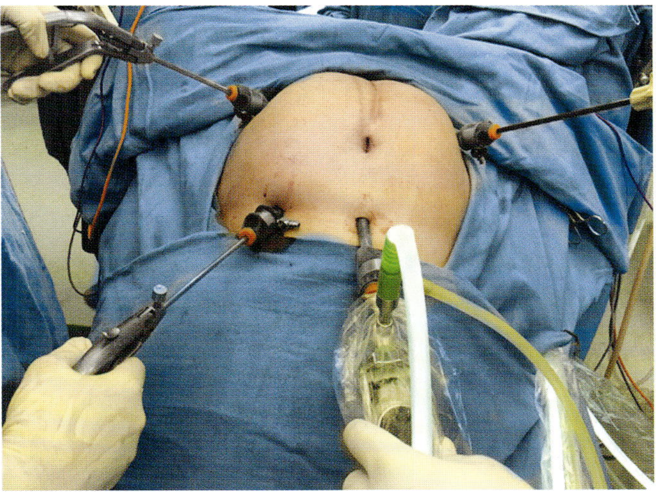

Fig. 3: Ports positioning after using Palmer's point entry.

Veress needle is removed and a 5 mm trocar is inserted into the peritoneal cavity using the same point. The laparoscope is then advanced and intra-abdominal placement is confirmed. Anterior abdominal wall adhesions are visualized and rest of the ports placed according to convenience.

DISCUSSION

Many authors have described the left upper quadrant as arguably the safest alternative insertion site for peritoneal access in women having undergone earlier laparotomies.[12-14]

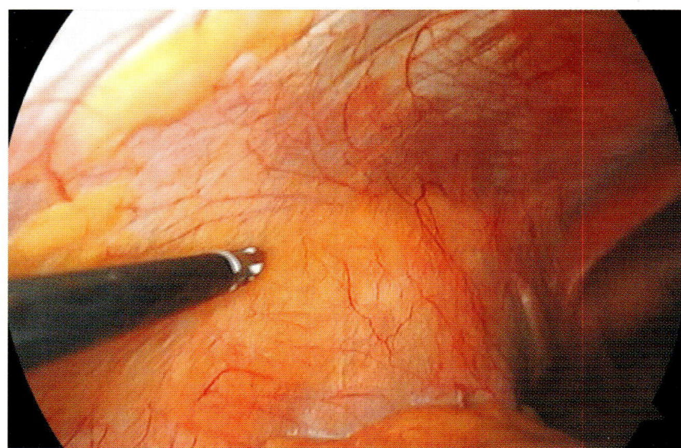

Fig. 4: Palmer's point entry; free of adhesions.

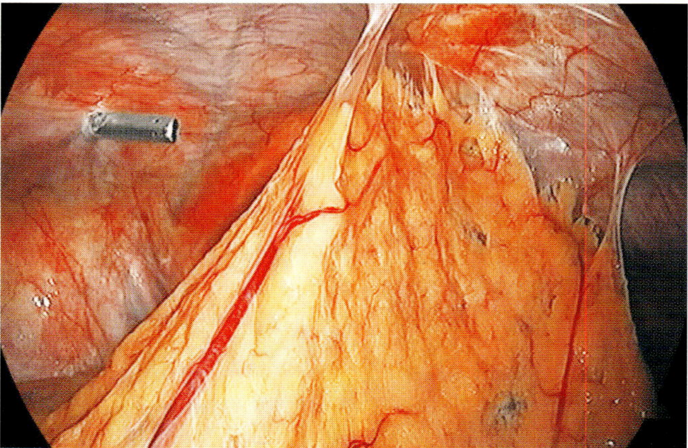

Fig. 5: Palmer's point entry with midline abdominal wall adhesions.

Marcello Granata et al. conducted a study at University College Hospital, London, United Kingdom on 385 patients undergoing laparoscopy using umbilical entry in 249 (64.6%) and Palmer's entry in 136 (35.4%). In almost three-fourths of cases, the indications for using Palmer's point were previous laparotomy or the presence of large uterine fibroids. The next most common reasons for choosing Palmer's point were known documentation of intra-abdominal adhesions from prior laparoscopies, large ovarian cysts, and hernias or hernia repairs. Entry via Palmer's point was successful in all except two cases (98.5%), and there were no entry-related complications.[9]

In another study, by GSS Mohapatra et al. on 1,324 patients who underwent laparoscopic surgery using different entry points conclusion was made that Palmer's point proved to be one of the safest modes of entry for operative laparoscopy with no significant entry related, intraoperative or postoperative complications.[15]

William K Johnston III et al. conducted a survey amongst urologists of two urological societies regarding the access point used by them for robot-assisted radical prostatectomy and associated complications. He reported that majority of the surgeons were using umbilical entry and one in five was facing a vascular complication. Palmers point, less commonly used by urologists, being away from major vasculature may reduce the morbidity for access in robot-assisted radical prostatectomy and warrants further awareness.[16]

In a study on 41 patients, who were at high risk for subumbilical adhesions (previous midline incisions or umbilical hernias), laparoscopic surgery was performed. Insufflation was done using Veress in the left upper quadrant in the ninth intercostal space and the primary trocar was placed in the left upper quadrant adjacent to the subcostal margin. Joel M Childers et al. reported 68% (28/41) of patients had subumbilical adhesions. One patient required laparotomy because of an enterotomy created when an 11 mm trocar was used. There were no complications in the remaining 40 patients, in whom smaller primary trocars were used.

He thus concluded that left upper quadrant is a safe location for primary trocar placement in patients at high risk for subumbilical adhesions, provided certain guidelines are followed.[17]

Bruce Patsner performed laparoscopy and operative pelviscopy in 90 women with a history of gynecologic cancer and at least one laparotomy using the left upper quadrant as a single entry site for the Veress needle and primary laparoscopy port. In 88 women it was performed without complication. One woman experienced transverse colon injury from primary port insertion and other had a rectosigmoid injury.

The study was concluded deeming the left upper quadrant approach as safe in patients with advanced gynecologic malignancy.[18]

Thus it can be concluded that Palmer's point is one of the *safe and effective* alternate entry site most commonly used for Veress needle and port insertion by surgeons.

REFERENCES

1. Deziel DJ. Avoiding laparoscopic complications. Int Surg. 1994;79:361-4.
2. Lekawa M, Shapiro S, Gordon LA, et al. The laparoscopic learning curve. Surg Laparosc Endosc. 1995;5:455-8.
3. Batemen BG, Kolp LA, Hoeger K. Complications of laparoscopy—operative or diagnostic. Fertil Steril. 1996;66:30-5.
4. Jansen FW, Kapiteyn K, Trimbos-Kemper T, et al. Complications of laparoscopy: a prospective multicentre observational study. Br J Obstet Gynaecol. 1997;104:595-600.
5. Chandler JG, Corson SL, Way LW. Three spectra of laparoscopic entry access injuries. J Am Coll Surg. 2001;192:478-91.

6. Palmer R. Safety in laparoscopy. J Repro Med. 1974;13(1):1-5.
7. Palmer R. (1949): Gynk. et Obstit.. 48, 206.7
8. Agarwala N, Liu CY. Safe entry techniques during laparoscopy: left upper quadrant entry using the ninth intercostal space—a review of 918 procedures. J Minim Invasive Gynecol. 2005;12(1):55-61.
9. Granata M, Tsimpanakos I, Moeity F, et al. Are we underutilizing Palmer's point entry in gynecological laparoscopy? Fertil Steril. 2010;94(7):2716-9.
10. RCOG (2008) Preventing entry-related gynaecological laparoscopic injuries; Gree-Top Guideline No. 49. RCOG, London.
11. Schwartz ML, Drew RL, Andersen JN. Induction of pneumoperitoneum in morbidly obese patients. Obes Surg. 2003;13:601-4.
12. Loffer FD. Endoscopy in high-risk patients. In: Martin DC (Ed). Manual of Endoscopy. Santa Fe Springs, CA: American Association of Gynecologic Laparoscopists; 1990. p. 43.
13. McDougall E, Figenshau RS, Clayman RV, et al. Laparoscopic pneumoperitoneum: impact of body habitus. J Laparoendosc Surg. 1994;4(6):385-91.
14. Phillips G, Garry R, Kumar C, et al. How much gas is required for initial insufflation at laparoscopy? Gynaecol Endosc. 1999;8:369-74.
15. Mahapatra GSS, Bhushan B. Comparative study of different entry sites in laparoscopic surgery: which is safest? IOSR J Dent Med Sci. 2017;16(1):64-6.
16. Johnston WK 3rd, Linsell S, Miller D, et al. Survey of abdominal access and associated morbidity for robot-assisted radical prostatectomy: does Palmer's Point warrant further awareness and study? J Endourol. 2017;31(3):283-8.
17. Childers JM, Brzechffa PR, Surwit EA. Laparoscopy using the left upper quadrant as the primary trocar site. Gynecol Oncol. 1993;50(2):221-5.
18. Patsner B. Laparoscopy using the left upper quadrant approach. J Am Assoc Gynecol Laparosc. 1999;6(3):323-5.

Lee-Huang Point

Rhythm Bhalla, Nutan Jain

■ INTRODUCTION

Endoscopy is the most recent development in the field of surgery that most contemporary gynecologists intend to master. It requires utmost skill and precision to gain primary access to the abdomen in minimally invasive surgery, because most dreadful complications occur during primary trocar entry. The recent available literature regarding primary access during endoscopic surgery has described many safe points of entry. Of these, the umbilicus has been traditionally the most preferred point, where the Veress needle is inserted. Alternative sites for Veress insertion need to be speculated, especially for patients with previous laparotomies who are suspected to have periumbilical adhesions or in cases of two successive failed insufflation attempts.

In 1993, Dr Chyi-Long Lee, a Gynecological Endoscopic Surgeon, and Dr Kuan-Gen Huang, a Gynecologist, teamed up to upgrade the use of endoscopic surgery for treatment of gynecologic malignancies in Taiwan. Their main aim was to device a laparoscopic technique for para-aortic lymphadenectomy in advanced cervical cancer. Together they described the Lee-Huang point, which is the site of primary trocar insertion in the upper abdomen (in the midline), midway between the xiphoid process and the umbilicus.[1] Since then, the Lee-Huang point has been extensively used in various gynecological endoscopy procedures.

■ LEE-HUANG POINT: A CRITICAL REVIEW

The Lee-Huang point has been widely accepted in performing para-aortic lymph node dissection in laparoscopic oncologic surgery. In this procedure, lymph nodes along the common iliac artery, abdominal aorta, and inferior vena cava are dissected and retrieved up to the level of the third part of duodenum, inferior mesenteric artery, and left renal vein. This procedure requires adequate distance between the primary trocar and the intended operative target, which should be wide enough to allow adequate view and working space in the operating field. Conventionally, umbilicus was considered to be the preferred point of entry in patients without previous surgeries. Its disadvantage is the limited view of the superior boundaries of dissection which lie in the upper abdomen. For patients with previous surgery, the primary trocar is placed at the Palmer's point (which is about 3 cm below the left subcostal margin on the midclavicular line). In comparison to umbilicus, the Palmer's point provides a higher but lateral view of the operative field. Thus there is a loss of central vision, which may disorient the surgeon during laparoscopy. A central view is of utmost importance in para-aortic lymphadenectomy because the operative target lies on either side of the major vessels, which thus allows the surgeon to approach both sides of the operative field easily.[2] Therefore, the Lee-Huang point has three advantages, it provides a higher operative view, a wider working space, and central vision rather than a lateral one, due to its midline position.

Lee-Huang point has been extensively used in patients with previous laparotomies and previous laparoscopic umbilical entry. Primary trocar entry is the most critical step in laparoscopy, which is associated with injuries to the gastrointestinal tract and major blood vessels, and about 50% of these occur prior to performing the actual surgery.[3] According to Royal College of Obstetricians and Gynaecologists (RCOG), the incidence of umbilical adhesions is 50% in previous midline vertical scars and 23% in previous low transverse incisions **(Fig. 1)**. RCOG has thus opined that umbilicus may not be the safest site of primary trocar insertion following previous surgery. The higher location of the Lee-Huang point avoids these periumbilical adhesions. Another advantage of Lee-Huang point is that, being in midline it provides entry through the avascular linea alba that gives very less resistance to trocar

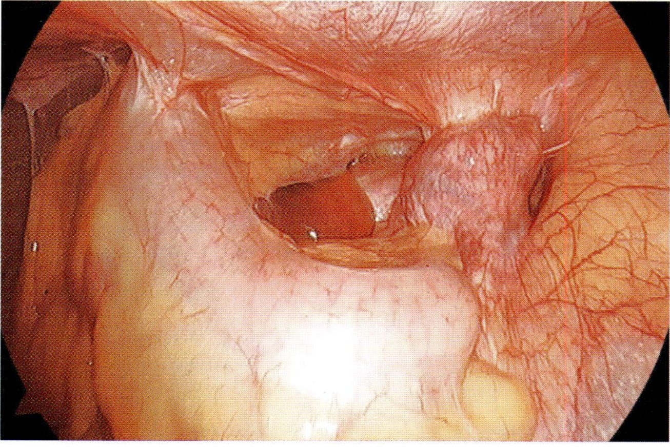

Fig. 1: Bowel adherent to anterior abdominal wall.

entry when compared to the Palmer's point. For primary trocar insertion through the Palmer's point, the surgeon has to traverse the abdominal muscles of the left upper quadrant. Excessive force is required to overcome resistance, which could lead to visceral or vascular injury in inexperienced hands. Therefore, primary abdominal access through Lee-Huang point is much safer than Palmer's point.[4] It is important to mention here that an important contraindication to using the Lee-Huang point insertion is a patient who has had previous surgery at the supraumbilical region.

The Lee-Huang point and Palmer's point have been extensively used in previous failed attempts at peritoneal insufflation. Complication rates increase with repeated umbilical entry, which have been reported in literature to be 0.8–16% at one attempt, 16–37% at two attempts, 44–64% at three attempts, and 84–100% in more than three attempts.[5] The complications reported were extraperitoneal insufflation, omental emphysema, visceral injuries, and failed laparoscopy. Due to significant increase in complication rates with multiple attempts, alternative entry such as at the Palmer's point or the Lee-Huang point should be resorted to after two failed insufflation attempts at the umbilicus. In patients with contraindications to these points or continued failed attempts, switching to the Hasson (open) technique or optical trocar access (under direct vision) is recommended. Relative contraindications to the Lee-Huang point include a previous midline vertical incision, hepatomegaly, splenomegaly, and previous history of intestinal obstruction. Now with Jain point, which is constantly noted to be free of adhesions **(Fig. 2)**, the 10 mm trocar can be inserted under direct vision of the Jain point port. Therefore, this new nonumbilical blind entry point (Jain point) can be effectively used in the above mentioned contraindications.

The Lee-Huang point has proved to be advantageous in cases of large abdominal-pelvic masses. Its higher location allows a wider view of the

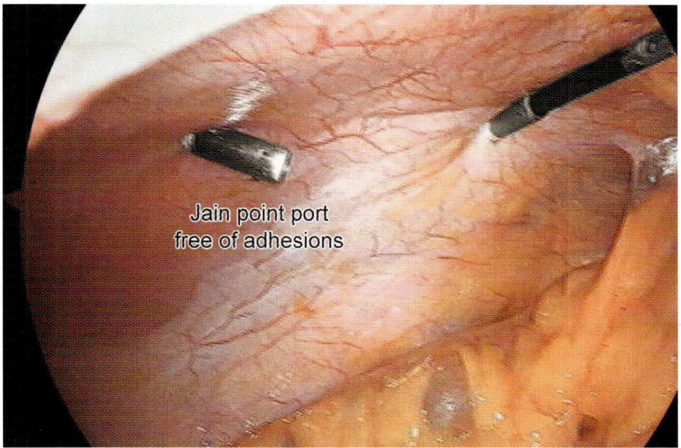

Fig. 2: Jain point port of entry free of adhesions.

operative field, avoids restricted movement of instruments, provides sufficient working space for the surgeon, and favors easy manipulation and retrieval of the specimen. The Lee-Huang point is also beneficial in performing laparoscopic procedures in morbidly obese patients where there is loss of anatomical landmarks, making primary trocar entry very difficult. The umbilicus migrates caudally in relation to the aortic bifurcation as body mass index (BMI) increases. In nonobese patients (BMI <25 kg/m^2) the umbilicus is about 0.4 cm below the aortic bifurcation, in overweight (BMI 25–30 kg/m^2) and obese (BMI >35 kg/m^2) patients, the umbilicus is about 2.4 cm and 2.9 cm below the aortic bifurcation, respectively.[6] In these circumstances the Lee-Huang point proves to be a stable vantage point in comparison to the conventional umbilical point of insertion. Another favorable advantage of Lee-Huang point is in cases of laparoscopic ovarian transposition, in patients receiving pelvic irradiation, due to its higher location. It allows both ovaries to be easily relocated to a high anterolateral position, about 3–4 cm above the level of umbilicus.[7]

With the evolution in minimally invasive surgery techniques, the Lee-Huang point has proven to be useful in the contemporary robotic-assisted surgeries, where it subdues the bulky arms of the robotic da Vinci machine, and provides an adequate view of the operative field and sufficient working space for large abdominal-pelvic masses and gynecologic cancer staging. Therefore, the use of Lee-Huang point has certainly evolved and considerably grown since its conception in 1993. Considering its contraindications, there is a desperate need to develop a technique that is simple, yet consistent, that can be universally accepted and used without any major complications.

SUGGESTED TECHNIQUE

Over the last decade, at our center, we have been performing numerous surgeries using the Jain point as the site of primary trocar access into the abdomen. The Jain point is located in the left paraumbilical region at the level of umbilicus, on a straight line drawn vertically upwards from a point 2.5 cm medial to anterior superior iliac spine (ASIS). The Veress needle is inserted at this point without lifting the abdomen, with index finger as a guard placed according to the anticipated thickness of the abdominal wall. Pneumoperitoneum created and then 5 mm telescope inserted and abdomen inspected 360°. Then 10 mm telescope is inserted under visual guidance of this 5 mm port. Other secondary ports are inserted under vision of this 10 mm telescope **(Figs. 3 to 6)**. By resorting to this novel entry technique, we can safely overcome all contraindications of Lee-Huang point discussed above, and perform major laparoscopic surgeries without the apprehensions of visceral or vascular injuries, which will be discussed in detail in the coming chapters.

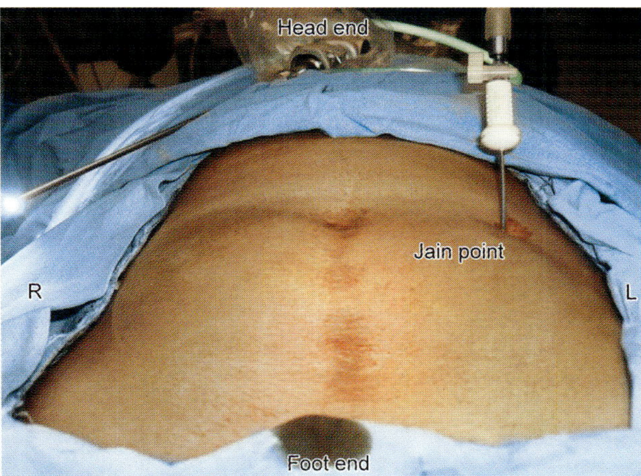

Fig. 3: Veress needle entry at Jain point.

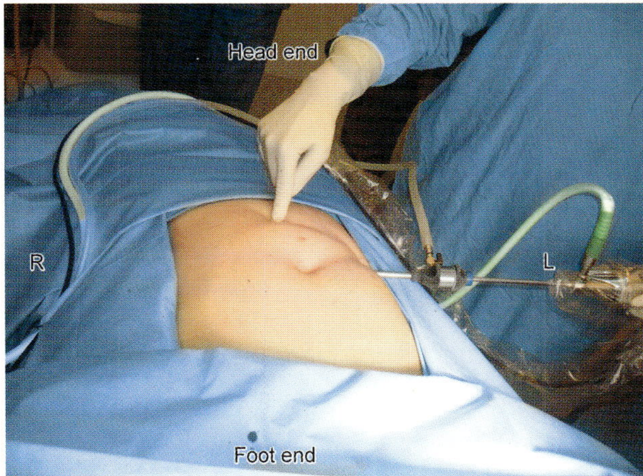

Fig. 4: Primary port entry at Jain point, finger pointing at Lee-Huang point.

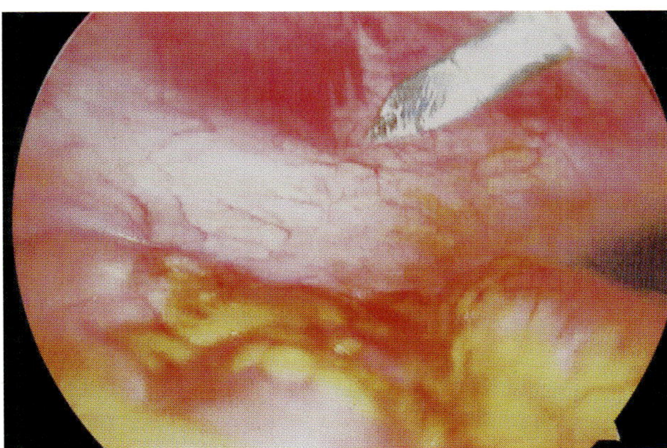

Fig. 5: Entry of 10 mm port at Lee-Huang point under vision of Jain point port.

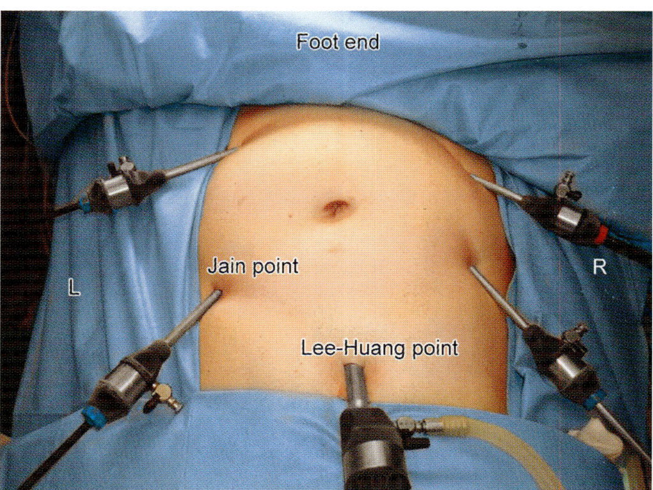

Fig. 6: Final port placement for surgery.

◼ REFERENCES

1. Lai CH, Huang KG, Hong JH, et al. Randomized trial of surgical staging (extraperitoneal or laparoscopic) versus clinical staging in locally advanced cervical cancer. Gynecol Oncol. 2003;89:160-7.
2. Lee CL, Huang KG. Total laparoscopic radical hysterectomy using Lee–Huang portal and McCartney transvaginal tube. J Am Assoc Gynecol Laparosc. 2002;9: 536-40.
3. Jansen FW, Kapiteyn K, Trimbos-Kemper T, et al. Complications of laparoscopy: a prospective multicentre observational study. Br J Obstet Gynaecol. 1997;104:595-600.
4. Lee CL, Huang KG, Jain S, et al. A new portal for laparoscopic gynecologic procedures: experience in 188 cases. J Am Assoc Gynecol Laparosc. 2001;8:147-50.
5. Richardson RF, Sutton CJG. Complications of first entry: a prospective laparoscopic audit. Gynaecol Endosc. 1999;8:327-34.
6. Hurd WW. The relationship of the umbilicus to the aortic bifurcation: implications for laparoscopic technique. Obstet Gynecol. 1992;80:48-51.
7. Huang KG, Lee CL, Tsai CS, et al. A new approach for laparoscopic ovarian transposition before pelvic irradiation. Gynecol Oncol. 2007;105:234-7.

5

Hasson Open Entry Technique

Swati Dubey, Nutan Jain

INTRODUCTION

In the course of the most recent two decades, fast advances have made laparoscopic procedure an entrenched method. Laparoscopy is presently broadly utilized in the practice of medicine, for both diagnostic and therapeutic purposes. Since laparoscopy is moderately new, despite everything it excites discussion, especially as to the best method for making the pneumoperitoneum. The initial step in laparoscopic surgery is to build up a pneumoperitoneum, which is the most dangerous step[1-4] and most of the complications happens at this step, with a death rate of 0.05–0.2%. There are various diverse methods accessible to the specialist for it. However, clearly laparoscopic surgeries are not risk free. Access in the abdominal cavity is related with injuries to the gastrointestinal tract and significant vessels and 50% of these real complications happen before initiation of the proposed medical procedure. Champault et al. have shown that 83% of vascular injuries, 75% of bowel injuries, and 50% of local hemorrhage injuries were caused during primary trocar insertion.[5] The incidence of these types of injuries may be higher in patients with previous abdominal surgeries and suspected adhesions. Although there is no accord in regards to the best strategy for accessing the peritoneal cavity to make pneumoperitoneum, Veress needle insertion is the most frequently used method by gynecologists around the world. The dangers of visceral or vascular injury can be diminished by imagining the peritoneal cavity before any instrument is introduced. This technique is known as open laparoscopy. Open laparoscopy was first described by Dr Harrith Hasson of Chicago, Illinois, who published this technique in the *American Journal of Obstetrics and Gynecology* in 1971.[6] Thereafter, this procedure of open laparoscopy has turned out to be generally acknowledged and is continually being modified to improve its training. Open laparoscopy ports vary from standard closed ports. Most distinct is their absence of bladed or sharp trocars. Trocar used in open laparoscopy is blunt and consist of framework where abdominal fascia can be attached to the port by stay sutures, thereby balancing and stabilizing the port to the patient. Hasson open laparoscopy port is an outstanding example of this framework.

TECHNIQUE[7,8]

For carrying out open laparoscopy, different techniques are available. Entry into the peritoneal cavity through sharp dissection of abdominal wall layers is the common factor/requirement. The skin, deep fascia, and parietal peritoneum of the anterior abdominal wall are in close proximity in the center of the umbilicus. Hence, it is the preferred site for skin incision. Most common technique is as follows:

- Both the surgeon and the assistant grasp the umbilical fold on each side by Allis forceps and stretch it anteriorly.
- Make a vertical incision in the center of the umbilicus from the base of the umbilicus using scalpel.
- Skin on either side is retracted using two Langenbeck retractors to view the underlying subcutaneous fat which is then cut to expose the rectus sheath.
- The surgeon catches this rectus sheath on one side using Kochers clamp. The same to be done on other side by the assistant. Now the rectus sheath to be elevated anteriorly by pulling these two Kochers clamp on each side and a vertical incision is given using scalpel. This incision excises the fascia and peritoneum and exposes the intraperitoneal cavity.
- If peritoneal cavity could not be entered previously, then it can be elevated using any blunt artery forcep and opened sharply.
- Use Metzenbaum scissors, or any other thin blunt-tipped instrument, to confirm entrance into the intraperitoneal cavity.
- Stay sutures are given on either side of the fascia before placement of the trocar.
- At last, a blunt trocar (Hasson blunt tip trocar)**(Fig. 1)** is introduced through this incision and pneumoperitoneum created. Now introduce the camera to confirm the location and create other accessory ports.
- In case stay suture cannot be placed on fascia then it can be given on skin.
- In case of gas leakage purse string type of suture can be placed.
- If there is evidence of bowel injury, extend the incision. Small bowel can be pulled out through that incision, repaired and placed back in the abdomen.

BENEFITS AND LIMITATIONS

The most favorable benefit of open laparoscopy is that the technique takes into account error free controlled entry into the abdominal cavity. Regardless, the data is yet uncertain as to superiority of open technique over closed laparoscopy. Another advantage of open technique is less likelihood of technical failures and thus less laparotomies encountered. As the incision

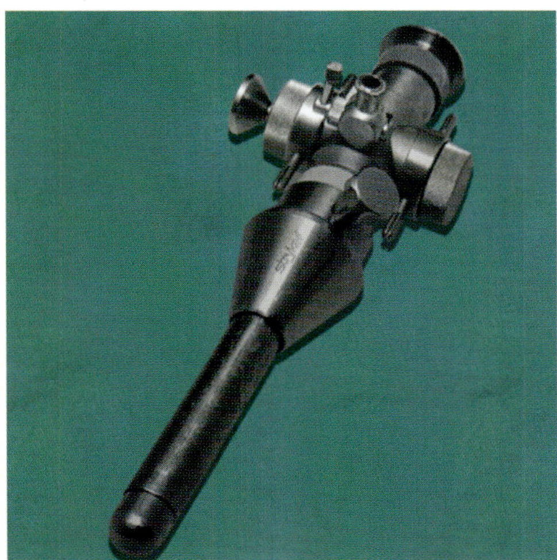

Fig. 1: Hasson blunt tip trocar.

is given through all layers of abdomen in open laparoscopy including peritoneum, gas escapes out more effectively at the end of the procedure. Later, the rectus sheath is closed with a figure of eight suture, using 2-0 polyglycolic acid polymer to prevent herniation.

A meta-analysis of 760,890 closed laparoscopy and 22,465 open laparoscopy cases reported that the incidence of vascular injury rate in closed laparoscopy was 0.44% compared with 0% in open laparoscopy.[9] The incidence of bowel injury was 0.7% compared to 0.5%, respectively. The authors concluded that the open (Hasson) technique eliminates the risk of vascular injury and gas embolism and reduces the risk of bowel injury and recommend the open technique to be embraced for primary laparoscopic entry.[9] But according to the data published in Cochrane database, there is no evidence that open technique is much safer than Veress needle closed technique.[10]

Normal time to create the pneumoperitoneum with open technique is 2–3 minutes. This is an ideal time to achieve pneumoperitoneum which is comparable to other published studies[11,12] as well as to the time taken to achieve pneumoperitoneum by blind insertion of the Veress needle and then the trocar.

Compared to closed laparoscopy, open technique has the advantage of retrieving specimen from the abdominal cavity easily. Hasson port might be removed anytime amidst the procedure and if required fascial incision can be extended and later sutured to the size (extent) of an occluder on the port before reinsertion of Hasson port.

Two of the downsides of open laparoscopy are potential for leakage of CO_2 gas and trouble in accomplishing pneumoperitoneum.

A published multivariate study revealed that open technique was associated with lower morbidity rate, in contrast with the closed technique, where morbidity related to umbilical trocar insertion was considered. As a matter of fact, closed laparoscopy was the main factor related with some of the specific complications like abdominal wall hematoma, umbilical hernia, wound contamination, and penetrating injury.

In conclusion, open laparoscopy is a safe, and easy to learn technique. It does not require costly, disposable instruments, in this way it is financially savvy. It might avoid laparotomies with their related discomfort and expenses. The technique involves a slightly bigger scar but gas leak can easily be relieved by using a purse string suture around the trocar or using towel clips over the skin edges.

REFERENCES

1. Mac Cordick C, Lecuru F, Rizk E, et al. Morbidity in laparoscopic gynecological surgery: results of a prospective single-center study. Surg Endosc. 1999;13(1):57-61.
2. Yuzpe AA. Pneumoperitoneum needle and trocar injuries in laparoscopy. A survey on possible contributing factors and prevention. J Reprod Med. 1990;35(5):485-90.
3. Corson SL, Chandler JG, Way LW. Survey of laparoscopic entry injuries provoking litigation. J Am Assoc Gynecol Laparosc. 2001;8(3):341-7.
4. Chapron CM, Pierre F, Lacroix S, et al. Major vascular injuries during gynecologic laparoscopy. J Am Coll Surg. 1997;185(5):461-5.
5. Champault G, Cazacu F, Taffinder N. Serious trocar accidents in laparoscopic surgery: a French survey of 103,852 operations. Surg Laparosc Endosc. 1996;6(5):367-70.
6. Hasson HM. A modified instrument and method for laparoscopy. Am J Obstet Gynecol. 1971;110(6):886-7.
7. Hibner M, Desai N. (2008). Open Laparoscopy. [online] Available from http://editorial.glowm.com/?p=glowm.cml/section_view&articleid=90 [Last accessed November, 2019].
8. Pickersgill A, Slade RJ, Falconer GF, et al. Open laparoscopy: the way forward. Br J Obstet Gynaecol. 1999;106(11):1116-9.
9. Larobina M, Nottle P. Complete evidence regarding major vascular injuries during laparoscopic access. Surg Laparosc Endosc Percutan Tech. 2005;15(3):119-23.
10. Ahmad G, Duffy JM, Phillips K, et al. Laparoscopic entry techniques. Cochrane Database Syst Rev. 2008;(2):CD006583.
11. Ballem RV, Rudomanski J. Techniques of pneumoperitoneum. Surg Laparosc Endosc. 1993;3(1):42-3.
12. Hurd WW, Randolph JF Jr, Holmberg RA, et al. Open laparoscopy without special instruments or sutures. Comparison with a closed technique. J Reprod Med. 1994;39(5):393-7.

6

Nonumbilical Midline Entry: A Modified Hasson Technique

Rooma Sinha, Rupa B

INTRODUCTION

The entry into the abdominal cavity by the primary port is the most important and crucial step in minimal access surgery. It is crucial because one cannot progress till the primary optical port with the camera is established. It is a step that requires the utmost attention of the surgeon as about half of the laparoscopic injuries occur at this phase.[1,2] The two most common techniques used for achieving initial access into the abdominal cavity are either closed or open techniques. The open-entry technique has a low complication rate with respect to vascular lesions.[3]

In patients who have a significantly high risk of intraperitoneal adhesions, seen in women with previous history of abdominal surgery including cesarean section, there is a need for a nonumbilical entry. Women with large fibroid uterus, large ovarian cysts, or an umbilical hernia or failed umbilical entry also need nonumbilical entry. The common point of such nonumbilical entry is described as Palmer's point or the Lee-Huang point. We described the technique of nonumbilical open entry used during Robotic surgery. The primary port during the minimal access surgery using robotic platform (DaVinci Si) is different from the regular laparoscopy surgery in two aspects. One the primary port for the camera needs to be in the midline (as described by Lee-Huang) and it should be 12 mm instead of 10 mm. This technique requires incising the skin of the abdominal wall and subsequently inserting a 12-mm XL trocar (Ethicon Endo-Surgery). The open-entry technique was initially described by an American gynecologist Hasson and we describe the modification of the same.[4]

TECHNIQUE

The point of primary port entry is identified about 7–8 cm above the target organ. As this becomes a distance of more than 10 cm when the pneumoperitoneum is achieved **(Fig. 1)**. The skin is incised longitudinally for a length of approximately 12–14 mm in the midline **(Fig. 2)**. The skin is then held and raised with the use of two Allis forceps. A blunt dissection is made using a sharp artery forceps in the subcutaneous fatty tissue to reach up to the rectus sheath **(Fig. 3)**. With the help of two small Kocher-Langenbeck skin retractors, rectus sheath is exposed **(Fig. 4)**. Next step is to hold the rectus sheath with two straight Kocher clamps or two Allis forceps. A small incision is made on the rectus sheath under vision using a scalpel with 11 mm blade **(Fig. 5)**. Two stay sutures through the fascia are then placed on both sides with the port closure Vicryl suture. After the procedure, these sutures are used to close the

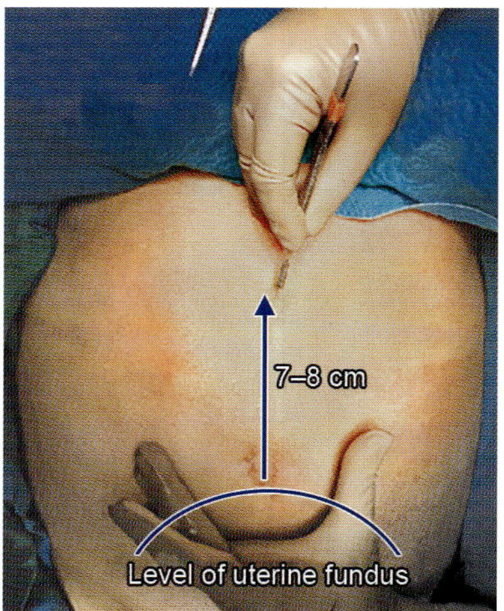

Fig. 1: Point of entry.

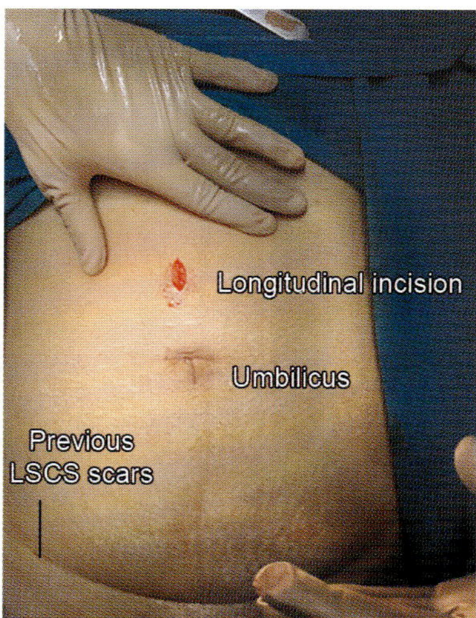

Fig 2: Longitudinal incision in midline.

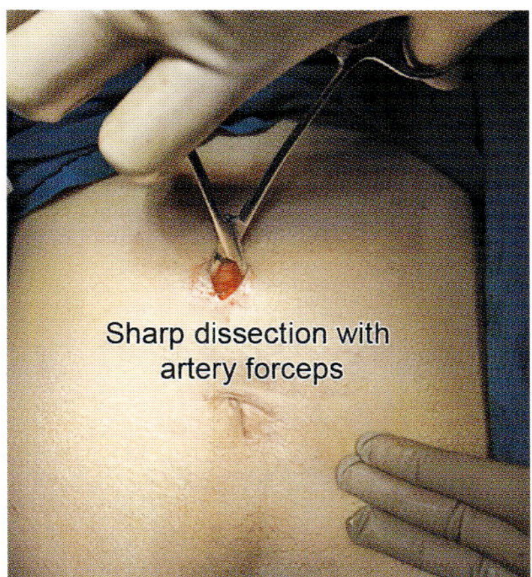

Fig. 3: Sharp dissection with artery forceps.

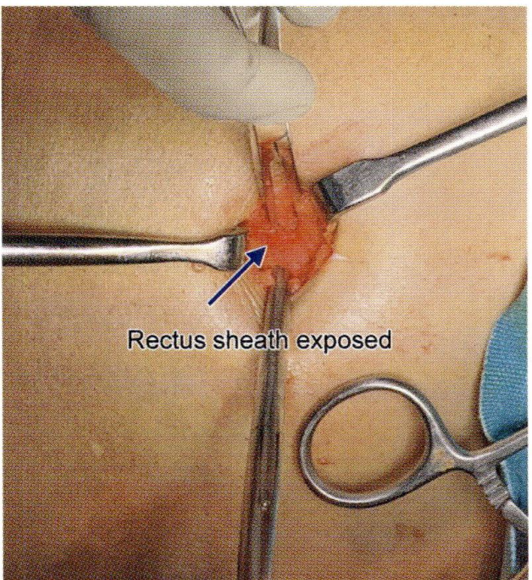

Fig. 4: Rectus exposed with the help of two skin retractors.

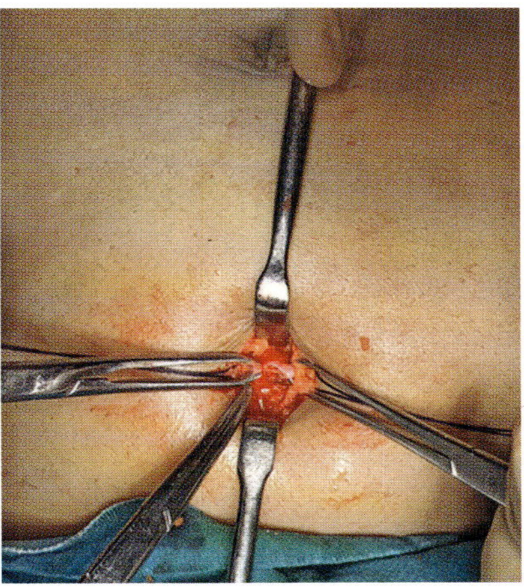

Fig. 5: Incision on the rectus sheath.

created fascia defect **(Fig. 6)**. This incision is gradually dilated with the help of sharp artery forceps **(Fig. 7)**. By this step the posterior sheath of peritoneum is exposed and is then sharply perforated with the help of the artery forceps **(Fig. 8)**. At times the posterior sheath is thick. In this situation the posterior sheath is held with the help of two artery forceps and excised. This enables the entry into the peritoneal cavity with all layers opened under vision **(Fig. 9)**. Now a 12 mm XL trocar (Ethicon Endo-Surgery) is introduced into the cavity and the pneumoinsufflator is connected **(Fig. 10)**.

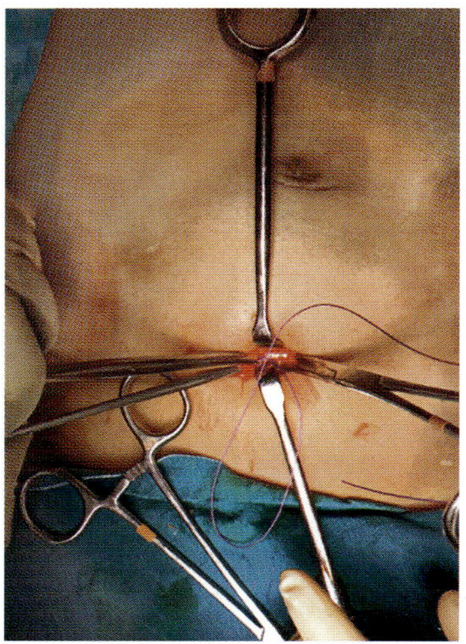

Fig. 6: Suture taken at both ends of excised rectus sheath.

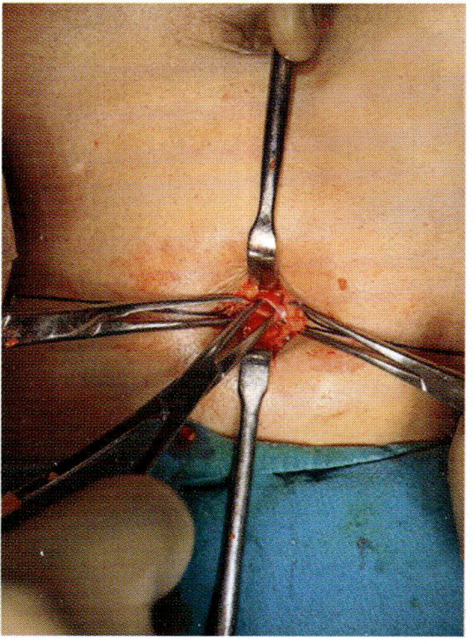

Fig. 7: Rectus sheath entry is gradually dilated.

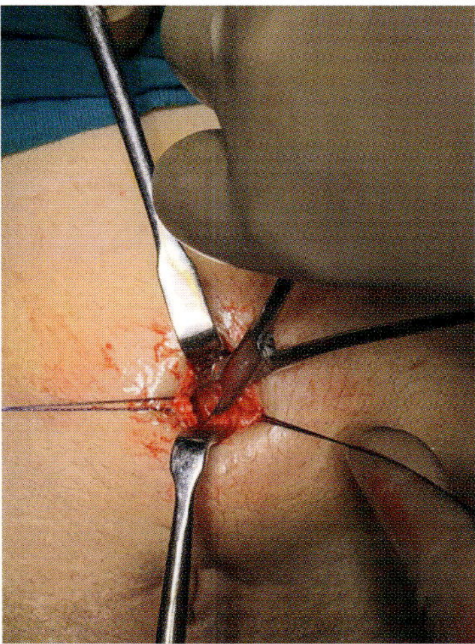

Fig. 8: Posterior peritoneal sheath is sharply perforated.

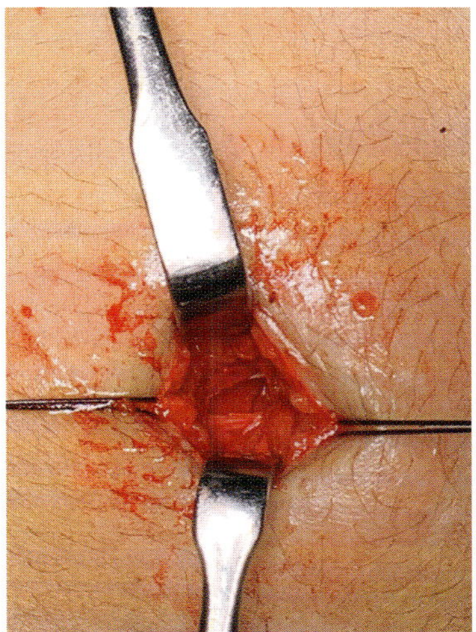

Fig. 9: All layers are opened under vision.

The pressure of <5 mm confirms intraperitoneal placement of trocar. Additionally this is also confirmed by introducing the telescope and documenting the correct entry.

With this modified Hasson open method, we aimed to reduce the disadvantages of open-entry technique. We have over the years standardized to the 10 steps mentioned above and are easily reproducible. The incision we made at the entry port is smaller than the open (Hasson) technique and a 12-mm trocar fits snugly avoiding escape of gas. Additionally, the fascia is fixed with sutures in the beginning and then the trocar was placed, these sutures

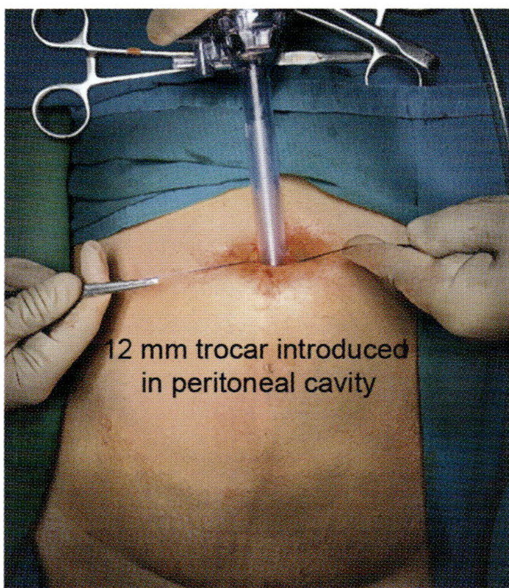

Fig. 10: A 12 mm disposable trocar introduced into peritoneal cavity.

can be tied around it to prevent gas leakage. The same technique and steps are applicable for the umbilical entry also.

CONCLUSION

Despite a variety of methods described for creating pneumoperitoneum, still there is no consensus on the most appropriate entry technique. The practicing laparoscopic surgeon should be familiar with at least more than one entry technique. Each surgeon should be well trained in whichever is their preferred technique and familiarity with alternative sites and techniques of laparoscopic entry. The challenge for laparoscopic surgeons today is to individualize aspects of surgery, such as laparoscopic entry, in order to minimize the risk of complications. Since our technique is a modified open access method, it offers an advantage of reproducibility in the steps mentioned and can detect complications early.

REFERENCES

1. Molloy D, Kaloo PD, Cooper M, et al. Laparoscopic entry: a literature review and analysis of techniques and complications of primary port entry. Aust NZJ Obstet Gynecol. 2002;3:246-54.
2. Jansen FW, Kapiteyn K, Trimbos-Kemper GCM, et al. Complications of laparoscopy: a prospective multicenter observational study. BJOG. 1997;104:595-600.
3. Bonjer HJ, Hazebroek EJ, Kazemier G, et al. Open versus closed establishment of pneumoperitoneum in laparoscopic surgery. Br J Surg. 1997;84:599-602.
4. Hasson HM. A modified instrument and method for laparoscopy. Am J Obstet Gynecol. 1971;110:886-7.

Establishment of Pneumoperitoneum through the Left Ninth Intercostal Space

Harry Reich, Jonathan M Reich

INTRODUCTION

To be honest when discussing laparoscopic entry sites for Veress needle insertion to establish pneumoperitoneum, we must admit that I have always been partial to the intraumbilical approach. We like to incorporate the place where skin, deep fascia, and parietal peritoneum meet, i.e., inside the umbilicus. *If normal pelvic examination, we will consider this spot. But this site may be contraindicated in previous surgeries, and suspected periumbilical adhesions, and then we need to know other nonumbilical sites.*

The choice of laparoscopic entry sites should be guided by basic anatomic considerations as well as history of prior abdominal surgeries. Areas free from vessels that may be injured and where there is less likelihood of perforating intra-abdominal organs are safest. Patients with prior lower abdominal surgeries frequently have bowel adherent to the anterior abdominal wall making the insertion of sharp instruments through the umbilicus risky. The right upper quadrant and epigastric regions should be avoided because of the presence of the liver and greater curvature of the stomach. The left upper quadrant region rarely is affected by adhesions from prior abdominal surgery, and the only contraindication to use of this route would be an enlarged spleen.

Injuries associated with pneumoperitoneum needle and trocar insertion during laparoscopy still occur even when experienced surgeons use new technological safeguards. To reduce the risk of injury and when umbilical insufflation fails, the laparoscopist must be comfortable with use of more than one entry site.

Palmer's point has always mystified me. It looks to be in the midclavicular line and 2–3 cm inferior to the left subcostal margin. The left ninth intercostal space (ICS) entry site has several advantages.[1,2] Technically, the left upper quadrant is easily accessible without rearranging the standard operating room laparoscopic set up or operator's position standing on the supine patient's left side if right-handed. The peritoneum in this area is firmly fixed to the undersurface of the ribs. This makes penetration with the pneumoperitoneum needle easy and subcutaneous emphysema rare. If prior surgery was in lower abdomen, the left upper quadrant is usually free of intra-abdominal lesions. Lastly, unlike the right upper quadrant where the liver and stomach might be injured, the left upper quadrant is a relatively safe area for needle and trocar insertion.

Nonumbilical veress needle insertion was used in over 100 cases as either an initial port of entry or after umbilical insertion failure, usually from adhesions or tenting of the parietal peritoneum away from the needle in obese patients. No complications of vessel or bowel injury occurred. Three failures of insufflation occurred early in the series before my confidence level in the ninth ICS approach was confirmed and were probably due to omentum surrounding the needle tip. Successful lysis of adhesions and completion of the intended laparoscopic procedure was accomplished in all cases. The left ninth ICS port of entry is safe and should be considered for patients who have had multiple prior laparotomies and/or who are suspected to have dense intra-abdominal adhesions.

TECHNIQUE (FIG. 1)

Under general anesthesia with endotracheal intubation and orogastric tube for stomach decompression, the lowest ICS is identified in the anterior axillary line region on the left. This is usually the ninth ICS, but occasionally the eighth. The ICS is spread with the surgeon's index finger, and a 1 mm stab wound made in the middle of the ICS. The pneumoperitoneum needle is held firmly near its tip to control all movement and to feel the penetration of the ICS layers. A firm but controlled push perpendicular to the skin and then away from the

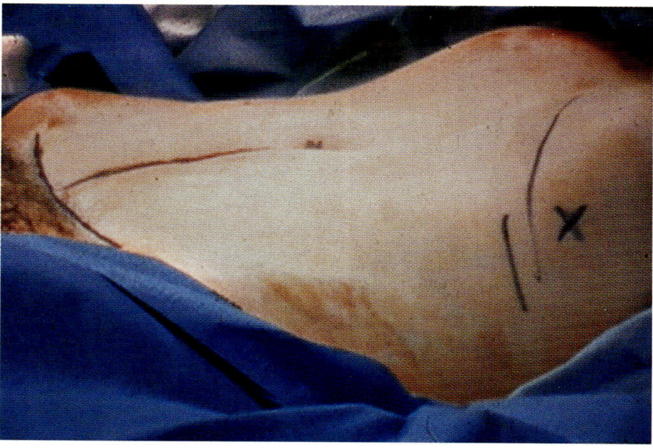

Fig. 1: Surface marking of ninth intercostal space.

upper costal margin and toward the superior aspect of the lower rib is used to penetrate the skin, muscle, fascia, and adherent peritoneum, after which a distinctive loss of resistance indicates intraperitoneal placement. In the average patient only 1–2 cm of wall is traversed to attain this position. Insufflation of CO_2 is begun and continued until pneumoperitoneum to 25–30 mm Hg is obtained. If initial flow is at high pressure, the needle is twisted to free it from surrounding omentum.

With experience, I discovered that as the peritoneal cavity filled with CO_2 gas, the 1 mm incision made for the veress needle would migrate downward from the 9th ICS to the subcostal region. If I made a 5 mm incision at the 9th ICS site of veress needle insertion, I could insert the laparoscopic trocar in the same incision.

Nonumbilical insufflation needle entry was used in over 100 cases as either an initial port of entry or after umbilical insertion failure, usually from tenting of the parietal peritoneum away from the needle in obese patients. No bowel injury was incurred. In one case there was bleeding from a subcostal arterial vessel, and this was easily coagulated with micro bipolar forceps. (We could not believe how easy this was to do!) Remember that there are vessels at the inferior subcostal margin of each rib (from above downward: vein, artery, nerve).

CONCLUSION

The left ninth intercostal space port of entry is safe and should be considered for patients who have had multiple prior laparotomies and/or who are suspected to have dense intra-abdominal adhesions. The technique is simple and adds safety to laparoscopy in patients at risk for anterior abdominal wall adhesions and entry site flexibility when umbilical insufflation fails.

LEARNING POINTS

- Ninth intercostal space is a safe entry point for patients with midline vertical and low pfannenstiel incisions.
- Exact surface marking is needed before proceeding for Veress needle entry.
- One should adhere to the methodology described in the text above.
- It will be good to be well conversant with this technique, as, it has been found to be safe in large case series.
- A 5 mm incision at 9th ICS site of Veress needle insertion, to avoid migration downward to subcostal region.

REFERENCES

1. Reich H, Levie M, McGlynn F, Sekel L. Establishment of pneumoperitoneum through the left ninth intercostal space. Gynecol Endosc. 199;4:141-3.
2. Reich H. Laparoscopic bowel injury. Surg Laparosc Endosc. 1992;2:74-8.

Challenges in Entry

8

Hazards of First Blind Port Umbilical Entry

Anadeep Chandi, Nutan Jain

Access into the abdomen is the foremost challenge of any laparoscopic surgery. The first entry into the abdomen is the most crucial and dangerous step in laparoscopic surgery as it is blind, thus amounting for complications like injuries to the gastrointestinal tract and major blood vessels. A large multicentric prospective study from 72 hospitals of the Netherlands revealed that the intestinal injuries and major complications during laparoscopy occur in 5.7/1,000 procedures. Approximately 70% of these are related to the primary port entry. The overall incidence of laparoscopic entry injuries is 3.3/1,000 with gastrointestinal damage occurring in 1.3/1,000 and abdominal vessel injuries in 1.05/1,000.[1] At least 50% of the major complications occur prior to commencement of the intended surgery.[1,2]

Laparoscopic entry injuries may be classified into two types. Type 1 injuries include damage to major blood vessels or the bowel in a normal location and are caused by entering with the Veress needle or the primary trocars (0.1–0.4%). Type 2 injuries lead to damage to vessels in the abdominal wall and to the bowel adherent to the abdominal wall and both can be caused by the Veress needle or the primary trocar. Complications associated with laparoscopy vary, depending on the experience of the surgeon and the medical staff as well as the wide range of operational demands.[3]

The umbilicus being a relatively weak point in the anterior abdominal wall has been the preferred site for creating the pneumoperitoneum and entering into the abdominal cavity since more than 70 years. Also known as "navel", it is considered the best site for insertion of the Veress needle or primary trocar as the skin is attached to the fascia and anterior peritoneum with minimal intervening muscle or fat **(Fig. 1)**. It lies typically at the level of the highest points of the iliac crests, opposite the disc between the 3rd and 4th lumbar vertebrae or opposite the 4th lumbar vertebra with a variable range between 3rd and 5th lumbar vertebrae among different individuals. The aortic bifurcation in most of the individuals, also rests between the 4th and 5th lumbar vertebrae

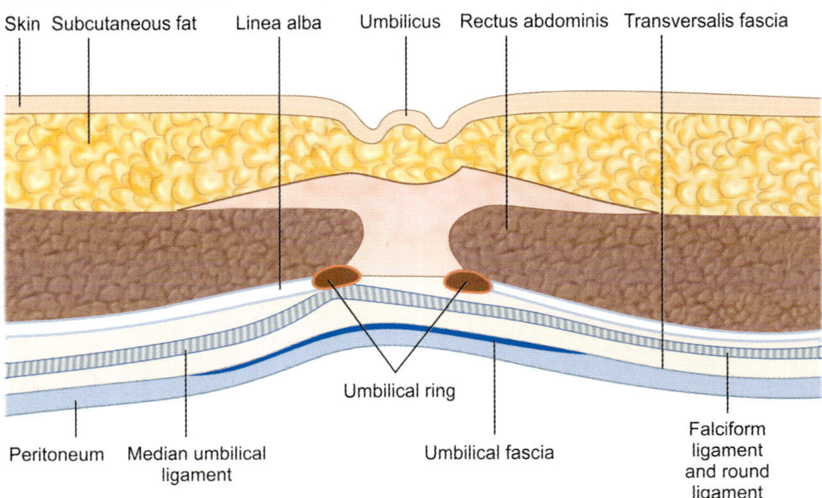

Fig. 1: Diagrammatic presentation of anatomy of umbilicus.

and within 1.25 cm above or below the highest points of the iliac crests.[4] However, the position of the umbilicus in relation to this bifurcation is quite variable and it should not be used to mark the aortic bifurcation's location.[5] Thus, the relation of this retroperitoneal vasculature to the insertion site must be very carefully considered before starting any laparoscopic surgery.

The radio imaging observations of the relationship of umbilicus and the bifurcation of aorta done by 106 abdominal computed topography (CT) scans revealed that the umbilicus lies -6.3 ± 26.5 mm from the aortic bifurcation.[6] Nezhat et al. determined the cephalocaudal relationship between the umbilicus and aortic bifurcation in 97 patients by direct measurement during laparoscopy in both supine and Trendelenburg positions with a marked suction-irrigator probe. The position of the bifurcation was quite variable, ranging from 5 cm cephalad to 3 cm caudal to the umbilicus in supine position, and from 3 cm cephalad to 3 cm caudal in Trendelenburg. The risk of vascular injury below the bifurcation was highlighted by their observation that the space between the common iliac arteries was always at least partially occupied by the left common iliac vein, and was completely filled by this vessel in 28% of the cases studied. They concluded that the presumed location of aortic bifurcation can be misleading during Veress needle or primary cannula insertion, and a more reliable guide is necessary for this procedure to avoid major retroperitoneal vascular injury.[7]

Umbilical-aortic bifurcation relationship is particularly even more important in patients with very thin and extremely obese body habitus where the normal relationship between the abdominal wall and the vasculature is altered. Hurd et al. observed the relationship of umbilicus to aortic bifurcation using magnetic resonance imaging (MRI) and CT and found that nonobese patients weighing < 160 lb (73 kg) and body mass index (BMI) of < 25 kg/m^2 had their umbilicus 0.4 cm caudal to aortic bifurcation with skin to peritoneum distance of 2 cm. In overweight patients weighing between 160 lb and 200 lb (73–91 kg) and BMI between 25 kg/m^2 and 30 kg/m^2, umbilicus was 2.4 cm caudal to aortic bifurcation, with skin to peritoneum distance of 2 cm. In extreme obese patients weighing > 200 lb (91 kg) or BMI > 30 kg/m^2, the umbilicus was located 2.9 cm caudal to aortic bifurcation, with skin to peritoneum median distance of 12 cm. The authors concluded that Veress needle insertion in nonobese patients should be at an angle of 45° from the horizontal. In obese patients, the Veress needle should be inserted at 90° angle from the horizontal because of increased distance to the peritoneum in such patients. In overweight patients, an angle between 45–90° from the horizontal would be satisfactory for intraperitoneal placement of Veress needle.[8] Attwell et al. also found that increasing subcutaneous fat thickness was associated with a more caudal position of the umbilicus relative to the aortic bifurcation.[6] On contrary, very thin woman, especially one with an android pelvis and prominent sacral promontory, presents specific hazards, as the depth of the umbilicus lies within 1–2 cm of the anterior surface of the aorta.[9] Anaise found that in thin patients, the distance between the abdominal wall and the retroperitoneal vessels may be less than 2 cm. Also, the distal aorta and right common iliac artery are particularly vulnerable to injury since the junction of these two vessels is directly below the umbilicus.[10] An intraoperatively finding of retroperitoneal hematoma noticed after Veress needle insertion through umbilical site is shown in **Figure 2**. This hematoma occurred due to injury to median sacral artery. Retroperitoneal hematomas require keen observation

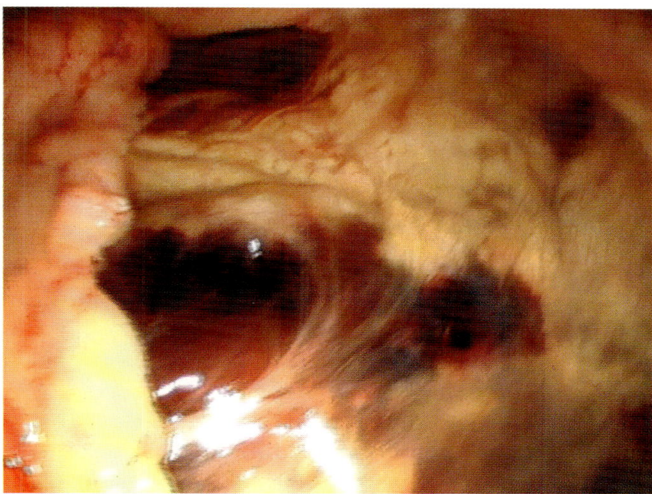

Fig. 2: A retroperitoneal hematoma after Veress needle insertion through umbilical site.

throughout the surgery so as to look for its extent and to know whether it is increasing or has become self-limiting.

A rare though hazardous complication of blind umbilical entry was reported by Richard et al., when iatrogenic vascular penetration presented as CO_2 embolism during insufflation, led to death from exsanguination due to delayed recognition.[11]

The resting position of the patient while entering into the abdomen during any laparoscopic surgery is also important. Premature Trendelenburg position can precariously shift the position of the bifurcation cephalad to rest directly below and closer to the umbilicus, making it vulnerable to injury with the target insertion angle of 45°, regardless of BMI.[7,12] It was found that the aortic bifurcation was located caudal to the umbilicus in only 11% of women undergoing laparoscopy when supine, compared with 33% in Trendelenburg position.[7] Thus, the Veress needle or primary trocar should ideally be inserted while the patient is maintained in an unaltered supine position.

Also, while entering blindly into the abdomen through umbilicus, the potential risk of adhesions between the intra-abdominal contents and the abdominal wall should be kept into consideration **(Figs. 3 and 4)**. The rates of adhesions could vary from 0% to 0.68% in those without any previous abdominal surgery, 0% to 15% in those with previous laparoscopy, 20% to 30% in those with previous laparotomy through a low transverse incision and 30% to 50% in those with a previous midline laparotomy.[13,14] According to Ellis and Liakakos et al., postsurgical adhesions are seen in 67–93% patients after general surgical operations and 70–95% patients undergoing major gynecologic surgery.[15,16] Another study reported subumbilical adhesions in 57% of patients after one low transverse laparotomy, 66% after two, and 92% after a midline laparotomy.[17]

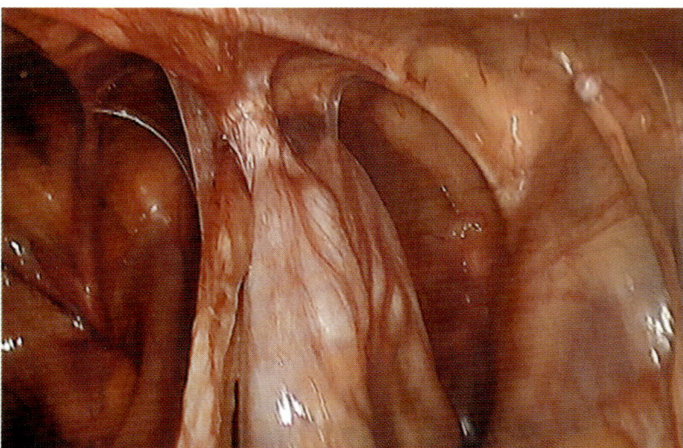

Fig. 3: Small intestine adherent to anterior abdominal wall in a patient with previous one infraumbilical midline laparotomy.

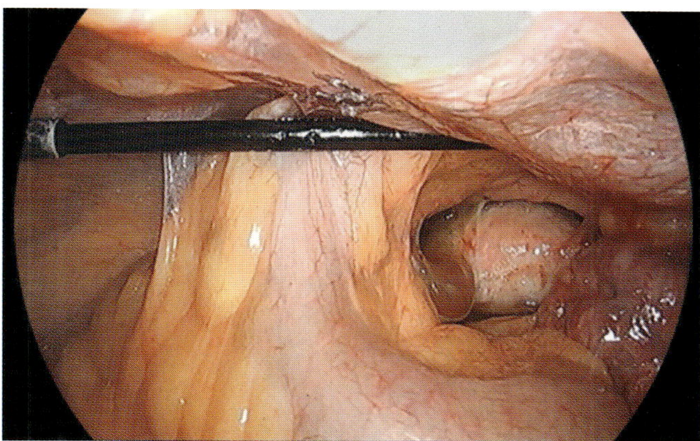

Fig. 4: Gut loops seen adherent to periumbilical region in patient with previous three cesarean sections. Abdominal entry was done through Jain point.

The open technique introduced by Hasson[18] would less likely cause major vessel injury than the closed method of Veress and if a segment of adherent bowel is injured, it might be more likely that this would be recognized at the same time, allowing immediate repair. However, a survey of 18 board-certified gynecologists who had performed a total of 10,840 open laparoscopies revealed eighteen instances of wound infection and six cases of bowel damage (0.6/1,000), four of which were recognized immediately but, in two of them, the diagnosis was late and reparative surgery was delayed.[19]

The other common cases where difficulty in entering the abdomen through umbilicus can be faced, is in women with large pelvic masses for whom Veress insertion could be impossible due to resistance offered directly by the mass reaching close to the umbilicus or if at all entered into the abdomen, would bring the telescope extremely close to the pelvic mass, thereby impacting the ease of surgery by hindering the operator's field of vision.[20-22] Also, Veress needle through umbilical site may enter into the large cystic mass reaching the periumbilical region, thereby causing accidental surgical spillage, that may worsen the prognosis especially in malignant cases.[23]

Despite many technical advances in laparoscopic surgery equipment and the extensive experience of many surgeons, there is still a number of injuries and deaths each year from insertion of trocars and Veress needles. The creation of a pneumoperitoneum along with insertion of trocars remains the source of significant injuries to intra-abdominal viscera and both intra- and retroperitoneal vessels.[24] Unfortunately, 30–50% of the bowel injuries and 15–50% of the vascular injuries are not diagnosed at the time of injury.[25] This delay has contributed to mortality rates of 3–30% for bowel and vascular injuries.[25,26]

A recent Dutch study analyzed 133 insurance claims filed after gynecological laparoscopic surgeries over past 20 years. Of the majority of claims being filed,

82% accounted for visceral and/or vascular injuries, specifically to the bowel (40%), ureters (20%) and vessels (11%). More than one-third of these injuries were entry related (38.3%). A delay in diagnosing the injuries was the primary reason for financial compensation (33.3%) and €12,000 was the median sum paid to patients. Also, it was observed that the number of claims remained relatively constant over the time. Hence, entering the abdominal cavity during laparoscopy continues to be a potential dangerous step.[27] This invites the need to shift to a nonumbilical site for Veress as well as the blind port insertion during laparoscopic surgeries.

REFERENCES

1. Jansen FW, Kapiteyn K, Trimbos-Kemper T, et al. Complications of laparoscopy: a prospective multicentre observational study. Br J Obstet Gynaecol. 1997;104:595-600.
2. Jansen FW, Kolkman W, Bakkum EA, et al. Complications of laparoscopy: an inquiry about closed versus open-entry technique. Am J Obstet Gynecol. 2004;190:634-8.
3. Alkatout I. Complications of laparoscopy in connection with entry techniques. J Gynecol Surg. 2017;33(3):81-91.
4. Gray H, Goss CM. Anatomy of the Human Body, 28th edition. Philadelphia: Lea and Febiger; 1966. pp. 646-7.
5. Pelosi MA III, Pelosi MA. Alignment of the umbilical axis: an effective maneuver for laparoscopic entry in the obese patient. Obstet Gynecol. 1998;92:869-72.
6. Attwell L, Rosen S, Upadhyay B, et al. The umbilicus: a reliable surface landmark for the aortic bifurcation? Surg Radiol Anat. 2015;37:1239-42.
7. Nezhat F, Brill AI, Nezhat CH, et al. Laparoscopic appraisal of the anatomic relationship of the umbilicus to the aortic bifurcation. J Am Assoc Gynecol Laparosc. 1998;5:135-40.
8. Hurd WW, Bude RO, DeLancey JO, et al. The relationship of the umbilicus to the aortic bifurcation: implications for laparoscopic technique. Obstet Gynecol. 1992;80(1):48-51.
9. Corson SL. Major vessel injury during laparoscopy. Am J Obstet Gynecol. 1980;138:589-90.
10. Anaise D. Vascular and bowel injuries during laparoscopy. [online] Available from www.danaise.com/vascular_and_bowel_injuries_duri.htm [Last accessed December, 2019].
11. Hanney RM, Alle KM, Cregan PC. Major vascular injury and laparoscopy. Aust N Z J Surg. 1995;65:533-5.
12. Lynn SC, Katz AR, Ross PJ. Aortic perforation sustained at laparoscopy. J Reprod Med. 1982;27:217-9.
13. Audebert AJ. The role of microlaparoscopy for safer wall entry: incidence of umbilical adhesions according to past surgical history. Gynaecol Endosc. 1999;8:363-7.
14. Vilos GA, Ternamian A, Dempter J, et al. Laparoscopic entry: a review of techniques, technologies, and complications. J Obstet Gynaecol Can. 2007;29(5):433-47.
15. Ellis H. The magnitude of adhesion related problems. Ann Chir Gynaecol. 1998;87:9-11.
16. Liakakos T, Thomakos N, Fine PM, et al. Peritoneal adhesions: etiology, pathophysiology, and clinical significance. Recent advances in prevention and management. Dig Surg. 2001;18:260-73.

17. Davis CJ. Prospective use of Palmer's point entry for therapeutic laparoscopy in women with previous abdominal surgery. J Minim Invasive Gynecol. 2005;12(5 Suppl):65.

18. Hasson HM. A modified instrument and method for laparoscopy. Am J Obstet Gynecol. 1971;110(6):886-7.

19. Penfield AJ. How to prevent complications of open laparoscopy. J Reprod Med. 1985;30(9):660-3.

20. Hurst BS, Matthews ML, Marshburn PB. Laparoscopic myomectomy for symptomatic uterine myomas. Fertil Steril. 2005;83(1)1-23.

21. Sinha R, Hegde A, Mahajan C, et al. Laparoscopic myomectomy: do size, number, and location of the myomas form limiting factors for laparoscopic myomectomy? J Minim Invasive Gynecol. 2008;15:292-300.

22. Granata M, Tsimpanakos I, Moeity F, et al. Are we underutilizing Palmer's point entry in gynecologic laparoscopy? Fertil Steril. 2010;94(7):2716-9.

23. Karthik S, Augustine AJ, Shibumon MM, et al. Analysis of laparoscopic port site complications: a descriptive study. J Minim Access Surg. 2013;9(2):59-64.

24. Kim HS, Ahn JH, Chung HH, et al. Impact of intraoperative rupture of the ovarian capsule on prognosis in patients with early-stage epithelial ovarian cancer: a meta-analysis. Eur J Surg Oncol. 2013;39(3):279-89.

25. Vilos GA, Vilos AG, Abu-Rafea B, et al. Three simple steps during closed laparoscopic entry may minimize major injuries. Surg Endosc. 2009;23:758-64.

26. Wind J, Cremers J, van Berge Henegouwen MI, et al. Medical liability insurance claims on entry-related complications in laparoscopy. Surg Endosc. 2007;21:2094-9.

27. Sandberg EM, Bordewijk EM, Klemann D, et al. Medical malpractice claims in laparoscopic gynecologic surgery: a Dutch overview of 20 years. Surg Endosc. 2017;31:5418-26.

Nutan Jain, Vandana Jain

Limitations and Contraindications of Palmer's Point

Palmer's point[1] was devised by a French gynecologist in the year 1974 with a first study published of 35 cases suggesting an alternate port of blind entry in cases where umbilical entry was deemed to be hazardous. This could be in cases of suspected umbilical adhesions[2,3] (**Fig. 1**) due to previous surgeries or previous infections. In his first paper, Palmer proposed a point which is in the midclavicular line three fingers breadth below the subcostal margin. It has been almost 70 years and since then all clinicians whether they are gynecologists, surgeons, and urologists, have all adhered to the Palmer's point entry (**Figs. 2A and B**) whenever there was need to change from the umbilical port.[4-6] It has a long safety profile enabling surgeons to make successful entry in cases of suspected adhesions. But over the years as the complexity of the cases is rising and surgical interventions in the population whether gynecological or general surgery or urology have been on a steady rise. In subsequent laparoscopies the laparoscopic surgeon is faced with the task of making the first blind entry in cases of multiple previous surgeries. In cases of suspected infections, or past

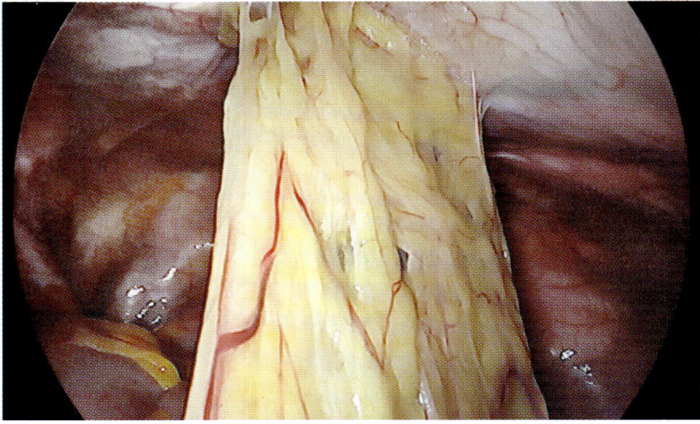

Fig. 1: Omental adhesion at umbilicus.

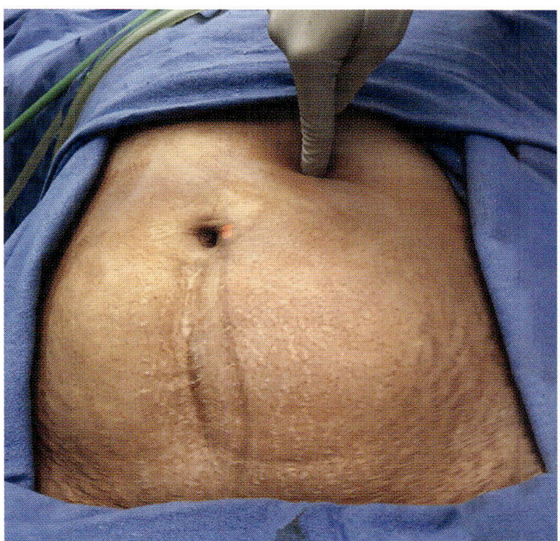

Fig. 2A: Finger pointing at Palmer's point.

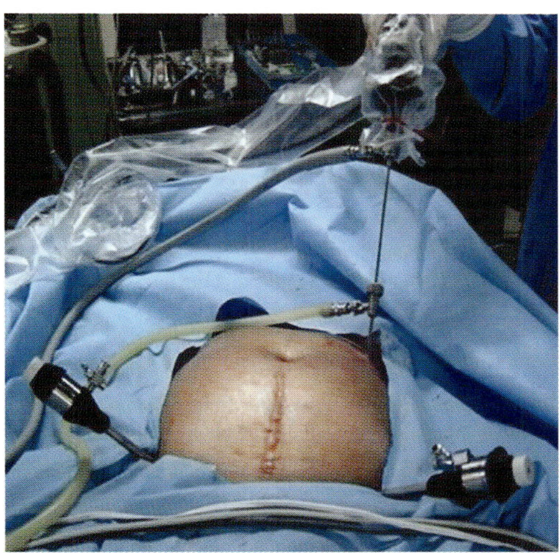

Fig. 2B: A 3 mm telescope at Palmer's point.

history of infectious disease, the challenge rises. As we practice in India, we face the daunting task rise of genital and abdominopelvic tuberculosis and this holds true for many developing nations in entire Asia and the Africas.[7-11] As Koch's is prevalent in infertile patients, it is often encountered in laparoscopies. And entry in these patients due to frequently encountered adhesions around the umbilicus and upper abdomen is always a challenge.[12-15]

As the epidemiology of the disease, prevalence of previous surgeries, and the disease pattern is changing over the years, there is constantly a need to have another alternate nonumbilical site to make entry. And not only because of the change in the disease pattern, also, because there are certain limitations to the use of Palmer's point. As we see by the surface anatomy, the Palmer's

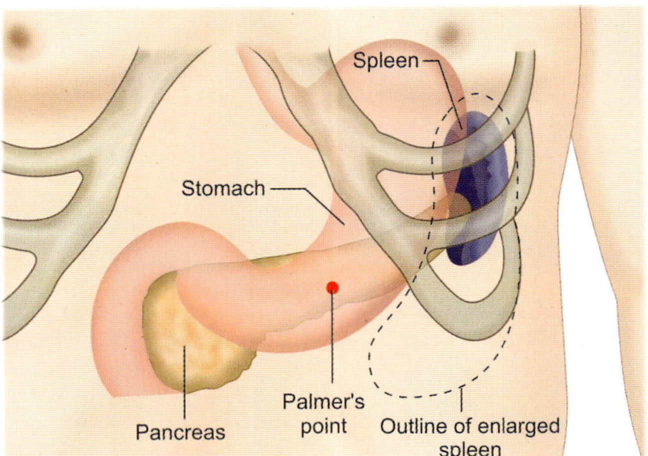

Fig. 3: Surface anatomy of Palmer's point.

point **(Fig. 3)** overlies exactly over the location of the stomach. If the bowel is well prepared and the patient is nil orally for last 6 hours, it is ok. But, if the stomach is bloated because of patient not adhering to the dietic instructions or may be because of a faulty placement of nasogastric tube, it can predispose for some entries into the stomach while making the entry through the Palmer's point.[16] Even I have one such **(Fig. 4)** unintended entry into the stomach while making the first blind entry in a case of previous surgeries. So this is the first contraindication that a full stomach or faulty placement of nasogastric tube makes a Palmer's point vulnerable for unintended gastroscopy (the surgeon's biggest nightmare, rather than seeing the omentum and bowel to see the inside of stomach).

Second contraindication to Palmer's point is in cases where the incisions are in the upper quadrant of the abdomen. These incisions in upper quadrant preclude the use of Palmer's point, as there could be adhesions at this point. We very often see the cases where the previous gallbladder surgery, before the advent of laparoscopic cholecystectomy **(Fig. 5)** has been done by a big Kocher's incision. At the time of repeat surgery there could be chances of adhesions at the Palmer's point also. So, this is another contraindication where we cannot use the Palmer's point. We recently reported our case of chevron incision **(Fig. 6)** in the Journal of Minimally Invasive Gynecology (JMIG) July/ August, 2018[17] wherein there was big Chevron incision from one end of the abdomen transversely till the other end of the abdomen for previous hydatid cyst of liver. So, when we put the finger on the incision **(Figs. 7A and B)** it was directly over the Palmer's point and done for a previous infectious pathology it definitely predisposes to adhesions in this surgery and here entry at the Palmer's point would become difficult or would meet with adhesions of the bowel and omentum.

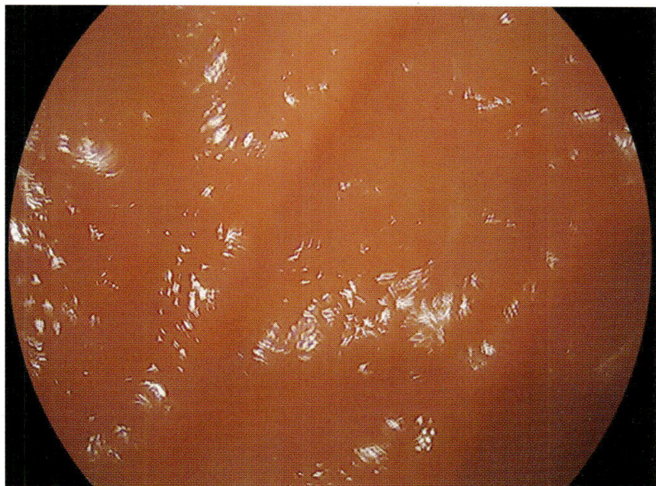

Fig. 4: Inside view of the bowel.

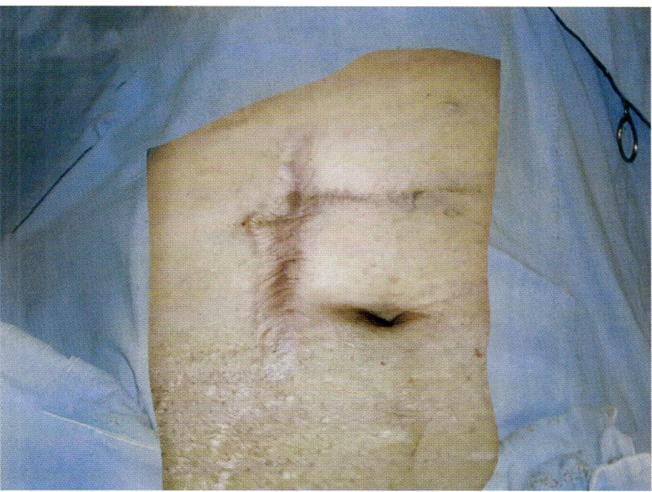

Fig. 5: Two big crisscrossing upper abdomen scars.

Previous surgeries in the upper quadrant totally contraindicate the use of Palmer's point. This is a very prevalent issue especially in general surgery or in cases of childhood surgeries, wherein the incisions tend to be long and at times vertical incision **(Fig. 8)**, going from the pubic symphysis to above the umbilicus reaching the upper quadrant of the abdomen. The previous nephrectomies, previous splenectomies, Chevron incisions, and previous open gallbladder incisions tend to be big and in upper quadrant. So, in all these cases the real need is to search for an alternate entry point.

Lastly the fourth contraindication for Palmer's point entry is big gastropancreatic masses, splenic enlargement[18] **(Fig. 9)**, portal hypertension,

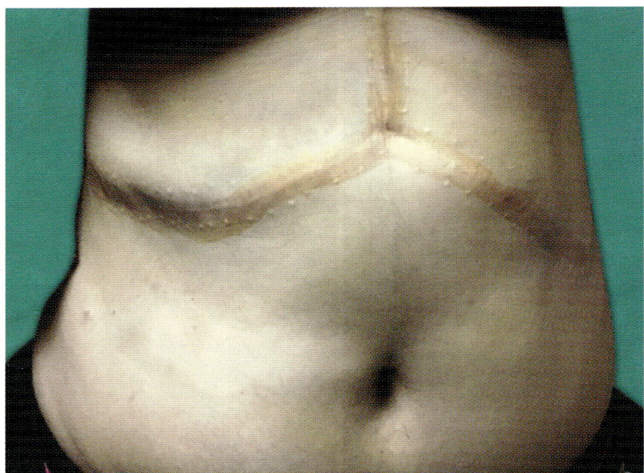

Fig. 6: Chevron incision (highlighted with Betadine solution).

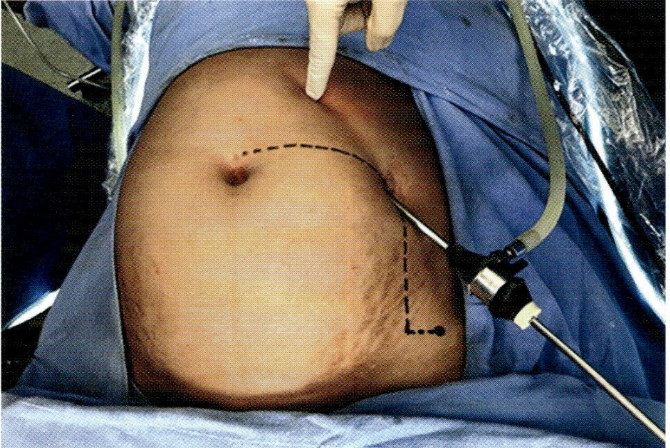

Fig. 7A: Finger pointing at Palmer's point.

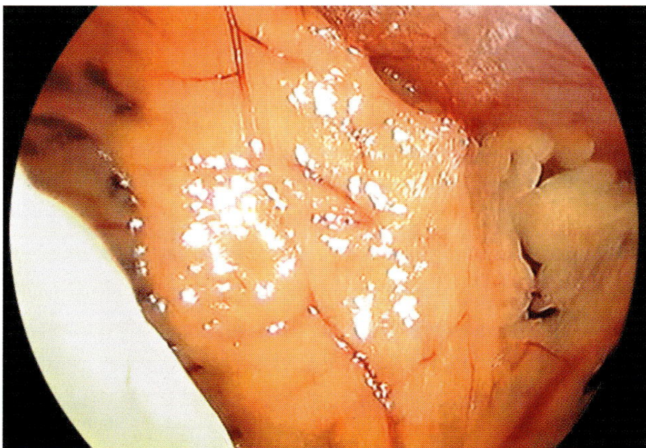

Fig. 7B: Adhesions at Palmer's point.

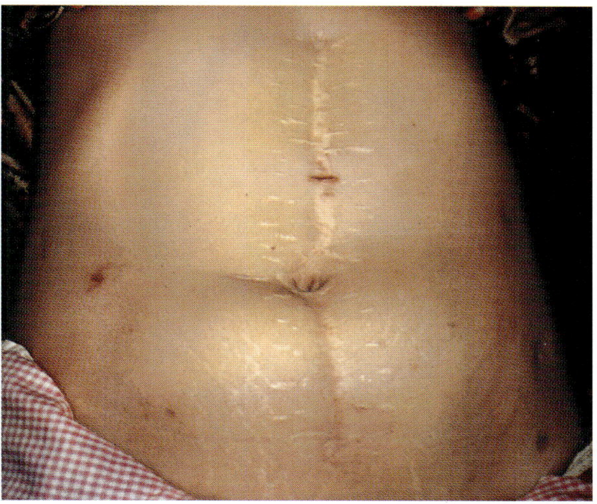

Fig. 8: Big vertical scar on abdomen.

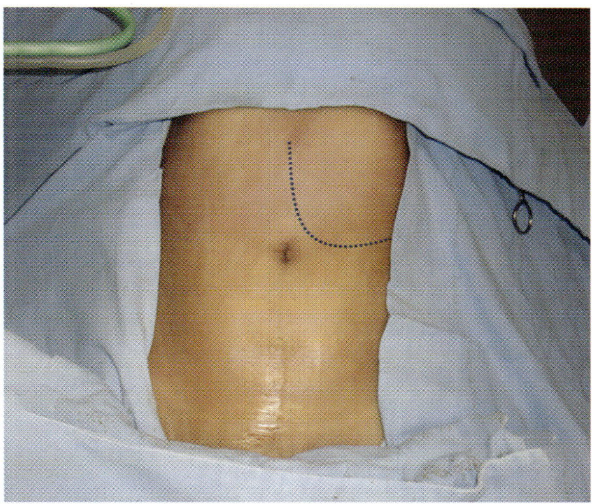

Fig. 9: Enlargement of spleen.

which also causes enlargement of the spleen and of the liver and thus negates a Palmer's point entry. In the gynecology whenever there is a big mass which is coming right up to the Palmer's point or even above it along with a previous surgery scar. So all these are the cases where we cannot use Palmer's point.

And in practice what we see every day, difficulty in making the surface marking of the Palmer's point with the well-draped patient. When the surgeon comes on the table the patient is usually fully painted and draped, and then locating the exact midclavicular line and marking three fingers breadth **(Fig. 10)** below the subcostal margin. Exact location of midclavicular line is not so precise, it could flay laterally or medially by a centimeter or so and this

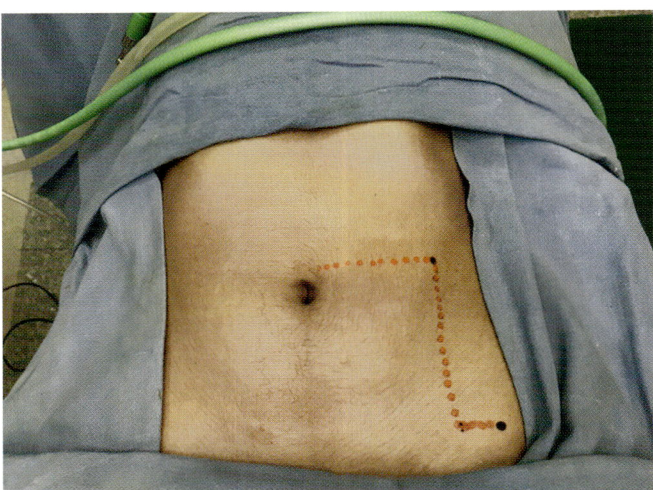

Fig. 10: Surface marking of Jain point.

could be disastrous in patients of diffuse previous infections pathologies like tuberculosis, previous septicemia, or any generalized condition which could predispose to adhesions from all over the abdomen or a frozen pelvis. So herein, we find the need to go for an alternate entry point. Hasson technique as discussed earlier does not totally negate bowel injury in spite of making an open laparoscopic entry.[19] There has still been incidences of entry into the bowel. The other entry that is Lee-Huang point[16] is again contraindicated in cases of upper abdominal incision or big abdominal gastropancreatic masses or enlarged liver, enlarged spleen which are in the upper quadrant. The 9th intercostal space[20] is another alternate entry point, but this generation of laparoscopic surgeons have hardly any exposure, as during their trainings, they have not seen their mentors using it. So, at this moment I feel that this entry point has become very less in use.

Lastly, the 9th intercostal space could not be used because of unfamiliar territory the risk of getting into the lungs and the risk of injuring the arteries at the lower edge of the rib.[21,22] All these preclude the liberal use of the 9th intercostal space. With all this discussion it remains that there is need to find another alternate site of entry which could be used when umbilicus is not the chosen site for entry and Palmer's point is contraindicated. Herein we will discuss in this book the need and the rationale, the evolution, and the technique of this new entry port which has been coined "The Jain point". It lies on straight line drawn 2.5 cm from the anterior superior iliac spine going right up to the upper margin of the umbilicus and we find more advantage of Jain point is that it can be used for all types of incisions including midline, upper abdomen, lower abdomen, and incisions on the right side which could be there because of appendicitis. It can be used in all patients of extremes of body weight, can be used in large masses, and the extra advantage that we find is that since it moves away from the umbilicus, it can be used for routine entry as a routine first blind port entry to avoid the major vessels which lies underneath the umbilical.

Another practical point which I feel is that surface marking of Jain point is easy on the patient. When the patient is fully painted and draped, still we can easily locate the anterior superior iliac spine, a bony landmark, which is in the sterile surgical field. Go 2.5 cm medial to anterior superior iliac spine (ASIS), then draw a line which comes at the upper margin of umbilicus and then draw a line from umbilicus, where these two lines intersect that is the Jain point. So, it is much easier done compared to locating the midclavicular line and then the Palmer's point in a fully painted and draped patient. Moreover a bony landmark is so much easier to locate and is constant point compared to three fingers breadth below the subcostal margin in midclavicular line to locate the Palmer's point. It is easier said than done. Soft tissue tend to move hitherto in a supine patient as especially in overweight, obese or flabby abdomen, and then marking the Palmer's point for entry is not so precise.

LEARNING POINTS

- Palmer's point is good for previous surgery cases, but has certain contraindications.
- Palmer's point cannot be used in upper abdominal scars.
- Palmer's point cannot be used with big gastropancreatic masses, or large pelvic masses coming beyond the Palmer's point.
- Splenic enlargement and portal hypertension are contraindications to its use.
- Bloated stomach predisposes to injury while entry by Palmer's point.
- Surface marking of Jain point is easier as it is from a fixed bony landmark, the ASIS and umbilicus, as they both are in the sterile undraped portion of patient's abdomen.

REFERENCES

1. Palmer R. Safety in laparoscopy. J Reprod Med. 1974;13:1-5.
2. Richardson RF, Sutton CJ. Complications of first entry: a prospective laparoscopic audit. Gynacol Endosc. 1999;8:327-34.
3. Royal College of Obstetricians and Gynaecologists. Preventing entry-related gynaecological laparoscopic injuries: Green-top Guideline No. 49. London: Royal College of Obstetricians and Gynaecologists; 2008.
4. Childers JM, Brzechffa PR, Surwit EA. Laparoscopy using the left upper quadrant as the primary trocar site. Gynecol Oncol. 1993;50:221-5.
5. Roy GM, Bazzurini L, Solima E, et al. Safe technique for laparoscopic entry into the abdominal cavity. J Am Assoc Gynecol Laparosc. 2001;8:519-28.
6. Corson SL, Brooks PG, Soderstrom RM. Safe technique for laparoscopic entry into the abdominal cavity. J Am Assoc Gynecol Laparosc. 2002;9:399.

7. Gupta N, Sharma JB, Mittal S, et al. Genital tuberculosis in Indian infertility patients. Int J Gynecol Obstet.2007;97(2):135-8.

8. Sharma JB, Pushparaj M, Gupta N, et al. Genital tuberculosis: an important cause of Ashermans' syndrome in India. Arch Gynecol Obstet. 2008;277:37-41.

9. World Health Organization. TB: a global emergency, WHO Report on the TB epidemic. Geneva: World Health Organization; 1994.

10. Dye C, Watt CJ, Bleed DM, et al. Evolution of tuberculosis control and prospects for reducing tuberculosis incidence, prevalence and deaths globally. JAMA. 2005;293:2790-3.

11. Sutherland AM. The changing pattern of tuberculosis of the female genital tract: a thirty-year survey. Arch Gynaecol. 1983;234:95-101.

12. Sharma JB, Roy KK, Gupta N, et al. High prevalence of Fitz-Hugh–Curtis Syndrome in genital tuberculosis. Int J Gynecol Obstet. 2007;99:62-3.

13. Sharma JB. Tuberculosis and obstetric and gynecological practice. In: Studd J, Tan SL, Chervenak FA (Eds). Progress in Obstetric and Gynaecology. Philadephia: Elsevier; 2008. pp. 395-427.

14. Sharma JB, Roy KK, Pushparaj M, et al. Laparoscopic finding in female genital tuberculosis. Arch Gynecol Obstet. 2008;278:359-64.

15. Sharma JB, Mohanraj P, Roy KK, et al. Increased complication rates associated with laparoscopic surgery among patients with genital tuberculosis. Int J Gynecol Obstet. 2010;109:242-4.

16. Lee CL, Huang KG, Jain S, et al. A new portal for gynecologic laparoscopy. J Am Assoc Gynecol Laparosc. 2001;8:147-50.

17. Jain N, Jain V, Aggarwal C. Left Lateral Port: Safe Laparoscopic Port Entry in Previous Large Upper Abdomen Laparotomy Scar. J Min Inv Gynaecol. 2019;26:973-6.

18. Jain N, Sareen S, Kanawa S, et al. Jain point: A new safe portal for laparoscopic entry in previous surgery cases. J Hum Reprod Sci. 2016;9(1):9-17.

19. Hasson HM. Open laparoscopy as a method of access in laparoscopic surgery. Gynaecol Endosc. 1999;8:353-62.

20. Agarwala N, Liu CY. Safe entry techniques during laparoscopy: Left upper quadrant entry using the ninth intercostal space—A review of 918 procedures. J Minim Invasive Gynecol. 2005;12:55-61.

21. Reich H. New laparoscopic techniques. In: Sutton C, Diamond M (Eds). Endoscopic Surgery for Gynaecologists. London: WB Saunders; 1993. p. 31.

22. Kumar S. Veress needle insertion through left lower intercostal space for creating pneumoperitoneum: Experience with 75 cases. J Minim Access Surg. 2012;8:85-9.

Introduction of Jain Point

10

What is Jain Point:
The Technique

Nutan Jain, Vandana Jain, Swati Kanawa

INTRODUCTION

With the recent advancements in minimally invasive surgery, many complicated and intricate procedures are being performed laparoscopically. In practice, it has been noticed that most catastrophic complications occur during primary access, which is thus considered to be the most challenging step in endoscopic surgery. Primary trocar entry is associated with injuries to the gastrointestinal tract[1] and major blood vessels,[1-8] and about 50% of these occur prior to performing the actual surgery.[9-13] This situation becomes more grave in the presence of previous surgeries. According to Royal College Of Obstetrics and Gynaecologists,[14] the incidence of umbilical adhesions is 50% in previous midline vertical scars and 23% in previous low transverse incisions. Royal College of Obstetrics and Gynaecologists has thus opined that umbilicus may not be the safest site of primary trocar insertion following previous surgery. Therefore, there is an emergent need to develop a new technique of primary access that does not utilize umbilicus as the first blind port to allow safe entry into the abdomen. And also in situations when laparoscopy is taken for cases with previous surgery and are associated with large masses and extremes of body mass index (BMI). Hence, we have devised a novel nonumbilical entry port technique over the years of practice. It is safe for novice and experienced alike. Over the years, it has been fondly coined as Jain point by our fellows.

WHAT IS JAIN POINT?

To avoid adhesions at umbilicus in previous surgery cases, most of the alternative entry ports are located in upper quadrant namely Lee Huang point, Palmer's point, and 9th intercostal space (**Fig. 1**). The Jain point lies in the left side of the abdomen at the level of umbilicus on a straight line drawn vertically upward from a point 2.5 cm medial to anterior superior iliac spine.[15-27] At the

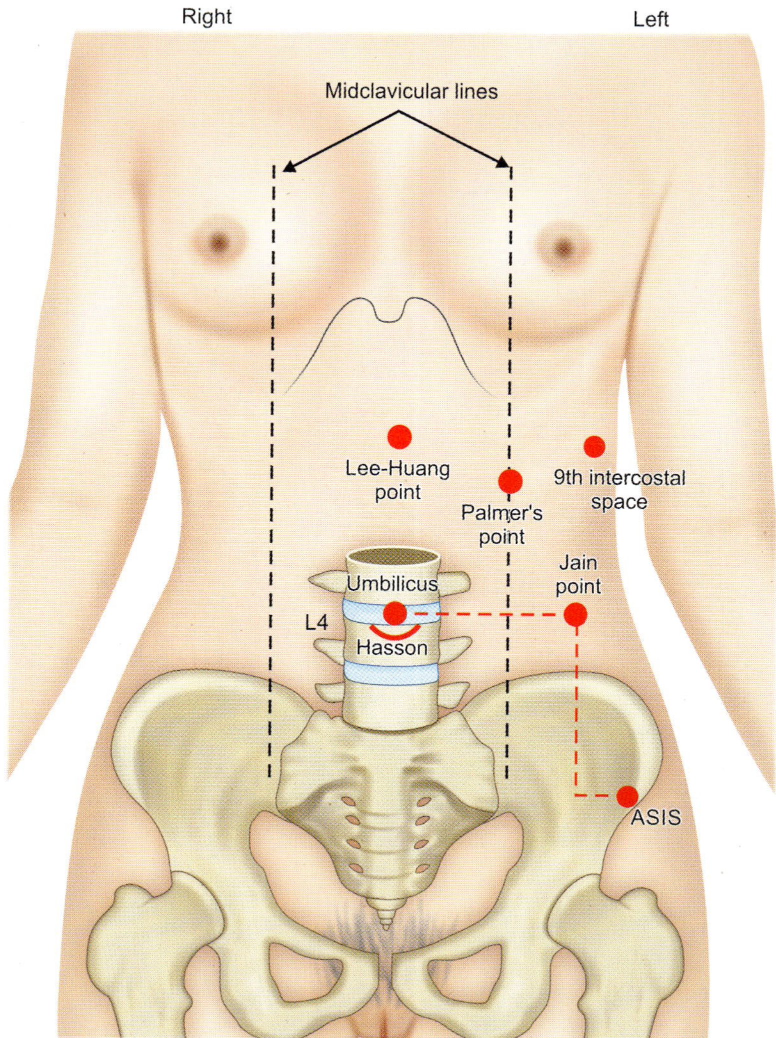

Fig. 1: Relative positions of all entry points. (ASIS: anterior superior iliac spine).

level of umbilicus, it lies at least 10–13 cm from the midpoint of umbilicus. This distance varies in this range according to the patient's weight, height, BMI, and presence of central obesity and other patient's variables. Basic aim is to avoid abdominal and umbilical adhesion and prevention of major retroperitoneal vessel injury.

SURFACE MARKING OF JAIN POINT

Jain point lies on a vertical line drawn 2.5 cm medial to anterior superior iliac spine (ASIS) at the level of umbilicus in the left paraumbilical region. It is roughly 10–13 cm lateral to the umbilicus, depending on the patient's body type **(Fig. 2)**.

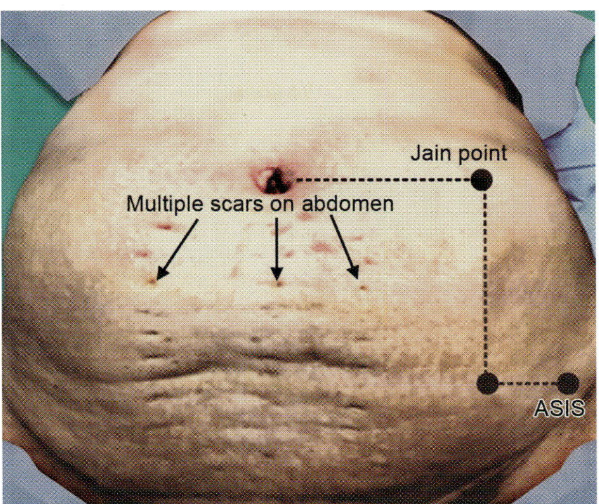

Fig. 2: Patient has three vertical scars. Jain point in the left paraumbilical region on a straight line drawn vertically upward from a point 2.5 cm medial to anterior superior iliac spine.

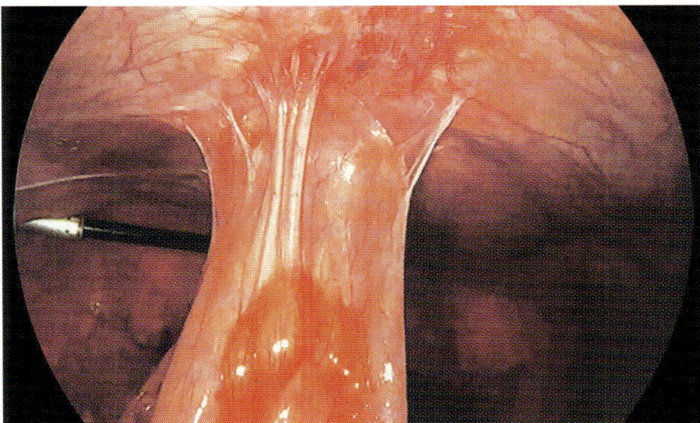

Fig. 3: 5 mm port at Jain point and left side free of adhesions, whereas bowel loops adherent at the umbilicus.

Jain point has a fixed bony point as reference point which makes the surface marking easy. This is an extra advantage compared to Palmer's point.

SURGICAL TECHNIQUE

When we enter the veress needle through umbilicus in a previous surgery case, an endoscopist's biggest nightmare is to avoid injury to adherent loop of bowel, omentum, and adhesions **(Fig. 3)**. To avoid these, we describe the entry technique from the Jain point. Jain point lies on a vertical line drawn 2.5 cm medial to ASIS at the level of umbilicus in the left paraumbilical region. It is roughly 10–13 cm lateral to the umbilicus, depending on the patient's body type.

Describing the Technique of Jain Point Entry (Figs. 4A to H)

For creating pneumoperitoneum, the preoperative preparation comprised of low residual diet for 48 hours prior to surgery. The stomach emptied of secretions and air by the use of orogastric tube by anesthetist, after endotracheal intubation. The operating table is laid in horizontal position. We make a very small 1–2 mm nick just enough for Veress needle entry. *By this step there is no chance of Veress needle flaying medially.* Veress needle is then inserted perpendicular to the abdominal wall in a vertical direction irrespective of patient being obese, average weight or thin. The abdominal wall is not lifted

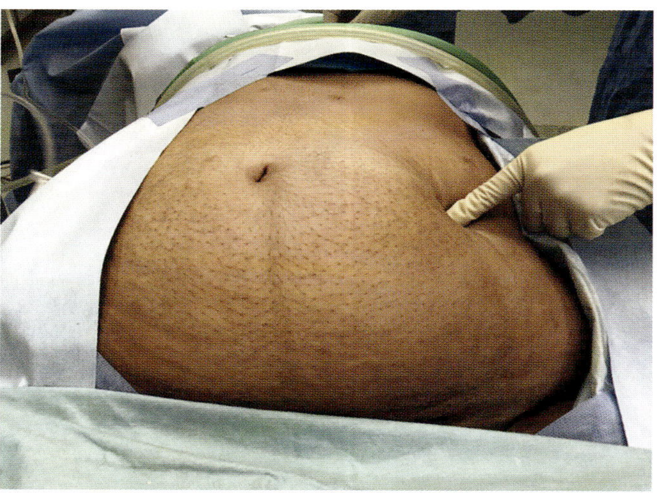

Fig. 4A: Finger pointing at the Jain point.

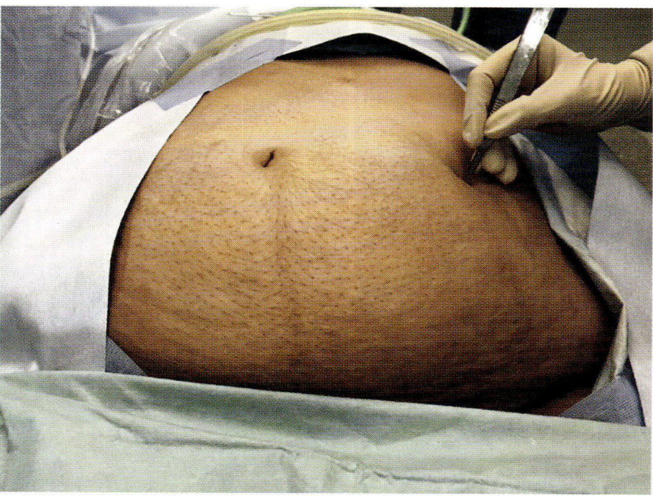

Fig. 4B: 1–2 mm nick given with 15 number surgical blade.

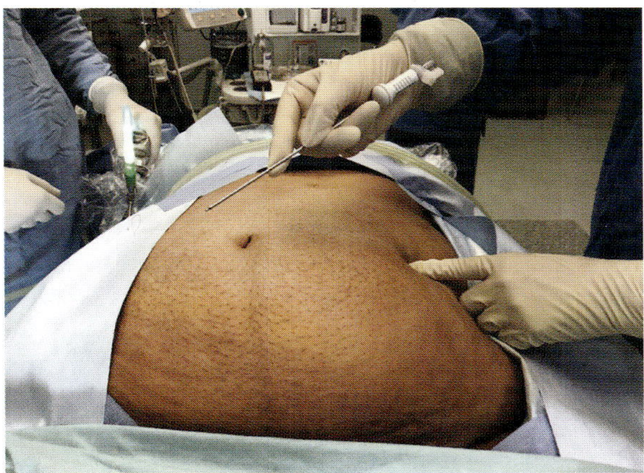

Fig. 4C: Holding the Veress needle with finger guard according to the anticipated thickness of abdominal wall.

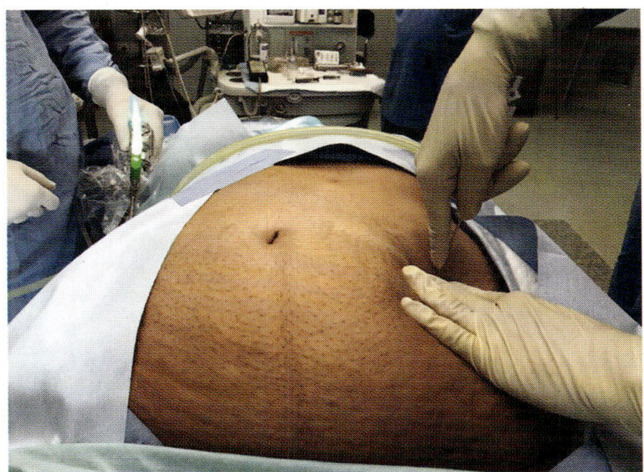

Fig. 4D: Veress needle is inserted perpendicular to the abdominal wall, in a vertical direction.

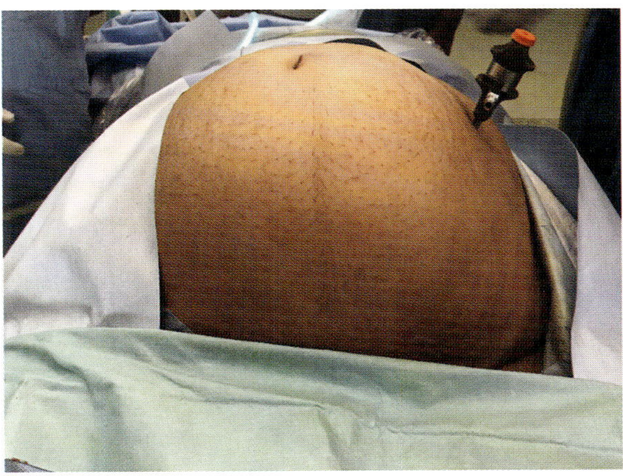

Fig. 4E: 5 mm trocar inserted at Jain point.

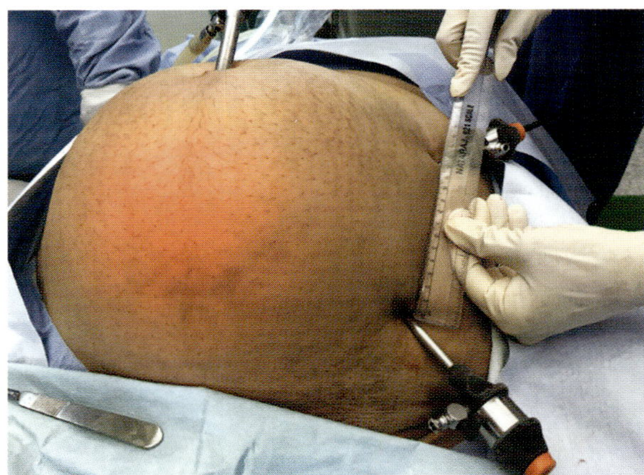

Fig. 4F: Distance between lower port and Jain point port.

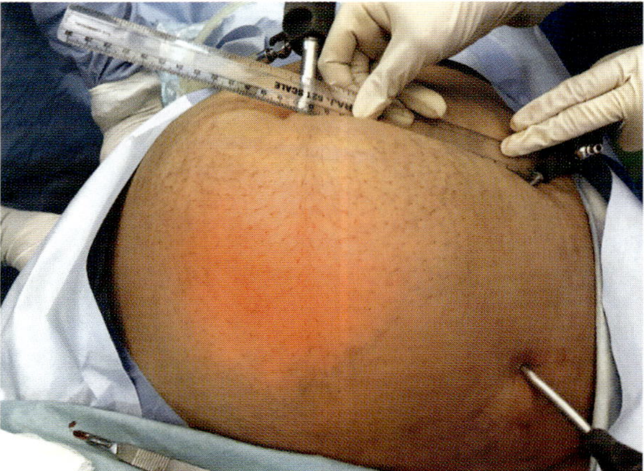

Fig. 4G: Distance between umbilicus and Jain point port.

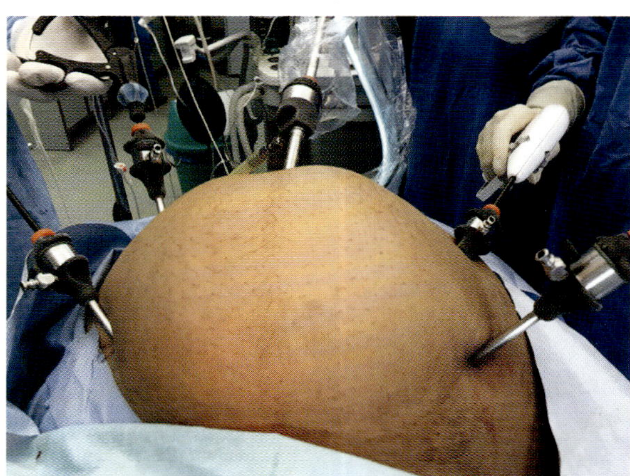

Fig. 4H: Final port placement.

and there is no change in direction of Veress *needle. This makes the insertion easy and simple.* We put a finger as a guard on the Veress needle according to the patient's BMI and flabby or thin abdominal wall. This is a very important safety feature. As we pass the Veress needle layer by layer, we feel two distinct pops. The first pop is at entry of Veress needle, as it passes through the aponeurosis of the external oblique muscle. The second pop is by the fused aponeurosis of internal oblique and transverses abdominis muscle aponeurosis. After this, the distinct feel of soft peritoneum and feeling of give way of resistance as the needle penetrates and enters the peritoneal cavity. This change in feel from the tough aponeurosis to soft peritoneum is the most important to confirm entry into peritoneal cavity.

In very thin **(Fig. 5A)** patients, this entry site is a boon as the risk of retroperitoneal vessel injury is negated and the layer by layer entry is very well defined due to good muscle tone.[28-30] In obese patients, a long Veress needle and 5 mm longer trocar is needed, though the technique remains same. In patients with flabby abdomen, as illustrated in **Figures 5B and C**, there is hardly any muscle tone so just a single prick with Veress needle on the skin easily tides it through the abdominal wall. The layer by layer entry is not delineated. This point is very important to remember as the depth of penetration cannot be judged due to practically no resistance offered during the needle passage through the layers of flabby abdomen. With large masses, the technique is the same but masses which are at or above the umbilicus are best entered by Jain point entry, as the Jain point lies 10–13 cm lateral to umbilicus, so the risk of hitting the mass or in case of a cyst, rupture, and spillage of contents is not there.[31]

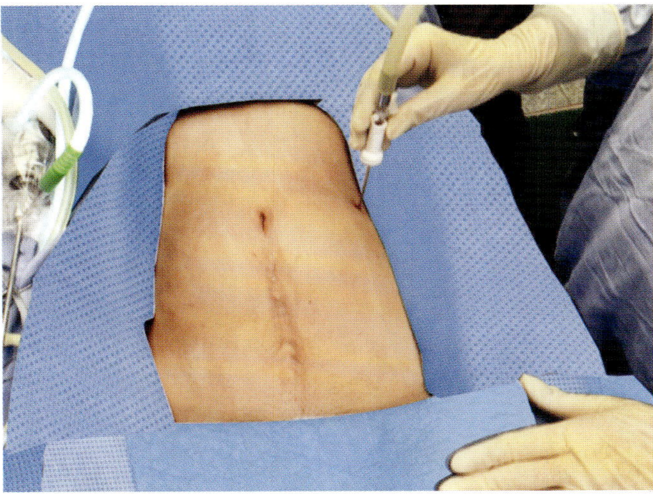

Fig. 5A: Veress needle in a very thin patient.

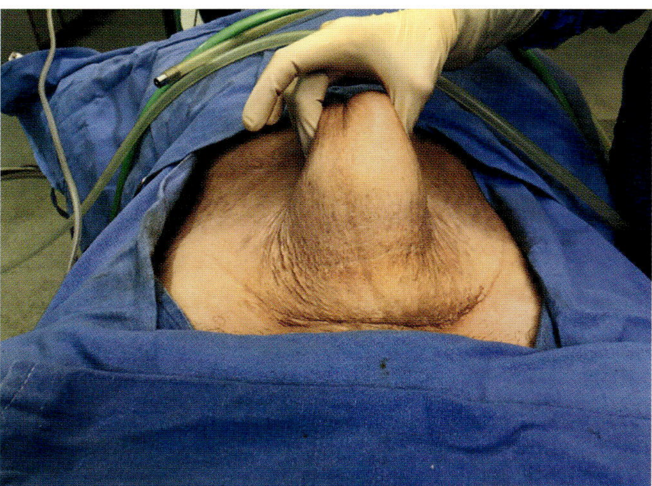

Fig. 5B: Flabby abdomen patient.

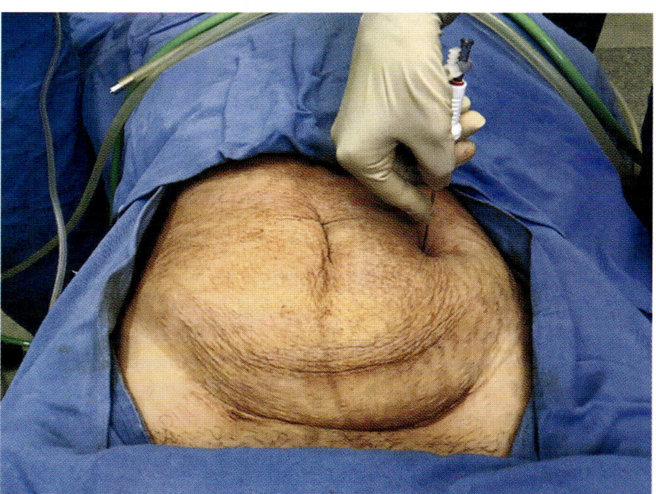

Fig. 5C: Veress needle in flabby abdomen patient.

The routine safety check of drop test and very initial intra-abdominal pressure (VIIP) test[32] are done and then CO_2 insufflation started. Once 3 liters of CO_2 has created a good pneumoperitoneum and abdomen duly tented with insufflation pressure of 25 mm Hg, then a 5 mm pyramidal tip reusable trocar is inserted. It is also inserted in a vertical direction, taking care not to flay laterally or medially towards sacral promontory. Then a 5 mm 0° telescope is inserted through Jain point to take a note of the pelvis and upper abdomen and adhesions which could be present due to previous surgery. A 360° check of whole abdomen is carried out and then the 10 mm port entry is optimized under direct vision. If it is a case of previous surgery, a note is made of adhesions and visually guided entry made by 10 mm telescope avoiding adhesions. So it becomes tailor-made according to the pathology, adhesions, and the patient type. Like if we are operating on a large pelvic mass, the 10 mm port can be placed much higher up under direct vision of the Jain point 5 mm port. After placing the 10 mm port, all other accessory ports are made according to the mandate of the case. Jain point port being lower and lateral at paraumbilical position becomes the main working port during the course of surgery. The distance between the Jain point port and ipsilateral left lower port is 10–12 cm which makes it very ergonomic for continuous working during course of surgery. Jain point thus has a dual benefit of being ergonomic main working port as well as first blind entry point. A case of TLH with large uterus is shown in **Figures 6 and 7**. TLH has been done using Jain point as main working port on the left side. 10 mm port is placed higher up with 30° telescope to show up the pathology better and carry out TLH in an easier manner without soiling the telescope repeatedly. Several demonstrations of live surgery workshops have continuously encouraged surgeons and gynecologists to use Jain point as the first blind port entry especially in patients with previously scarred abdomen.

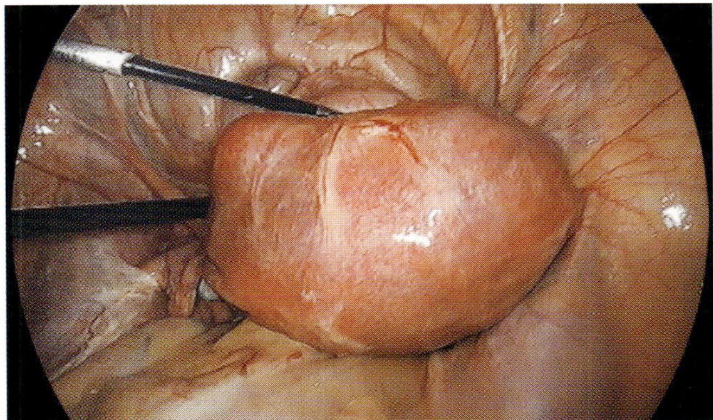

Fig. 6A: Fibroid uterus for total laparoscopic hysterectomy (TLH).

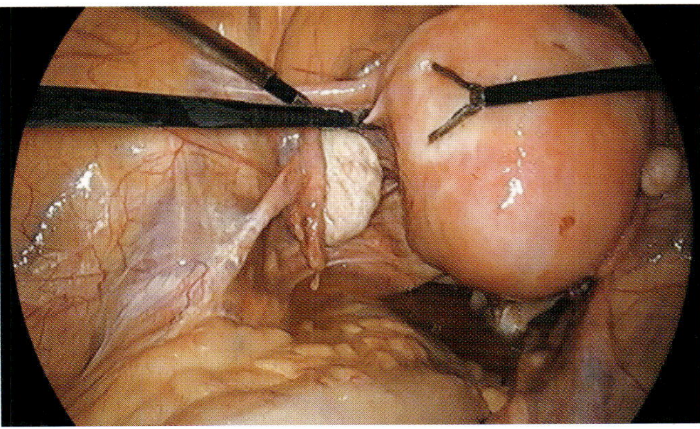

Fig. 6B: Coagulation and cutting of ovarian ligament.

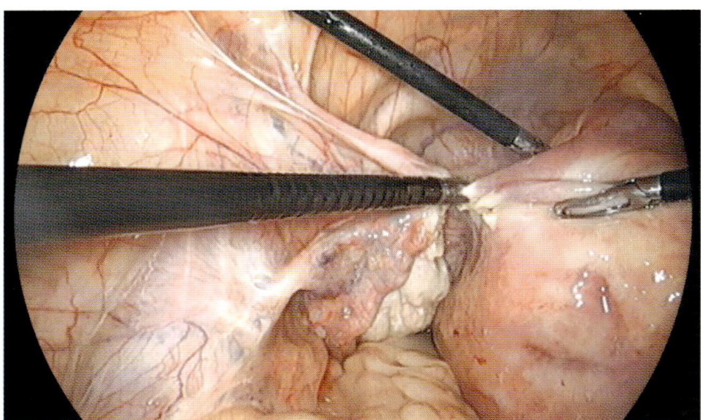

Fig. 6C: Coagulation and cutting of round ligament.

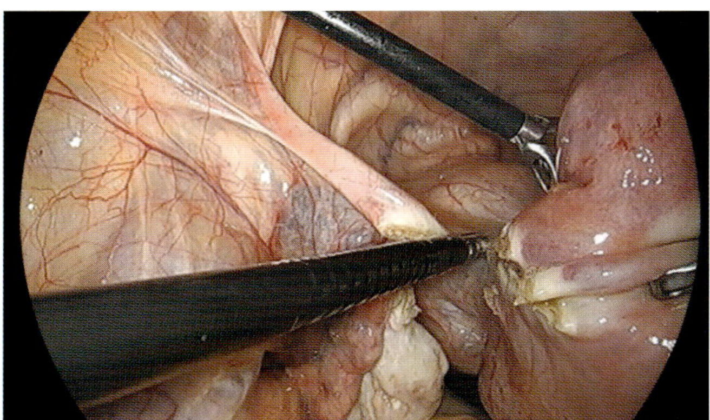

Fig. 6D: Coagulation and cutting to open up the broad ligament.

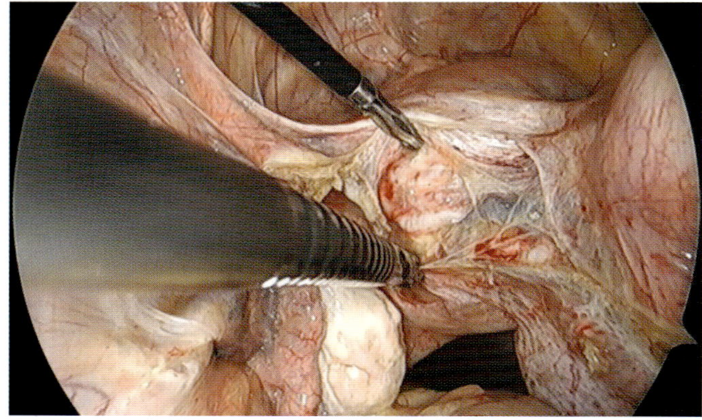

Fig. 6E: Uterine artery skeletonized.

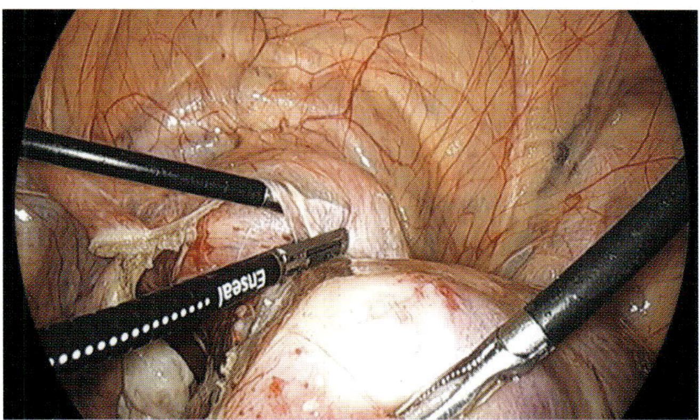

Fig. 6F: Cutting the uterovesical fold of peritoneum.

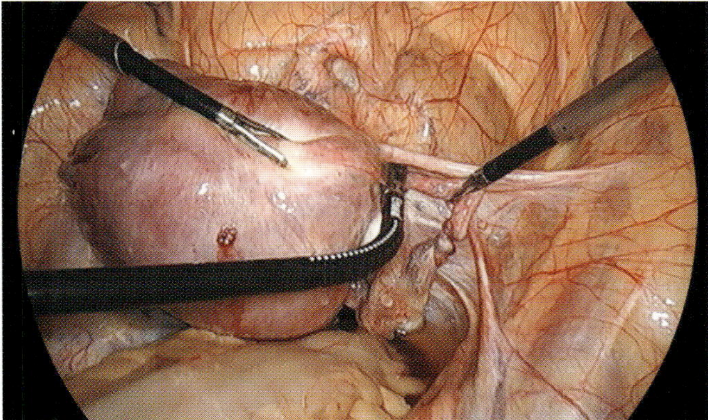

Fig. 7A: Coagulation and cutting of tubo-ovarian ligament using articulating Enseal.

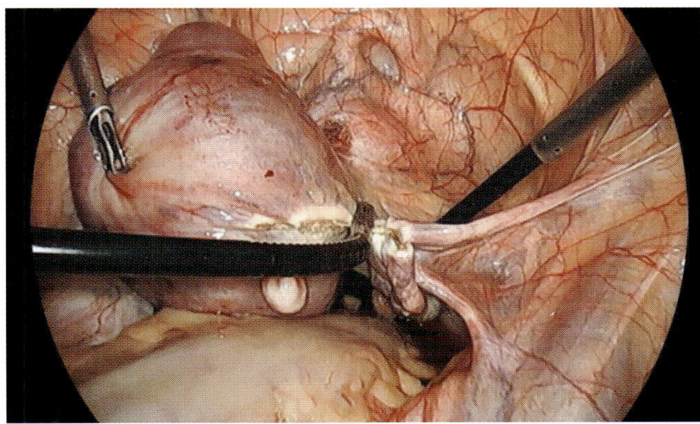

Fig. 7B: Coagulation and cutting of round ligament.

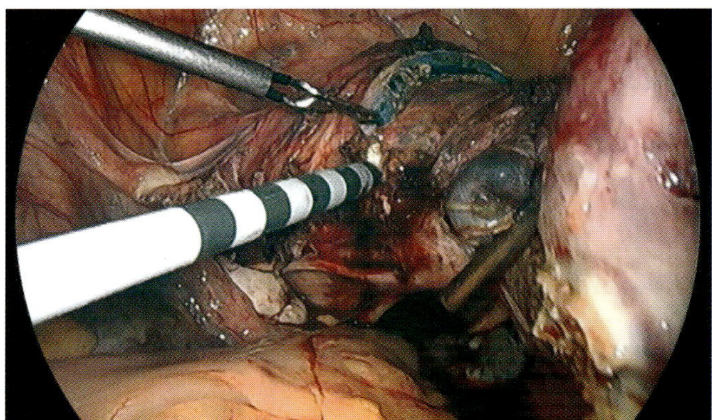

Fig. 7C: Colpotomy completed.

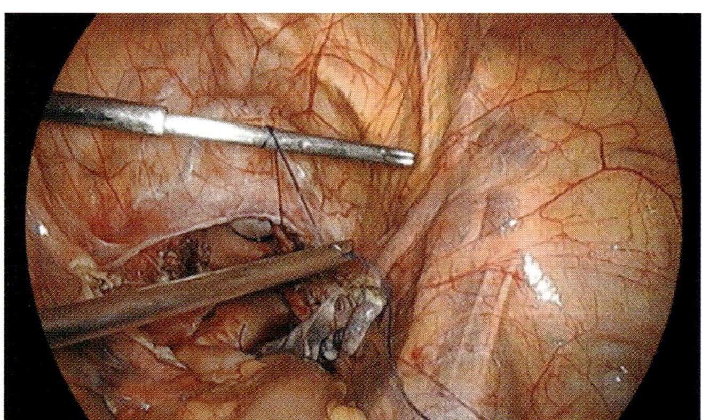

Fig. 7D: Securing the vaginal angle by 1.0 vicryl suture.

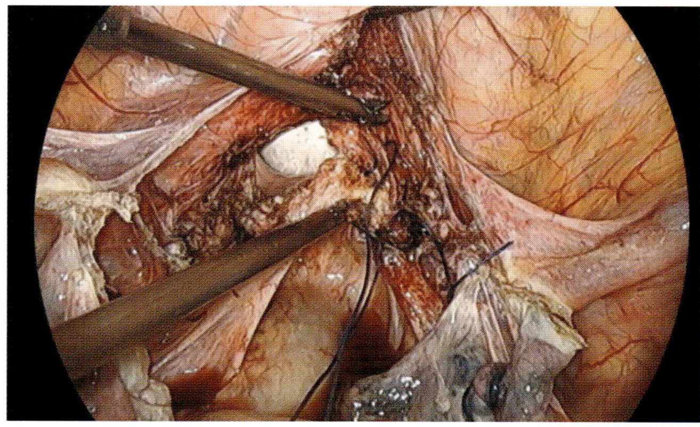

Fig. 7E: Closure of the vaginal vault.

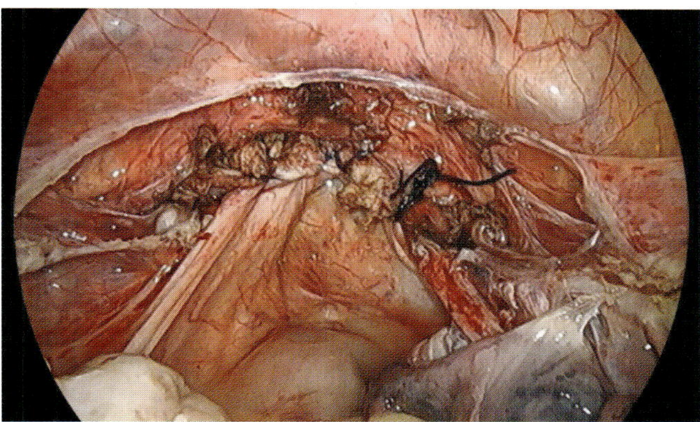

Fig. 7F: Vault closure completed.

LEARNING POINTS

- Patient should be in supine position, during insertion of Veress needle and first blind port.
- Nasogastric tube to be in proper place.
- Surface marking of Jain point to be made precisely.
- As the ASIS is easily felt, fixed bony point marking the Jain point is easy.
- Veress needle to be inserted perpendicularly.
- No lifting of the abdominal wall.

REFERENCES

1. Nordestgaard AG, Bodily KC, Osborne Jr RW, et al. Major vascular injuries during laparoscopic procedures. Am J Surg. 1995;169(5):543-5.
2. Larson GM, Vitale GC, Casey J, et al. Multipractice analysis of laparoscopic cholecystectomy in 1,983 patients. Am J Surg. 1992;163(2):221-6.
3. Leibl BJ, Schmedt C-G, Schwarz J, et al. A single institution's experience with transperitoneal laparoscopic hernia repair. Am J Surg. 1998;175(6):446-52.
4. McDonald PT, Rich NM, Collins Jr GJ, et al. Vascular trauma secondary to diagnostic and therapeutic procedures: laparoscopy. Am J Surg. 1978;135(5):651-5.
5. Mintz M. Risks and prophylaxis in laparoscopy: a survey of 100000 cases. J Reprod Med. 1977;18(5):269-72.
6. Yuzpe AA. Pneumoperitoneum needle and trocar injuries in laparoscopy. A survey on possible contributing factors and prevention. J Reprod Med. 1990;35(5):485-90.
7. Baadsgaard SE, Bille S, Egeblad K. Major vascular injury during gynecologic laparoscopy: report of a case and review of published cases. Acta Obstet Gynecol Scand. 1989;68(3):283-5.
8. Chapron C, Pierre F, Harchaoui Y, et al. Gastrointestinal injuries during gynaecological laparoscopy. Hum Reprod. 1999;14(2):333-7.
9. Magrina JF. Complications of laparoscopic surgery. Clin Obstet Gynecol. 2002;45(2):469-80.
10. Sigman HH, Fried GM, Garzon J, et al. Risks of blind versus open approach to celiotomy for laparoscopic surgery. Surg Laparosc Endosc. 1993;3(4):296-9.

11. Jansen FW, Kapiteyn K, Trimbos-Kemper T, et al. Complications of laparoscopy: a prospective multicentre observational study. Br J Obstet Gynaecol. 1997;104(5):595-600.

12. Harkki-Sirén P, Kurki T. A nationwide analysis of laparoscopic complications. Obstet Gynecol. 1997;89(1):108-12.

13. Härkki-Siren P, Sjöberg J, Kurki T. Major complications of laparoscopy: a follow-up Finnish study. Obstet Gynecol. 1999;94(1):94-8.

14. Royal College of Obstetricians and Gynaecologists. (2008). Preventing entry-related gynaecological laparoscopic injuries. Green-top Guideline Number 49. [online] Available from https://www.rcog.org.uk/en/guidelines-research-services/guidelines/gtg49/ [Last accessed January, 2020].

15. Jain N, Sareen S, Kanawa S, et al. Jain point: a new safe portal for laparoscopic entry in previous surgery cases. J Hum Reprod Sci. 2016;9(1):9-17.

16. Jain N, Mann S, Jain V. To study the safety of Jain point as an alternate to standard palmer's point in patients with previous surgeries. J Min Inv Gynaecol. 2014;21(6):S162.

17. Jain N, Jain V, Kanawa S. Standard technique of port placement by new laparoscopic entry port (The Jain point). In: Jain N (Ed). Comprehensive Video Atlas of Laparoscopic Surgery in Infertility and Gynecology. New Delhi: Jaypee Brothers Medical Publishers (P) Ltd; 2016. pp. 33-7.

18. Jain et al. presented lecture on "Jain point: a new safe portal for laparoscopic entry in previous surgery cases" at "26th Annual ESGE Congress" on 18th to 21st October, 2017, at Antalya, Turkey.

19. Jain et al. presented on "Jain point: a new safe portal for laparoscopic entry in previous surgery cases" at "International Workshop on Laparoscopic Endometriosis & Pelvic Anatomy" on 8th and 9th December, 2017, at Pune, India.

20. Jain et al. presented lecture on "Jain point: a new safe portal for laparoscopic entry in previous surgery cases" at "Beyond Gynecological Surgery from Imagination to Innovation & Education, AAGL Regional Meeting" on 4th to 6th April, 2018, at Clermont Ferrand, France.

21. Jain N, Jain V, Aggarwal C. Left lateral port: Safe laparoscopic port entry in previous large upper abdomen laparotomy scar. J Minim Invasive Gynecol. 2019;26(5):973-6.

22. Jain et al. presented on "Jain point: A new safe portal for laparoscopic entry in previous surgery cases" at "AAGL 2018 47th Global Congress on MIGS", on 11th to 15th November 2018 at Las Vegas, Nevada.

23. Jain et al. presented abstract on "New laparoscopic entry port for previous surgery cases: Jain point" at "AAGL 2019 48th Global Congress on MIGS", on 9th to 13th November 2019 at Vancouver, BC, Canada.

24. Hameed F, Iqbal MS, Iqbal Z, Liaqat K (2018) Safety of Direct Trocar Insertion for Laparoscopic Procedures. APMC 12:212-214.

25. Sharp HT. (2019). Overview of gynecologic laparoscopic surgery and non-umbilical entry sites. [online] Available from https://www.uptodate.com/contents/overview-of-gynecologic-laparoscopic-surgery-and-non-umbilical-entry-sites [Last accessed January, 2020].

26. Mulayim B, Aksoy O. Direct trocar entry from left lateral port (Jain point) in a case with previous surgeries. J Gynecol Surg. 2019.

27. Abdullah AA, Abdulmageed MU, Katoof FM. The efficacy of direct trocar versus veress needle method as a primary access technique in laparoscopic cholecystectomy. Mustansiriya Med J. 2019;18(1):47-50.

28. Hurd WH, Bude R, DeLancey J, et al. Abdominal wall characterization with magnetic resonance imaging and computed tomography. The effect of obesity on the laparoscopic approach. J Reprod Med. 1991;36(7):473-6.
29. Hurd WW, Bude RO, DeLancey J, et al. The relationship of the umbilicus to the aortic bifurcation: implications for laparoscopic technique. Obstet Gynecol. 1992;80(1):48-51.
30. Nezhat F, Brill AI, Nezhat CH, et al. Laparoscopic appraisal of the anatomic relationship of the umbilicus to the aortic bifurcation. J Am Assoc Gynecol Laparosc. 1998;5(2):135-40.
31. Detorakis S, Vlachos D, Athanasiou S, et al. Laparoscopic cystectomy in-a-bag of an intact cyst: is it feasible and spillage-free after all? Minim Invasive Surg. 2016;2016:8640871.
32. Vilos GA. The ABCs of a safer laparoscopic entry. JMIG. 2006;13(3):249-51.

Evolution of Jain Point

Nutan Jain, Shivam Vatsal, Monika Ranwa

We were doing laparoscopic surgeries since the early nineties, and in 1998 we converted to same side working and stopped using contralateral style of working and suturing. So, we found over due course, that the upper port on the left paraumbilical position was always found to be free of adhesions. This observation which was seen over couple of years prompted us to start using this port as a first blind entry port. In the beginning, we started putting the 5 mm port through this point and then optimized the 10 mm port according to the mandate of the case. As things progressed, gradually we found that using this port rather than the Palmer's point for first blind port entry in cases of previous surgery cases also kept on resulting in no bowel or omental adhesions, and we continued our journey of making the first blind port through this point. So, this was the beginning in the early 21st century that we found that this port can be used safely for entry, and during making our entries through this point we compared with the umbilical entry that here there was no risk of major retroperitoneal vessel injury. The biggest nightmare through umbilical entry is the risk of catastrophic bleeding from the major retroperitoneal vessels that are so close below the umbilicus. Beneath the upper left lateral port, the omentum and bowel adhesions were really not found. So, this observation over years prompted us to start using it routinely and then we evaluated its benefits compared to the Palmer's point. Whenever we were using the Palmer's point we saw that the Palmer's point port was usually remaining redundant after the first blind entry. In our practice also we had one direct entry into the stomach in a case of a bloated stomach where we tried the Palmer's point entry, so a bloated stomach becomes a contraindication for Palmer's point. As we progressed in our journey of laparoscopic surgery we converted from contralateral working pattern to same side working where in both working ports, come from the same side where the surgeon is standing. The upper port at paraumbilical position is "The Jain point," and the lower one is 2.5 cm medial and 1 cm above the anterior superior iliac spine. So, this was the evolution of the Jain point, wherein we started putting the first blind Veress needle and 5 mm port through the Jain point. We published our data in 2016, where in the fellows fondly coined the term Jain point. So, we have started using it after a long background of doing major laparoscopic surgeries since 1992 and diagnostic laparoscopies we were doing from our residency days way back during 1980–1981. During this long spell of doing surgeries and observations we saw that the upper paraumbilical port was always found to be free of adhesions. From here, we took the clue that this point could be used as the first blind port entry in previous surgery cases, where we have the biggest issue of bowel/omental adherence at the umbilicus. Then, the second nightmare specially for beginners and always a relief even for advanced endoscopic surgeons also is to see the first blind umbilical trocar gone in safely. Beneath the umbilicus lie all the major retroperitoneal vessels, so it was very clear to understand that since the Jain point is about 10–13 cm lateral to the umbilicus, there is no risk of major vessels injury when we enter through this point. So, with all these observations, coupled over an active teaching and learning unit, we had opportunity for this point to be tried by fresh trainees and fellows. We have had our fellowship programs since 1999, so that makes complete 20 years since when fellows and trainees were making the first blind port entry through this point **(Figs. 1 to 4)**. So it has been a long time since it is being used. Now, we have documented our results since 2011, from there in we started using Jain point exclusively as the first blind port for Veress as well as first 5 mm trocar and not the usual umbilical entry. From here comes a long-term safety profile of usage and the rationale of use of Jain point. This entry method can be further utilized for more challenging cases like previous surgeries, multiple previous scars, large masses, big cystic masses, and combinations of big masses and previous surgeries, obese or very thin

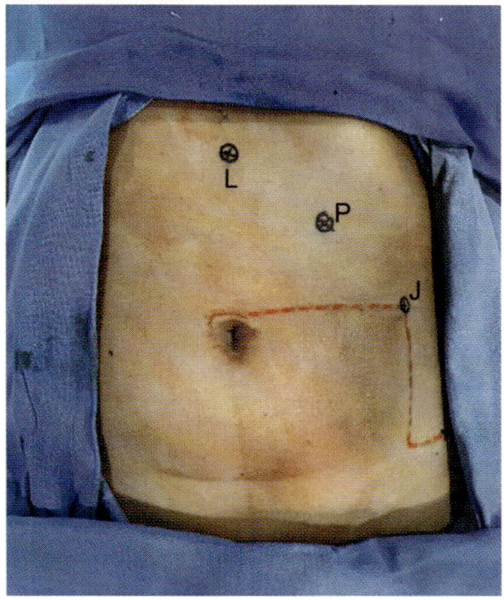

Fig. 1: Surface marking of Jain point. (L: Lee-Huang point; P: Palmer's point; J: JAIN POINT).

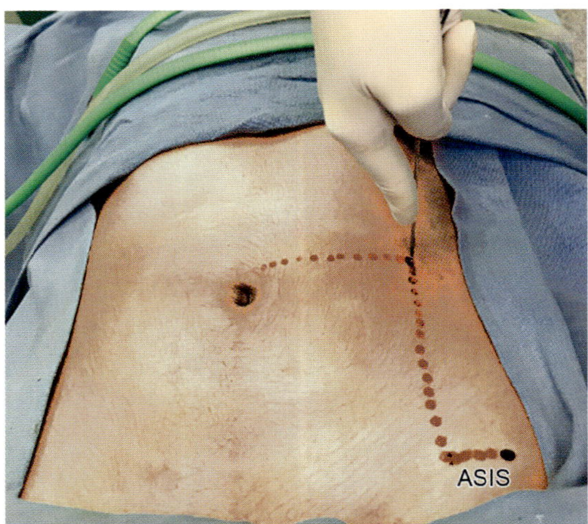

Fig. 2: Direction of the Veress needle.

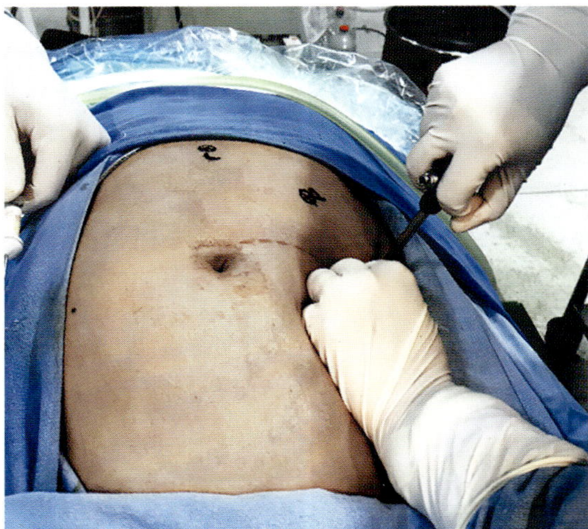

Fig. 3: A 5 mm trocar inserting at Jain point.

patients. In all such cases, the umbilical approach is deemed to be hazardous and here a nonumbilical approach is highly welcome. So, in this text and in the entire textbook we shall be focusing on the development, rationale, and the ergonomics of a nonumbilical port "The Jain point". Its usage in extremes of body mass index (BMI) and other complex clinical situations will be presented in coming chapters.

LEARNING POINTS

- Jain point entry moves away the primary port to a nonumbilical position avoiding catastrophic complications to vessels, viscera, and adhesions.

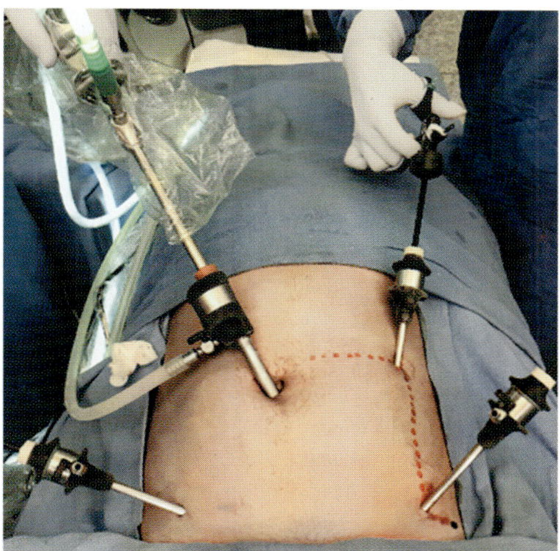

Fig. 4: Final port placement.

- Rather than being redundant it becomes the main working port in is due course of surgery.
- Easily replicable with a short learning course.
- Good for beginners and in previous surgery cases.
- Has easy landmarks umbilicus and anterior superior iliac spine (ASIS).

■ SUGGESTED READING

1. Jain et al. presented lecture on "Jain point: A New Safe Portal for Laparoscopic Entry in Previous Surgery Cases: Beyond Gynecological Surgery from Imagination to Innovation & Education" at AAGL Regional Meeting in Clermont Ferrand, France on 4th to 6th April 2018.
2. Jain et al. presented lecture on "Jain point: A New Safe Portal for Laparoscopic Entry in Previous Surgery Cases" at 26th Annual ESGE Congress in Antalya, Turkey on 18-21 October 2017.
3. Jain et al. presented lecture on "Jain point: A New Safe Portal for Laparoscopic Entry in Previous Surgery Cases" at International Workshop on Laparoscopic Endometriosis and Pelvic Anatomy on 8th and 9th Dec, 2017 at Pune, India.
4. Jain et al. presented lecture on "New Laparoscopic Entry Port for Previous Surgery Cases: Jain point" at AAGL 2019 48th Global Congress on MIGS in Vancouver, BC, Canada on 9th to 13th November 2019.
5. Jain et al. presented on "Jain point: A New Safe Portal for Laparoscopic Entry in Previous Surgery Cases" at AAGL 2018 47th Global Congress on MIGS in Las Vegas, NevaDa on 11th to 15th November 2018.
6. Jain N, Jain V, Aggarwal C. Left lateral port: safe laparoscopic port entry in previous large upper abdomen laparotomy scar. J Minim Invasive Gynecol. 2019;26(5):973-6.
7. Jain N, Jain V, Kanawa S. Standard technique of port placement by new laparoscopic entry port (the Jain point). Comprehensive video atlas of laparoscopic surgery in infertility and gynecology. 2016; 2:33-37.

8. Jain N, Mann S, Jain V. To study the safety of Jain point as an alternate to standard Palmar's point in patients with previous surgeries. J Min Inv Gynaecol. 2014;21(6 S):S162.

9. Jain N, Sareen S, Kanawa S, et al. Jain point: a new safe portal for laparoscopic entry in previous surgery cases. J Hum Reprod Sci. 2016;9:9-17.

10. Koh CH, Janik GM. Laparoscopic microsurgical tubal anastomosis. In: Adamson GD, Martin DC (Eds). Endoscopic Management of Gynecologic Disease. Philadelphia: Lippincott-Raven; 1996. pp. 119-45.

11. Koh CH, Janik GM. Laparoscopic microsuturing techniques. St Louis: Medical Video Productions; 1996.

12. Koh CH, Janik GM. Laparoscopic tubal reanastomosis. In: Tulandi T (Ed). Endoscopic Surgery for Gynecologists, 2nd edition. London: WB Saunders; 1997.

13. Mulayam B, Aksoy O. Direct trocar entry from left lateral port (Jain point) in a case with previous surgeries. J Gynec Surg. 2019. Published online, 22 Oct 2019.

14. Sharp HT. (2019). Overview of gynecologic laparoscopic surgery and non-umbilical entry sites. [online] Available from https://www.uptodate.com/contents/overview-of-gynecologic-laparoscopic-surgery-and-non-umbilical-entry-sites. [Last accessed January, 2020].

Rationale of Jain Point

Nutan Jain, Aruna Arya, Swati Varshney, Sonam Singh

INTRODUCTION

The anatomical rationale of using Jain point is to avoid retroperitoneal vessels which lie in deep proximity to the umbilicus, making the first umbilical entry hazardous in at least 50% of the laparoscopic entries. The major catastrophic injuries occur at the time of the blind umbilical port insertion.[1,2] So, there has constantly been a search to find a new safe port of entry which could avoid this catastrophic injury to the retroperitoneal vessels **(Fig. 1)**. Here, in the Jain point we hardly find any risk of injuring the major retroperitoneal vessels, which lie beneath the umbilicus. To make laparoscopy entry safer, a nonumbilical approach is being advocated to not only avoid the major vessels, also in suspected cases of periumbilical adhesions there could be a risk of injury to the viscera, bowel, and omental adhesions.[3,4]

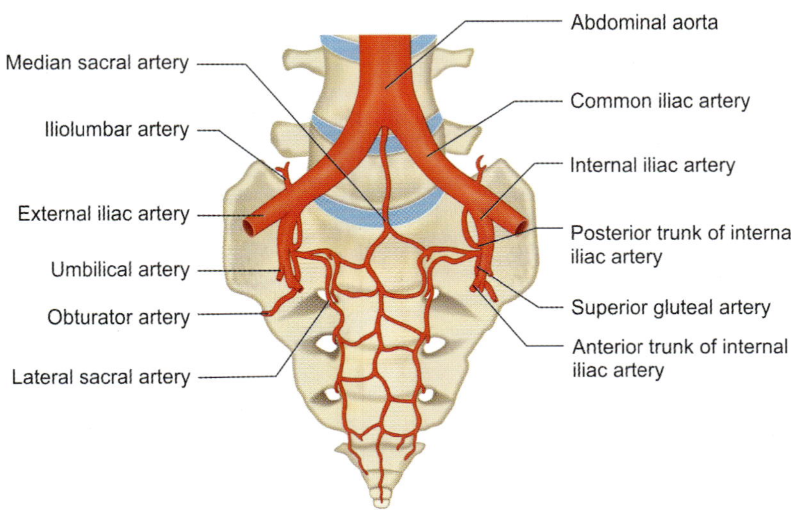

Fig. 1: Jain point free from the risk of major vessel injury.

Unsuspected bowel adhesions can also happen in previous surgeries and patients with previous infectious pathologies.[5,6] So, if we shift away the first blind entry point from the umbilicus to a nonumbilical entry point, then we can have protection against retroperitoneal vessel injury and also avoidance of injury to adherent loop of bowel **(Fig. 2)** or omentum in cases of previous surgery.[7-10]

Here we propose the Jain point, so that we can ensure or we can at least hope for more safer **(Fig. 3)**, smooth first blind entry. In our large period of study ranging for almost 10 years and more than 7,000 cases, there was just one injury to the bowel, and none to the major vessels. Trivial complications like omental emphysema and preperitoneal insufflation,[11] which are caused by a little over or under shoot of the Veress needle, are usually seen in the

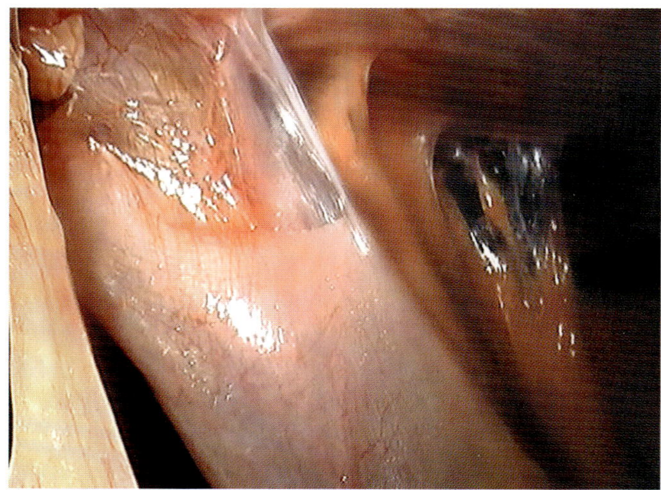

Fig. 2: Multiple bowel loops stuck.

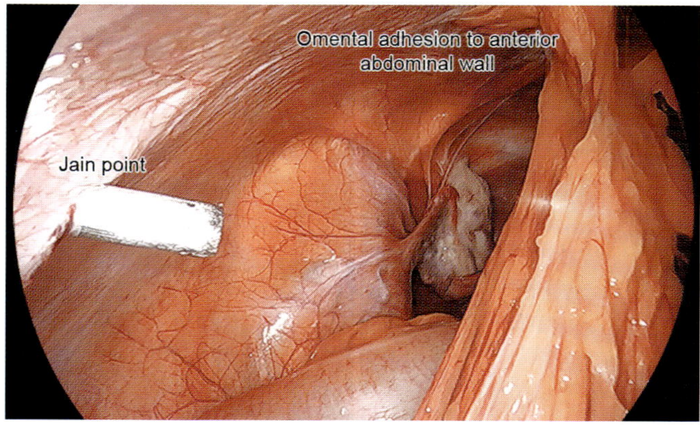

Fig. 3: Jain point totally free of adhesion.

first week of the fellow trying to make transition from the umbilical entry and once they understand the nuances and the technique and methodology of the Jain point insertion, the trivial complications like omental emphysema or preperitoneal placement are significantly reduced. Also, the failed insertions which are usually seen in the early learning curve of the Jain point technique are also reduced substantially after continued use of this method of insertion of the Veress needle and the first blind port. So, taking into account the need to make laparoscopy safer the first hurdle to laparoscopy is safe first blind port entry and accordingly we propose in this text the nonumbilical entry port.

Here, we also want to emphasize on the logical justification for Jain point being located in the left paraumbilical region on the left side rather than the right side. In our overall experience of 30 years in operative laparoscopy, we gradually started working with both working ports coming from the same side,[12,13] while standing on the left side of patient. It is discernibly observed that most adhesions are present in mid abdomen, upper abdomen, right side, and lower pelvis, whereas left side of pelvis is found consistently free of adhesions. The sigmoid colon adheres at the pelvic brim. From here, up to the level of spleen and kidney (at T10/T12–L1 position) there is a nascent area which is found consistently free of abdominal adhesions. In this area, we devised the Jain point at level of umbilicus **(Figs. 4A and B)**. Also, the intestinal pathologies are more common on right side of abdomen because of the distribution of Peyer's patches[14] which are aggregates of lymphoid nodules concentrated in wall of terminal ileum and cecum and constitute an important part of immune system. Hence, intestinal infections like chronic appendicitis, tuberculosis, and enteric infection occur in terminal ileum and lead to all type of adhesions in right side of abdomen.[15-18] Many times on inserting the first blind port we see lot of adhesions in the right side though there is no history of previous surgery **(Figs. 5 and 6)**.

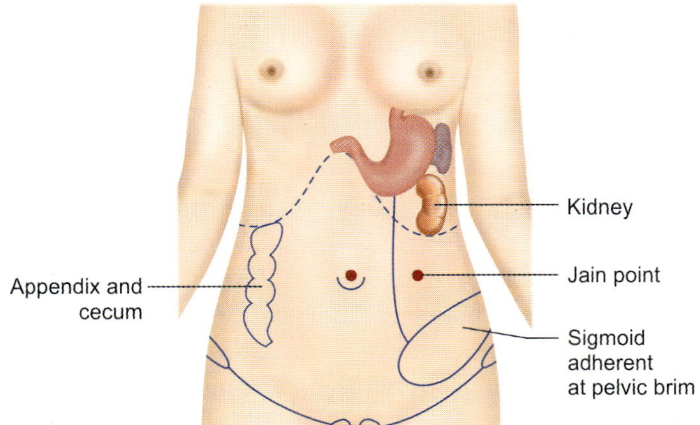

Fig. 4A: A diagrammatic representation of the Jain point port.

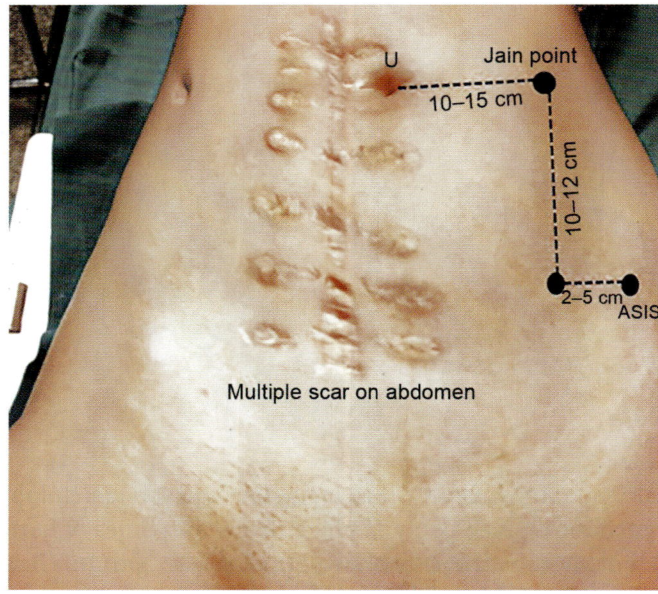

Fig. 4B: Jain point lies in the left paraumbilical region, in a straight line drawn vertically upward from a point 2.5 cm medial and 1 cm above anterior superior iliac spine (ASIS).

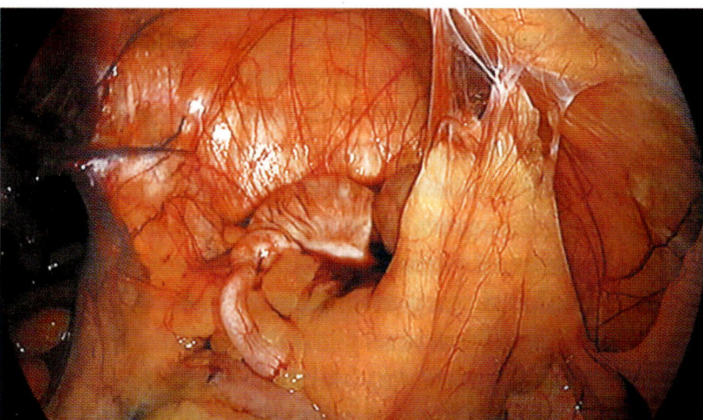

Fig. 5: Case without any previous surgery showing adhesions in mid abdomen. Appendix adhesion usually seen on right side.

One more reason of terminal ileum being exposed to brunt of intestinal infections could be terminal ileum getting narrowed and more horizontal in position just before the ileocecal valve, leading to more stasis and hence more prone to intestinal pathologies.[19] After this observation gradually we started utilizing left side of the abdomen for first blind port entry in previous surgery cases. Over the last decade, fellows named it Jain point. This has been first blind nonumbilical port of entry for all our cases. This anatomical rationale of the Jain point clearly justifies its use in intricate cases that require a meticulous

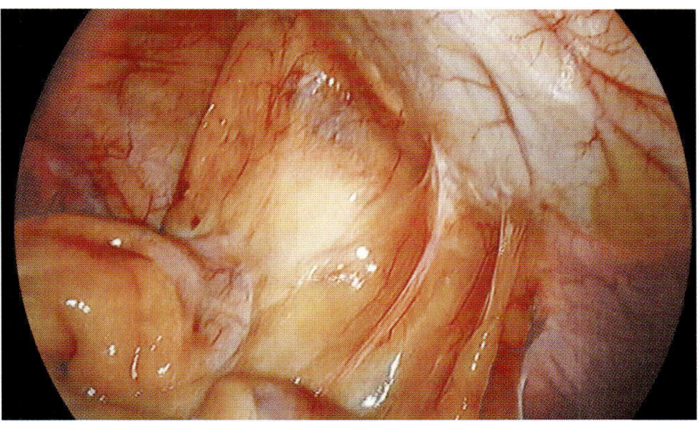

Fig. 6: Adhesions on right side without any previous surgery.

and heedful surgical approach, like cases with previous surgeries, big masses and extremes of BMI, pregnancy, previous mesh hernia repairs.[20-24] The crux of above all is to first make our routine laparoscopic entry safer and then as we take up more challenging cases the same method and technique works irrespective to the various challenges posed by complex clinical situations. Making safe laparoscopic access by a nonumbilical approach everyday will keep us in the routine and any challenges which come by previous surgery or extreme of BMI are all tackled in the similar manner.

LEARNING POINTS

- Primary port placement including Veress needle through umbilicus accounts for 40% of laparoscopic complications.
- Anatomy of Jain point is such that no superficial vessel or deep retroperitoneal vessels are directly under it as it is far away from sacral promontory.
- On the left side, no viscera from pelvic brim up to T10–T12 where spleen, stomach, and kidney are located.
- On the right side, usually adhesions of appendix and cecum noted due to episodes of subacute appendicitis and ileocecal Koch's.
- On the right side, gallbladder surgery or enlarged liver could preclude blind entry.
- Distance of Jain point from umbilicus is around 10–13 cm depending on obesity, body types, BMI, central or truncal obesity, but definitely being more lateral avoids midline vertical scars adhesions and big solid and cystic masses.

REFERENCES

1. Jansen FW, Kapiteyn K, Trimbos-Kemper T, et al. Complications of laparoscopy: a prospective multicentre observational study. Br J Obstet Gynaecol. 1997;104(5):595-600.

2. Jansen FW, Kolkman W, Bakkum EA, et al. Complications of laparoscopy: an inquiry about closed versus open-entry technique. Am J Obstet Gynecol. 2004;190:634-8.

3. Sharp HT. (2019). Overview of gynecologic laparoscopic surgery and non-umbilical entry sites. [online] Available from https://www.uptodate.com/contents/overview-of-gynecologic-laparoscopic-surgery-and-non-umbilical-entry-sites. [Last accessed January, 2020].

4. Royal College of Obstetricians and Gynaecologists. Preventing entry-related gynaecological laparoscopic injuries. Green-top guideline no. 49. London: RCOG; 2008.

5. Liakakos T, Thomakos N, Fine PM, et al. Peritoneal adhesions: etiology, pathophysiology, and clinical significance. Recent advances in prevention and management. Dig Surg. 2001;18(4):260-73.

6. Ellis H. The magnitude of adhesion related problems. Ann Chir Gynaecol. 1998;87(1):9-11.

7. Varma R, Gupta JK. Laparoscopic entry techniques: clinical guideline, national survey, and medicolegal ramifications. Surg Endosc. 2008;22(12):2686-97.

8. Tulikangas PK, Robinson DS, Falcone T. Left upper quadrant cannula insertion. Fertil Steril. 2003;79(2):411-2.

9. Chang FH, Chou HH, Lee CL, et al. Extraumbilical insertion of the operative laparoscope in patients with extensive intra-abdominal adhesions. J Am Assoc Gynecol Laparosc. 1995;2(3):335-7.

10. Kumakiri J, Takeuchi H, Sato Y, et al. A novel method of ninth-intercostal microlaparoscopic approach for patients with previous laparotomy. Acta Obstet Gynecol Scand. 2006;85:977-81.

11. Richardson RE, Sutton CJG. Complications of first entry: a prospective laparoscopy audit. Gynaecol Endosc. 1999;8:327-34.

12. Koh CH, Janik GM. Laparoscopic microsurgical tubal anastomosis. Obstetrics and Gynecology Clinics of North America. 1999;26(1):189-200.

13. Jain N, Jain V, Mann S, et al. The concept of ipsilateral suturing and clinical applications. In: State-of-the-Art Atlas and Textbook of Laparoscopic Suturing in Gynecology. New Delhi: Jaypee Brothers Medical Publishers (P) Ltd.; 2015. pp. 57-76.

14. Jung C, Hugot J-P, Barreau F. Peyer's patches: the immune sensors of the intestine. Int J Inflam. 2010;2010:823710.

15. Bhansali SK. Abdominal tuberculosis. Experiences with 300 cases. Am J Gastroenterol. 1977;67(4):324-37.

16. Joshi MJ. The surgical management of intestinal tuberculosis—a conservative approach. Indian J Surg. 1978;40:79-83.

17. Palmer KR, Patil DH, Basran S, et al. Abdominal tuberculosis in urban Britain—a common disease. Gut. 1985;26:1296-305.

18. Tandon RK, Sarin SK, Bose SL, et al. A clinico-radiological reappraisal of intestinal tuberculosis—changing profile? Gastroenterol Jpn. 1986;21(1):17-22.

19. Haskell H, Andrews CW Jr., Reddy SI, et al. Pathologic features and clinical significance of "backwash" ileitis in ulcerative colitis. Am J Surg Pathol. 2005;29(11):1472-1.

20. Childers JM, Brzechffa PR, Surwit EA. Laparoscopy using the left upper quadrant as the primary trocar site. Gynecol Oncol. 1993;50:221-5.

21. Roy GM, Bazzurini L, Solima E, et al. Safe technique for laparoscopic entry into the abdominal cavity. J Am Assoc Gynecol Laparosc. 2001;8:519-28.
22. Corson SL, Brooks PG, Soderstrom RM. Safe technique for laparoscopic entry into the abdominal cavity. J Am Assoc Gynecol Laparosc. 2002;9:399.
23. Tulikangas PK, Nicklas A, Falcone T, et al. Anatomy of the left upper quadrant for cannula insertion. J Am Assoc Gynecol Laparosc. 2000;7:211-4.
24. Jain N, Sareen S, Kanawa S, et al. Jain point: A new safe portal for laparoscopic entry in previous surgery cases. J Hum Reprod Sci. 2016;9(1):9-17.

Ergonomics of Jain Point

Nutan Jain, Bhumika Bansal, Kaustubh Srivastava

INTRODUCTION

Laparoscopy or minimally invasive surgery is a boon for the patients as they enjoy the comforts of early recovery and early return to routine normal activity. But, it does not give the same benefits to the surgeons. To make over for the lack of tactile feel, long working length of instruments and clumsy approach angles, the minimal access surgeon suffers severe musculoskeletal ailments ranging from neck pain, cervical spondylitis, and back pain. The other physical constraints reported are shoulder pain due to abduction of shoulder (chicken wing scapula) during laparoscopy termed as "laparoscopic shoulder", backache, hand finger joint pain, tenosynovitis, burning eyes, stress exhaustion, and hand muscle injury. In the initial years of starting laparoscopy, I myself suffered from tennis elbow due to the practice at that time of making accessory ports in the lower abdomen just above the pubic hairline within the safety triangle. It meant making the ports within 4 cm of the midline to avoid the superficial vessels just outside it. This meant a very awkward, acute angle of working and severe limitation in ergonomic working. Thanks to better understanding, we all gradually shifted to outside the safety triangle and started making the ports outside this limited territory of safety triangle. At that time the working was mainly by bringing the instruments from lower ports from the right and left side of the patient. This meant bending over to the contralateral **(Figs. 1A and B)** side and the concerned hand making a full extension at shoulder, inwards bending of elbow and then further rotation of wrist inward to execute the final surgical action. This meant severe stress on the surgeon's body and if he or she became a high volume surgeon meant poor ergonomics over long spells of working hours. Thankfully, the concept of working from the same side as the standing surgeon was popularized by Koh and Janik and saved many surgeons and especially the ones not enjoying a tall body from developing musculoskeletal ailments. I converted soon and enjoyed long spells of surgeries and suturing

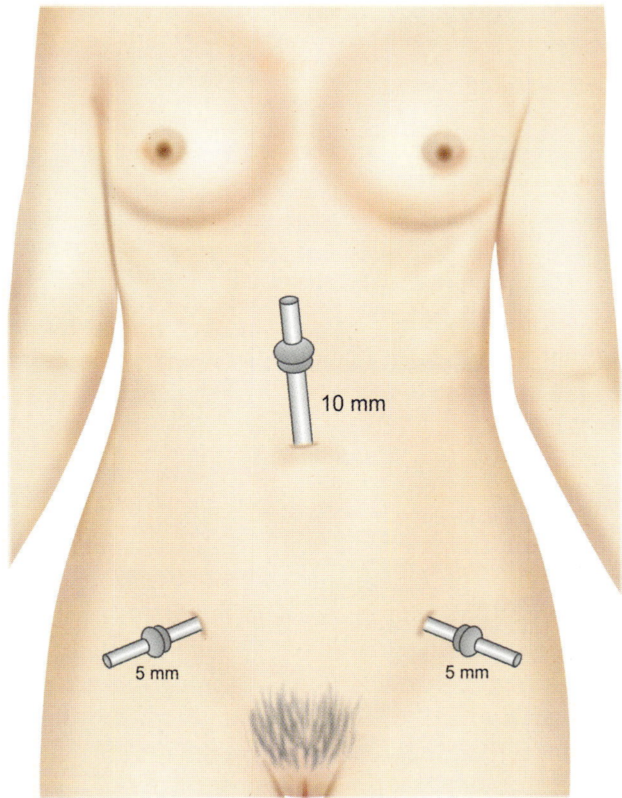

Fig. 1A: Contralateral ports placement.

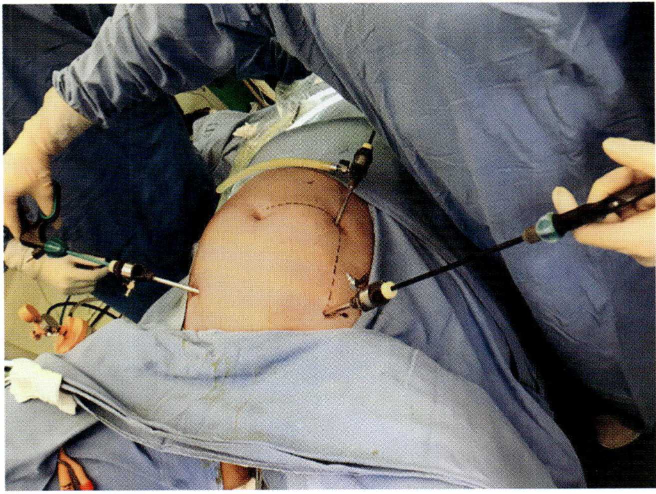

Fig. 1B: Surgeon learning over to other side for contralateral port working.

in laparoscopy. Most common reason for the inability of ergonomics to be applied optimally in the field of laparoscopy could be enumerated as the lack of complete awareness among surgeons, communication gap between the practitioners of laparoscopy and the designers of the instruments, inadequate knowledge of the potential problems for the users in the instruments created by the designers, and the contradictory expert advice which reduces the credibility of ergonomics as a science. Manasnayakorn et al. have tried to understand ergonomics; they have studied in animal models and have indicated that the best task efficiency and performance quality are obtained with an ideal manipulation angle between 45° and 60°. This can be achieved by correct placement of the ports. The 90° manipulation angle had the greatest muscle workload by the deltoid and trapezius muscles as in contralateral working. Manipulation angle ranging from 45° to 75° with equal azimuth angles is recommended. Manipulation angles below 45° or above 75° are accompanied by increased difficulty and decreased performance. Task efficiency was reported to be better with equal azimuth angles so hand and body maneuvers should be such to come close to these ideal situations. There exists a direct correlation between the manipulation and the elevation angles. This situation of shoulder and elbows is achieved while working with both the hands coming from the same side of patients as the standing surgeon. This gives the best manipulation and elevation **(Figs. 2A and B)**. The ergonomic layout for endoscopic surgery consists of a manipulation angle **(Fig. 3)** ranging from 45° to 75° with equal azimuth angles.

The suggested position of the arms is slight abduction, retroversion, and rotation inward at the shoulder level. If we see this is the ideal situation in which a classic open surgeon adopts while operating. A similar situation is in place when the endoscopic surgeon is working while standing on the same side of the patient and the dominant hand is coming from the upper paraumbilical position port and the left hand is about 10 cm below 2.5 cm medial to the anterior superior iliac spine (ASIS). So, ergonomically Jain point port is at the upper paraumbilical position giving precise, stress-free working over long hours **(Figs. 4A and B)**.

It gives the extra benefit of becoming highly ergonomic port which becomes a main working port after the first blind port entry and continuous to be used all through the surgery right from the first blind port to the finishing of suction irrigation and whatever the last step of the surgery. So, if we are using disposable trocars, it also adds a little to the reduction in one of the number of trocars. Since if we use the Palmer's Point for the first blind port it becomes redundant and usually does not remain feasible to be used all through the surgery. In ergonomics we have to conclude these two points that Jain point is at the level of the umbilicus about the 10–13 cm away from the umbilicus and more importantly the distance between the two upper and lower ports made on the left side is 10–12 cm **(Figs. 5A to C)**.

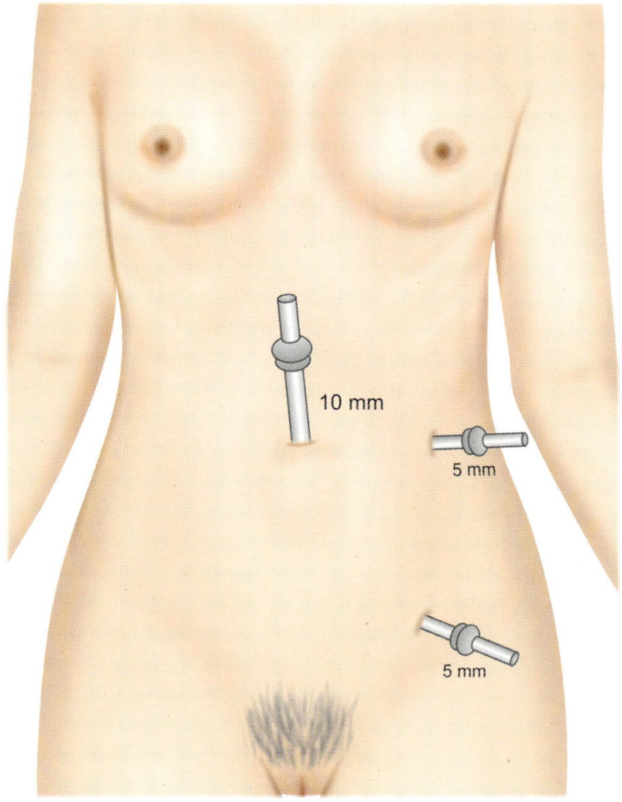

Fig. 2A: Ipsilateral port placement.

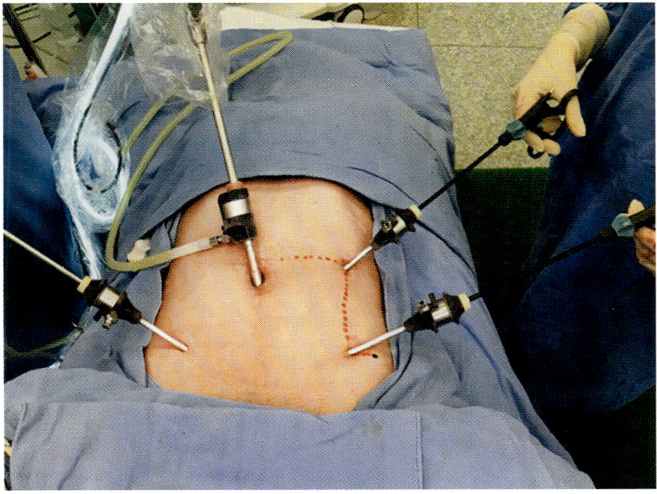

Fig. 2B: Ipsilateral port for the surgeon standing on the left of the patient.

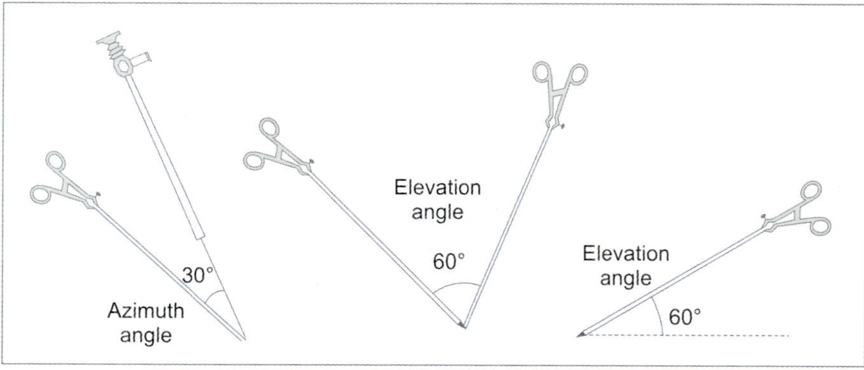

Fig. 3: Manipulation angle.

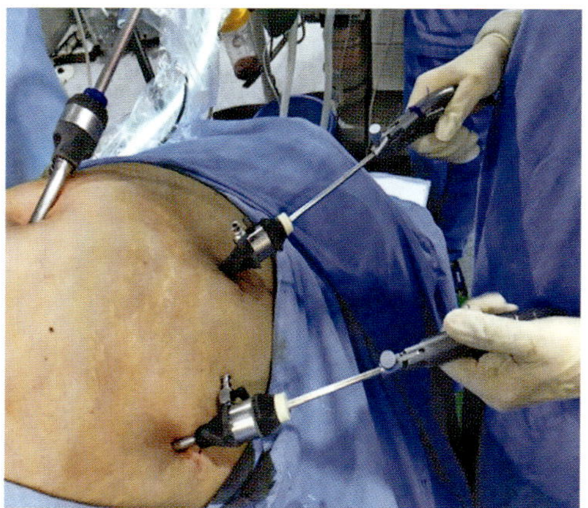

Fig. 4A: Ergonomics of Jain point.

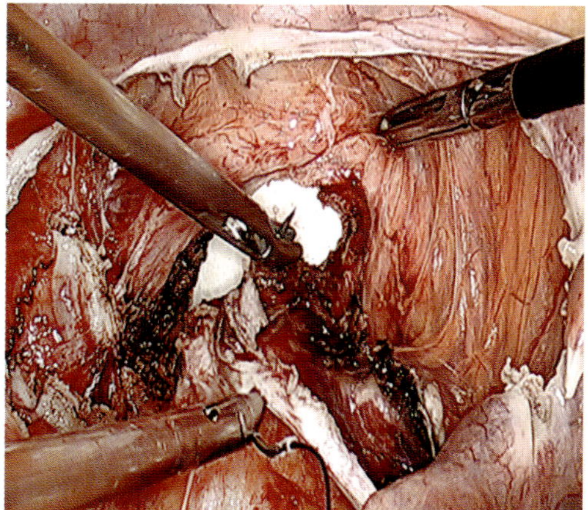

Fig. 4B: Suturing continues effortlessly due to ergonomic placement of Jain point and lower port.

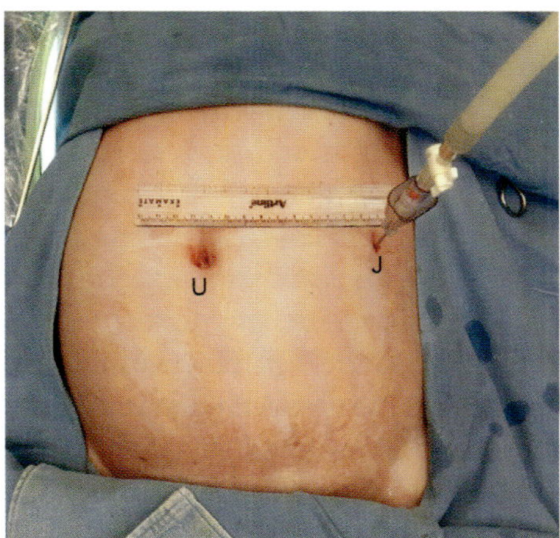

Fig. 5A: Distance from umbilicus to Jain point.

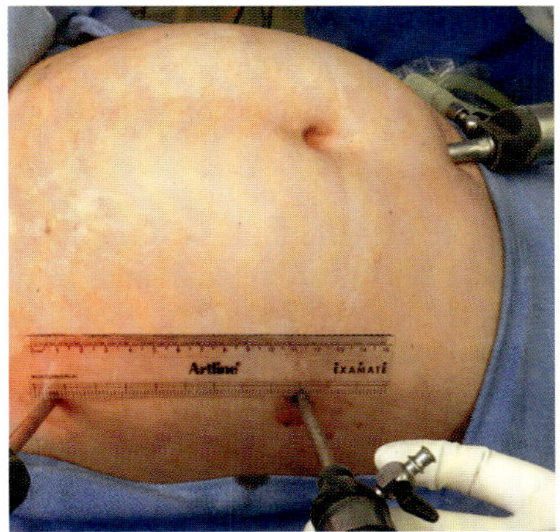

Fig. 5B: Distance from Jain point to left lower port.

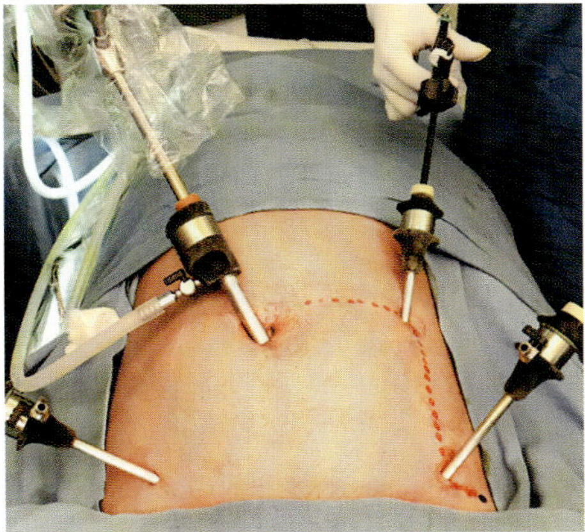

Fig. 5C: Jain point port converts to routine working port.

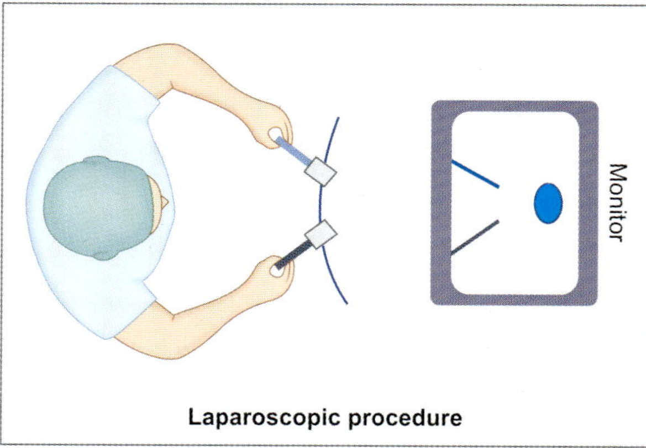

Fig. 6: Position of the monitor.

So, making it an easy workable situation where in left side two ports lie about 10–12 cm apart from each other making a good ergonomic working, do not have the chopstick effect. This is what we will emphasize all through during the book in the form of illustrations, pictures, snap shots from the surgeries, and also videos showing the normal ergonomic easy stress-free working by utilizing these two ports.

LEARNING POINTS

- Long surgeries need special attention to ergonomics.
- Keep the monitor at the level of your eyes **(Fig. 6)**.
- Table height to be adjusted according to the surgeon.
- When ports come from same side as the standing surgeon it gives stress-free precise working which is easily accomplished by port position made after entry with Jain point.
- Avoid the wide extension at shoulder as will be needed for contralateral working, this is the cause of maximum musculoskeletal stress and strains.
- Physical fitness of laparoscopic surgeons is most important.

SUGGESTED READING

1. Aggarwal R, Grantcharov T, Moorthy K, et al. Toward feasible, valid, and reliable video-based assessments of technical surgical skills in the operating room. Ann Surg. 2008;247:372-9.
2. Berguer R, Forkey DL, Smith WD. The effect of laparoscopic instrument working angle on surgeons' upper extremity workload. Surg Endosc. 2001;15:1027-9.
3. Berguer R, Rab GT, Abu-Ghaida H, et al. A comparison of surgeons' posture during laparoscopic and open surgical procedures. Surg Endosc. 1997;11:139-42.
4. De U. Ergonomics and Laparoscopy. Indian J Surg. 2005;67:164-6.
5. Forkey D, Smith W, Berguer R. 19th Annual International Conference of the IEEE Engineering in Medicine and Biology Society. A comparison of thumb and forearm

muscle effort required for laparoscopic and open surgery using an ergonomic measurement station. Chicago: IL; 1997. pp. 1705-8.

6. Hanna GB, Shimi SM, Cuschieri A. Task performance in endoscopic surgery is influenced by location of the image display. Ann Surg. 1998;227:481-4.

7. Hemal AK, Srinivas M, Charles AR. Ergonomic Problems Associated with laparoscopy. J Endourol. 2001;15:499-503.

8. Jain N, Jain V, Aggarwal C. Left Lateral Port: Safe Laparoscopic Port Entry in Previous Large Upper Abdomen Laparotomy Scar. J Minim Invasive Gynecol. 2019;26(5):973-6.

9. Jain N, Jain V, Kanawa S. Standard technique of port placement by new laparoscopic entry port (The Jain point). Comprehensive video atlas of laparoscopic surgery in infertility and gynecology. 2016;2:33-7.

10. Jain N, Mann S, Jain V. To Study the Safety of Jain point as an Alternate to Standard Palmar's Point in Patients with Previous Surgeries. J Minim Invasive Gynecol; 2014.

11. Jain N, Sareen S, Kanawa S, et al. Jain point: A new safe portal for laparoscopic entry in previous surgery cases. J Hum Reprod Sci. 2016;9:9-17.

12. Jain N, Sareen S, Kanawa S, et al. Presented abstract on New Laparoscopic Entry Port for Previous Surgery Cases: Jain point: AAGL 2019 48th Global Congress on MIGS, in Vancouver, B.C., Canada on 9th to 13th November 2019.

13. Jain N, Sareen S, Kanawa S, et al. presented lecture on Jain point: a new safe portal for laparoscopic entry in previous surgery cases: Beyond Gynecological Surgery from Imagination to Innovation & Education, AAGL regional meeting in Clermont Ferrand, France on 4th to 6th April 2018.

14. Jain N, Sareen S, Kanawa S, et al. presented on Jain point: A New Safe Portal for Laparoscopic Entry in Previous Surgery Cases: AAGL 2018 47th Global Congress on MIGS, in Las Vegas, Nevada on 11th to 15th November 2018.

15. Jain N, Sareen S, Mann S, et al. presented lecture on Jain point: a new safe portal for laparoscopic entry in previous surgery cases: 26th Annual ESGE Congress, in Antalya, Turkey on 18-21 October 2017.

16. Jain N, Sareen S, Mann S, et al. presented on Jain point: a new safe portal for laparoscopic entry in previous surgery cases: "International Workshop on Laparoscopic Endometriosis & Pelvic Anatomy" at Pune, India on 8th and 9th Dec, 2017.

17. Kant IJ, de Jong LC, van Rijssen-Moll M, et al. A survey of static and dynamic work postures of operating room staff. Int Arch Occup Environ Health. 1992;63:423-8.

18. Kilbom A. Measurement and assessment of dynamic work. In: Wilson EC Jr (Ed). Evaluation of human work: A practical ergonomics methodology. London: Taylor and Francis; 1990. pp. 641-61.

19. Koh CH, Janik GM. Laparoscopic microsurgical tubal anastomosis. In: Adamson GD, Martin DC (Eds). Endoscopic Management of Gynecologic Disease. Philadelphia: Lippin Cott-Raven; 1996. pp. 119-45.

20. Koh CH, Janik GM. Laparoscopic microsuturing techniques. St Louis: Medical Video Productions; 1996.

21. Koh CH, Janik GM. Laparoscopic tubal reanastomosis. In: Sutton C, Diamond M (Eds). Endoscopic Surgery for Gynecologists, 2nd edition. London, UK: WB Saunders; 1997.

22. Manasnayakorn S, Cuschieri A, Hanna GB. Ergonomic assessment of optimum operating table height for hand-assisted laparoscopic surgery. Surg Endosc. 2009;23:783-9.

23. Manasnayakorn S, Cuschieri A, Hanna GB. Ideal manipulation angle and instrument length in hand-assisted laparoscopic surgery. Surg Endosc. 2008;22:924-9.

24. Mattern U, Waller P. Instruments for minimally invasive surgery: Principles of ergonomic handles. Surg Endoscop. 1999;13:174-82.

25. Mulayam B, Aksoy O. (2019). Direct Trocar Entry from Left Lateral Port (Jain point) in a Case with Previous Surgeries. [online] Available from https://www.liebertpub.com/doi/abs/10.1089/gyn.2019.0077 [Last accessed January, 2020].

26. Nguyen NT, Ho HS, Smith WD, et al. An ergonomic evaluation of surgeons' axial skeletal and upper extremity movements during laparoscopic and open surgery. Am J Surg. 2001;182:720-4.

27. Patkin M, Isabel L. Ergonomics, engineering and surgery of endosurgical dissection. J Royal Coll Surg Edinburgh. 1995;40:120-32.

28. Sharp HT. (2019). Overview of gynecologic laparoscopic surgery and non-umbilical entry sites. [online] Available from https://www.uptodate.com/contents/overview-of-gynecologic-laparoscopic-surgery-and-non-umbilical-entry-sites [Last accessed January, 2020].

29. Van Veelen MA, Meiier DW. Ergonomics and design of laparoscopic instruments: results of a survey among laparoscopic surgeons. J Laparoendosc Adv Surg Tech A. 1999;9:481-9.

14

Role of Jain Point in Previous Surgery Cases

Nutan Jain, Swati Kanawa, Sonika Mann, Sunil Gupta

INTRODUCTION

The surgical indications in patients with previous surgeries are rising, like previous cesarean sections, infectious pathologies and genital tuberculosis, cystectomies, and myomectomies. So, whenever a patient with previous surgery approaches for laparoscopic surgery, the complication rates could rise because of the adhesions present at the first blind entry port namely the umbilicus **(Figs. 1A to D)**.[1]

Generally, the first blind entry is through the umbilicus, and in previous surgeries whether the scar is lower abdominal, midline, para median, or a big scar ranging from pelvis right up to the upper abdomen or other abdominal scars, umbilicus is the most common site to have adhesions.[2] 12% cases have umbilical adhesions, which could be omental or bowel or both.[2] So, we need

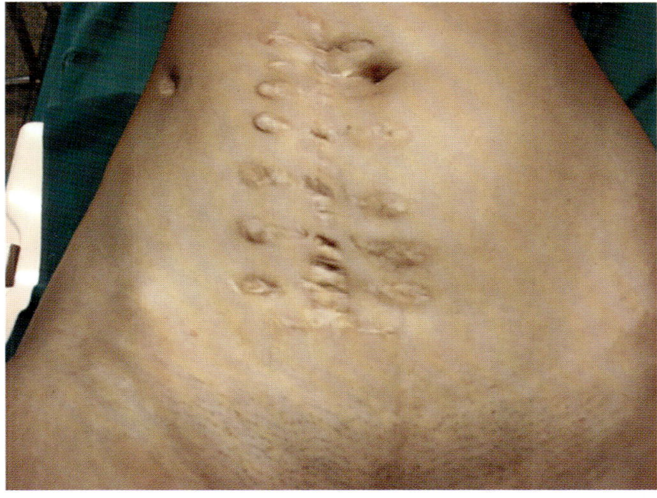

Fig. 1A: Multiple scar on abdomen.

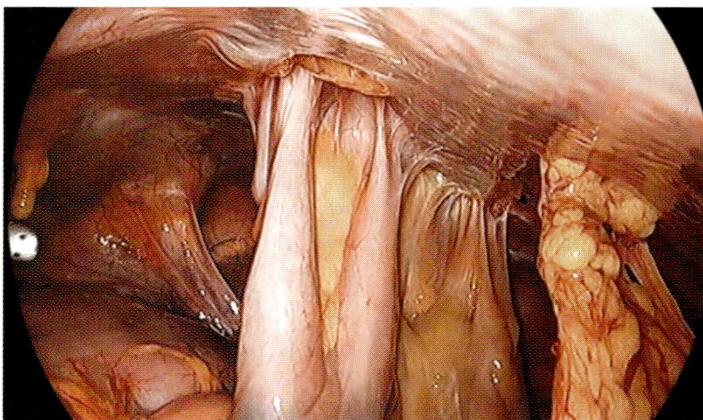

Fig. 1B: Surgical picture showing umbilical, bowel, and omental adhesions.

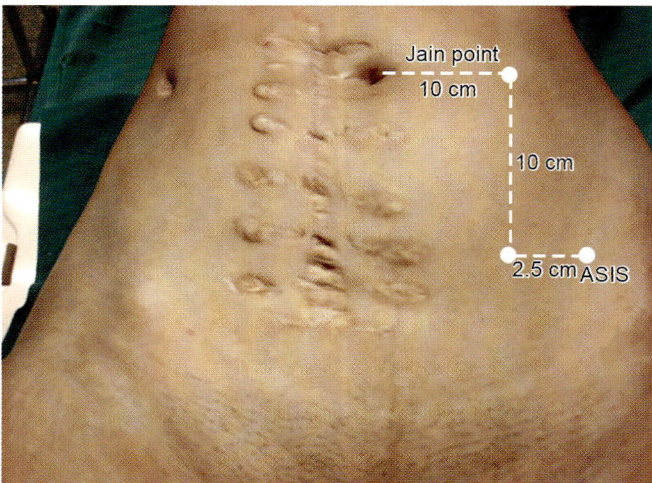

Fig. 1C: Surface marking of Jain point.

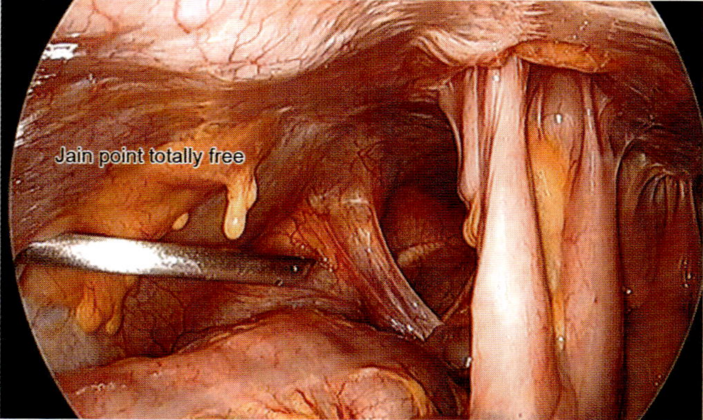

Fig. 1D: Multiple bowel loops stuck at anterior abdominal wall with left side abdomen totally free explaining the rationale of Jain point on left side mid abdomen.

to find an alternate nonumbilical site technique for the first blind port entry. The commonly available are the Palmer's point,[3] Lee Huang point,[4] the 9th intercostal space,[5] and the Hasson's open technique.[6] Preoperatively we can try to find out whether there would be adhesions below the umbilicus by the visceral slide test by preoperative ultrasound as described by Tu et al.[7] Nezhat et al.[8] have further demonstrated combining a novel saline infusion technique (PUGSI) with existing visceral slide test. It has proven to be an excellent approach in detecting patients at higher risk for visceral injury. P Lal et al. devised a modified open laparoscopy technique which is safe and easy to learn.[9,10] All these have been discussed in a separate chapter in the beginning of the book. But for a quick recap, the Palmer's point will remain the most common non umbilical port for the first blind entry, since it has a long safety profile of close to 45 years, as it was introduced first in 1974. The little concerns regarding Palmer's point is that it cannot be used in the left upper abdomen scars. Other contraindications are the cases of big gastropancreatic masses, hepatosplenomegaly, and a bloated stomach and a faulty placement of nasogastric tube, which will again lead to bloated stomach. So those situations, where Palmer's point is contraindicated, are quite commonly seen as in open gallbladder surgery (*cholecystectomy*) done by giving a big Kocher incision (before the advent of laparoscopy). Other scars in the upper abdomen, or other scars which could be because of any intestinal pathology and these usually have big midline vertical scar going above the umbilicus. So, these are the situations where we really have to look up for another nonumbilical site. The other one, the Lee-Huang point which is midway between the umbilicus and epigastrium can also be used but again the same concerns exists with Lee-Huang point which is mid way between umbilicus and epigastrium about the Palmer's point will remain with the Lee-Huang also, and moreover as the Lee-Huang point is higher up in upper abdomen, the novice who wants to change from Palmer's point may find it still more difficult to go through the Lee-Huang point, where potential risk of laceration of liver could be there, in an unfamiliar territory for first blind port entry. So, as an alternate site for previous surgeries Lee-Huang point has not found much favor. The 9th intercostal space described by Neena Aggarwala et al. also remained a little under-utilized since the risk of injury to the lung or intercostal nerve and vessels running in the costal groove at the lower border of rib also remains.

The Hasson's open technique has also not found much favor with the gynecologists who have under-utilized this technique. However, if we look at Hasson's technique, which if compare to all the other nonumbilical entry ports and Palmer's point also, has the least chances of complications. It has also been seen in bigger meta-analyses that the complication rates do not decrease with the use of Hasson's technique, but still this technique continues to enjoy favor with the general surgeons. The use of safety shields, optical trocars does not decrease the chances of injury. The threaded trocars by Artin Ternamian.[11-19]

This trocarless visual access cannula system (Endoscopic Threaded Imaging Port, ENDOTIP; Karl Storz Endoscop GMBH, Tuttlingen, Germany) has no crystal tip compressing and distorting monitor images at tissue-cannula interface. Therefore, interpretations of monitor images are easier and layered entry is more real-time and interactive. The threaded trocars, which are gradually introduced with the telescope inside them, have also been introduced to reduce the chances of complications or to detect a bowel loop when inserting the trocar. All these innovations came with the bang but again after long years of uses, it was found that they offer no further benefit over the usual metal reusable trocars, and the incidence of bowel injuries did not reduce, it was only recognized instantly the moment it occurred, because they had the provision of telescope along with the trocar going inside. So, with this scenario, that there is no perfect entry port, the industry and technological advancement have also not been able to reduce the chances of bowel and visceral injury, which could be at the umbilicus or at other site, the search for the newer entry port is always ongoing. Though there have been leaps and bounce of progress in laparoscopic surgery, but still the entry-related complications continue to be large and almost at the same percentage as they were about 30 years ago.[20] So we propose Jain point as a newer nonumbilical entry port which by its logic looks to be applicable in all situations of previous surgeries. It is advisable to be used in lower pfannenstiel incision, mid-line incisions, paramedian incisions, and also upper abdominal incisions. Compared to Palmer's point it is lower down and much lateral. So being lateral it is almost 10–13 cm from the umbilicus, and goes far lateral from the possibility of bowel loops adherent at the previous scar site. It also becomes applicable in the scenario of the upper abdominal scars, as it is much lower than the Palmar's point, being at the level of L4, it remains away from even a bloated stomach or the loops of bowel, which could be with the mid-line vertical incision, or the paramedian incision. The anatomical location of the Jain point makes it more suitable to be utilized in all types of incisions in the mid, lower, and the upper abdomen.[21-24]

Constantly doing laparoscopies for the last 30 years and then converting to ipsilateral style of working, we were utilizing paraumbilical port, and gradually this observation became constant that the left lateral paraumbilical site was free of adhesions and gradually it became our first port of entry. For last 10 years, we are continuously using this site as the first blind port entry and believe me it has taken away all the stress which use to be there earlier when there were multiple incisions in the abdomen. Now we are totally assured that the entry with the Jain point will land us safely into the peritoneal cavity in scarred abdomen of previous surgeries.

As I discussed earlier, the anatomical rationale is that it is lateral, lower at the level of L4. Then it came to mind, why there are lesser adhesions beneath it. So we just looked again into the anatomy and the surface marking of abdominal wall and also of all the viscera, and we saw that the spleen and the kidney come

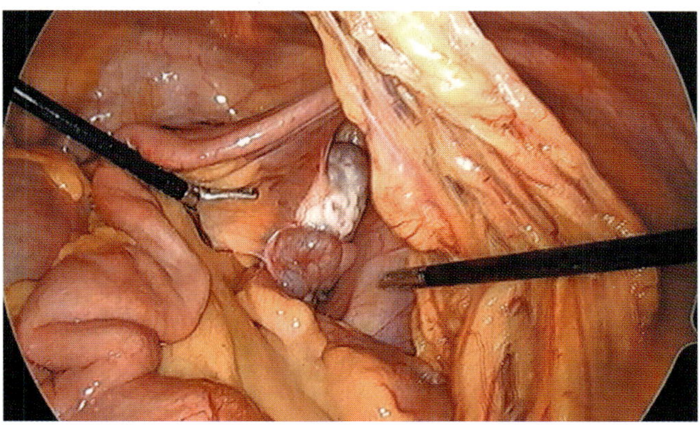

Fig. 2: Right side adhesions.

maximum up to the level of T12, L1. The descending colon is retroperitoneal and the sigmoid colon adheres over the pelvic brim, so that is why whole of the left mid abdomen from the pelvic brim up to the level of T12, L1 is the nascent area, where usually the bowel adhesions do not happen. If at all it is a frozen pelvis due to abdominogenital Koch's, we have found repeatedly and almost constantly that this site is free of adhesion. Jain point entry has taken away lot of stress and thought process in planning from where to make the entry in such type of cases. At our institution, constant use for the last 10 years by the senior consultant, by other consultants, trainees, fellows and even short-term trainees reveal that entry by Jain point tides over the difficult situations of entry in previous surgery cases. And why we have chosen to be on the left side, it is also a simple logical explanation that on the right side the ileocecal junction is the site of all types of bowel infections namely, the abdominal Koch's, appendicitis, ulcerative colitis, Crohn's disease, and repeated attacks of subacute appendicitis. They all couple up with the stasis of terminal ileum. So, the right-side mid abdomen **(Fig. 2)** becomes the seat of infection even without a previous surgery. So, it is better to go from the left side, but in cases where there are multiple scars and at the Jain point if there are previous drain sites, or small scars of burns, injuries or other marks, then we use the Jain point mirror image from the right side **(Figs. 3A and B)**. In cases of multiple scars, drain site scar, injuries burns scars at Jain point, we use mirror image of Jain point in right side of abdomen.

PREOPERATIVE WORK-UP OF A PATIENT WITH PREVIOUS SURGERIES

For all such cases, we first of all look at the patient's abdomen and make a note of all incisions, the location, and the type of incisions, kind of surgeries. At times we get totally bizarre incisions which could be due to emergency surgeries or in cases of infectious pathologies. Then we ask the patient's history of each and

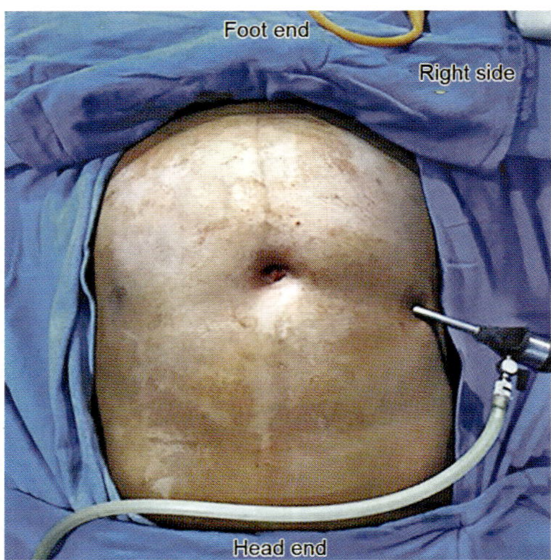

Fig. 3A: Right side mirror image.

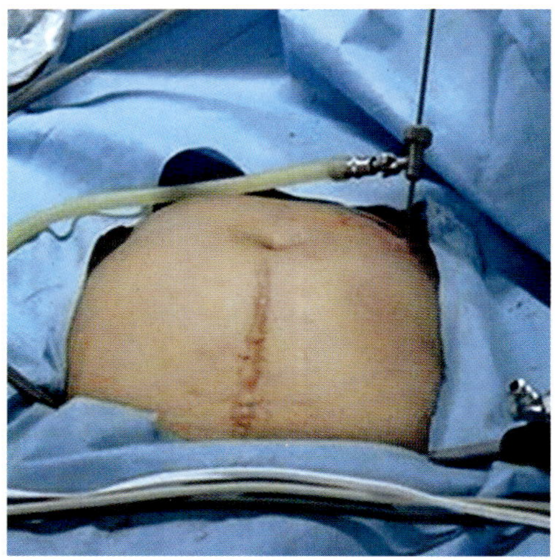

Fig. 3B: A 3 mm scope at Palmer's point.

every procedure—what was the length of hospital stay, how was the recovery, and what were the drain sites which were used. If at all the surgery has been done for hernia, we try to look into the operative notes to find out the size and the type of the mesh used. Particularly in cases of laparoscopic mesh hernia repair whether a composite mesh has been used. It is important to be very careful about the amount of adhesions that could be present on to the mesh. So, the size of the mesh is very important and usually the mesh used is of about 15 × 15 cm. So, on one side it will come maximum up to 7.5 cm and as we have stated the Jain point stays 10–13 cm outside the umbilicus. So, the Jain point port stays outside the mesh. In previous mesh hernia surgery, we cannot use

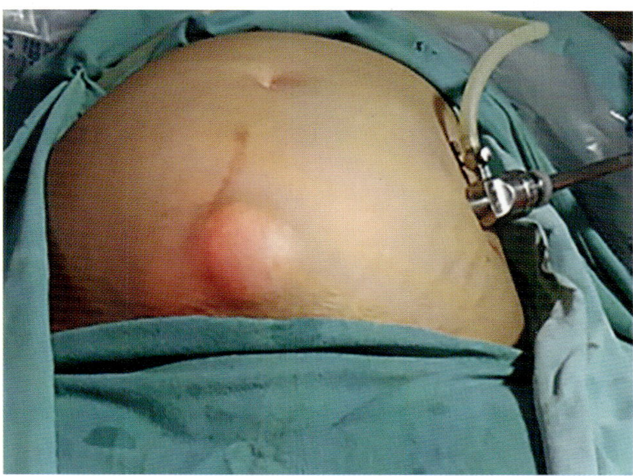

Fig. 4: A 5 mm Jain point port converted to 10 mm port.
Courtesy: Dr Medhavi Tomar.

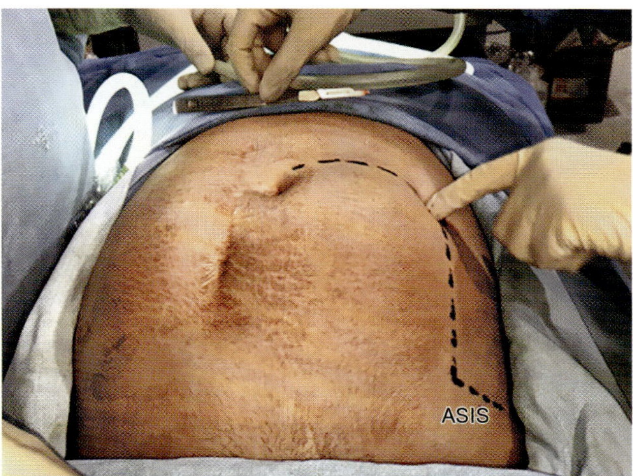

Fig. 5A: Finger pointing at Jain point.

umbilicus as primary entry point, hence Jain point offers a logical alternative site which later becomes the operative port **(Fig. 4)**.

After the history has been taken, all previous surgical sites have been noted, we take the patient for the surgery and on the table, it is prudent to mark the Jain point from anterior superior iliac spine (ASIS) and umbilicus as landmark. It is a positive feature in favor of Jain point that we have fixed bony landmark, hence, easier to mark.

TECHNIQUE OF ENTRY (FIGS. 5A TO F)

We hold and introduce the Veress needle after making a small 2 mm stab incision in a perfectly vertical direction perpendicular to the patient's abdomen.

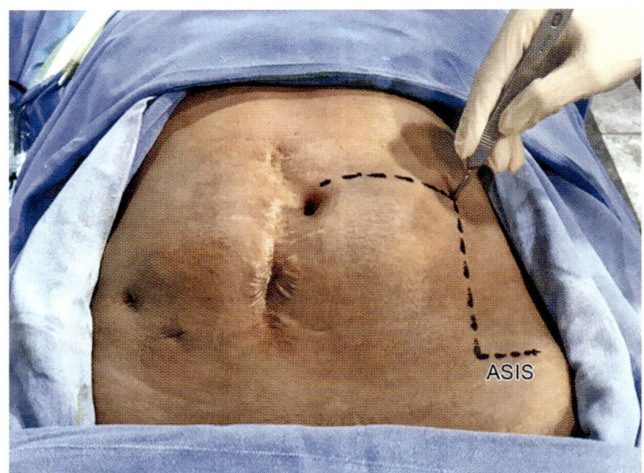

Fig. 5B: A 2 mm nick with 15 no. surgical blade at Jain point.

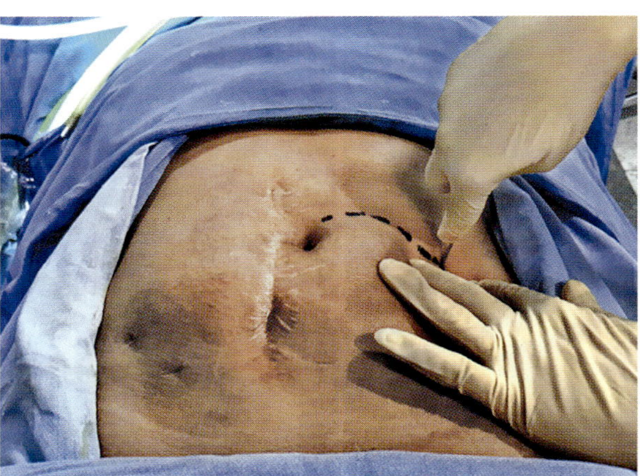

Fig. 5C: Inserting the Veress needle at Jain point in a vertical direction.

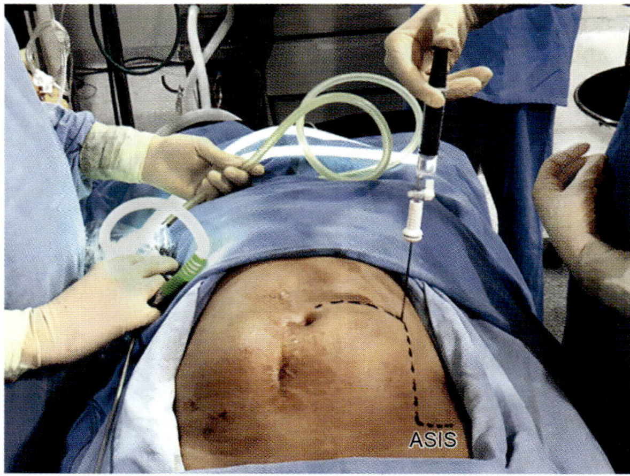

Fig. 5D: Saline aspiration test.

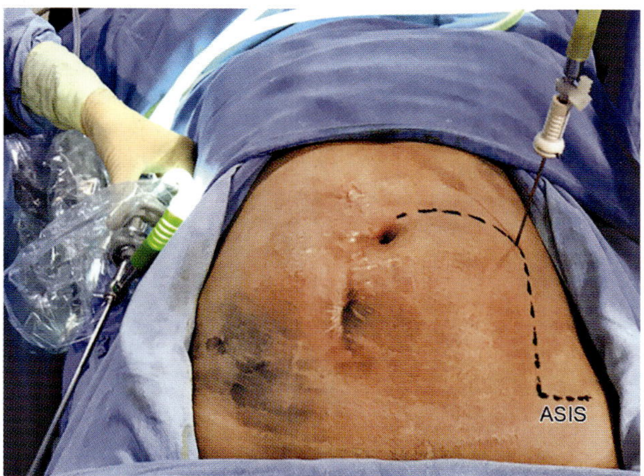

Fig. 5E: Veress needle connected to CO_2 gas pipe.

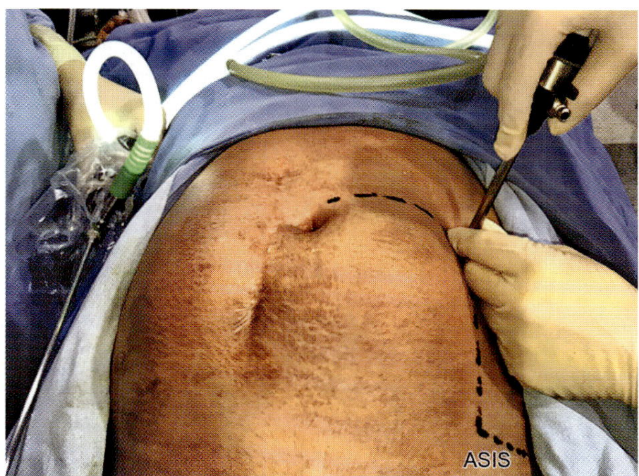

Fig. 5F: A 5 mm trocar inserting at Jain point.

We do not flay the needle in any direction, and there is no need to change it to 45° angle. It is simply introduced vertically and the surgeon feels and hears the pops. The first pop is at the entry through the external oblique aponeurosis. Second at the fused aponeurosis of transversus abdominis and internal oblique muscle and the third not a pop, rather, it is more of a feeling of a give way of resistance, as the needle passes through the tough aponeurosis to the soft peritoneum and goes freely without resistance into the peritoneal cavity. So that is why I say it is two pops and third is feeling of give way of resistance. Once we feel confident about the entry the two safety checks, the LIVIP[25] test and the drop test, are carried out and if the drop test is good but still we find a little higher pressure the needle is slightly withdrawn or then at that time abdominal wall is slightly lifted up. If the needle is touching any omentum, that is released. Hence, it is a very simple technique; there is no lifting of abdomen, simple one direction of the Veress needle in all subset of patients, whether they are obese, thin, flabby or with previous surgeries **(Figs. 6A to F)**. A 5 mm zero degree telescope is inserted through Jain point to take a note of the pelvis and upper abdomen and adhesions which could be present due to

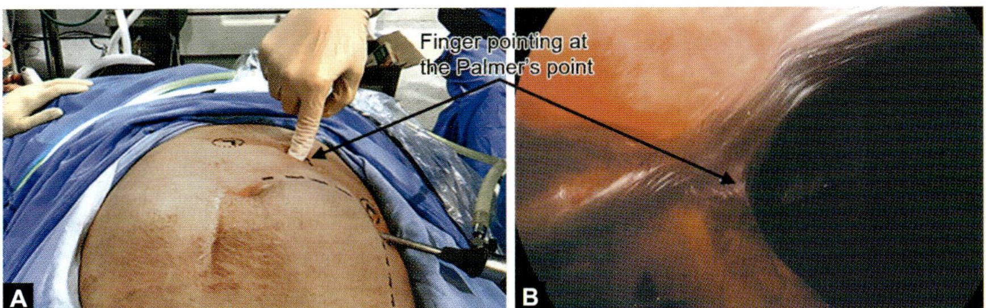

Figs. 6A and B: (A) Finger pointing at the Palmer's point; (B) Laparoscopic picture showing finger pointing at the Palmer's point where bowel and omentum are adherent.

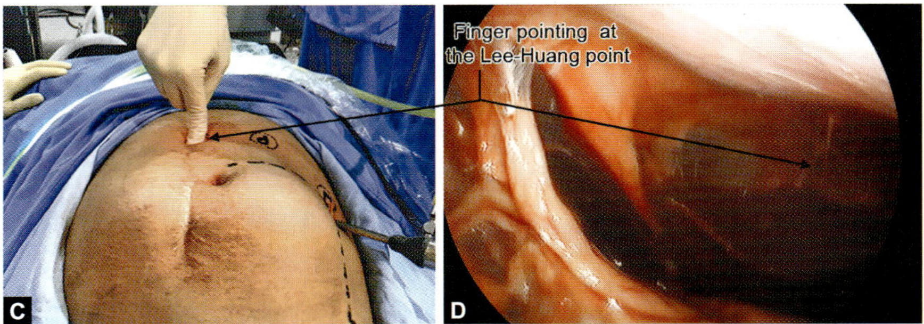

Figs. 6C and D: (C) Finger pointing at the Lee-Huang point; (D) Finger pointing at the Lee-Huang point, where gallbladder is adherent.

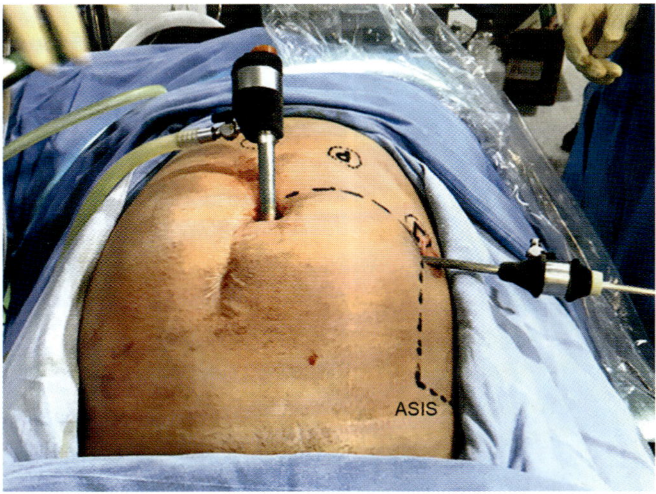

Fig. 6E: A 10 mm trocar inserted under direct vision of 5 mm telescope.

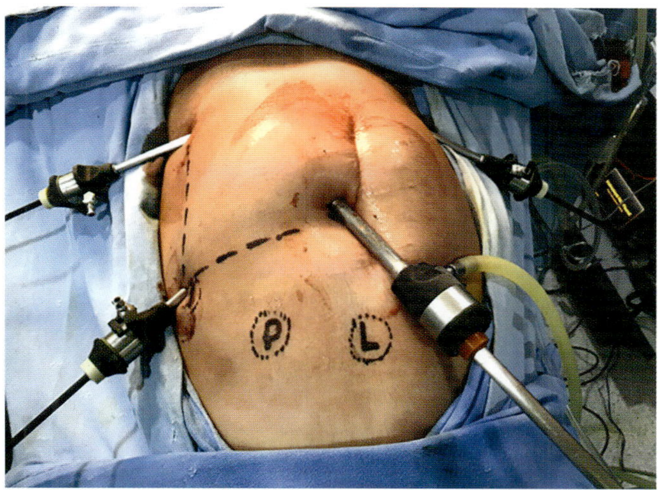

Fig. 6F: Final port placement.

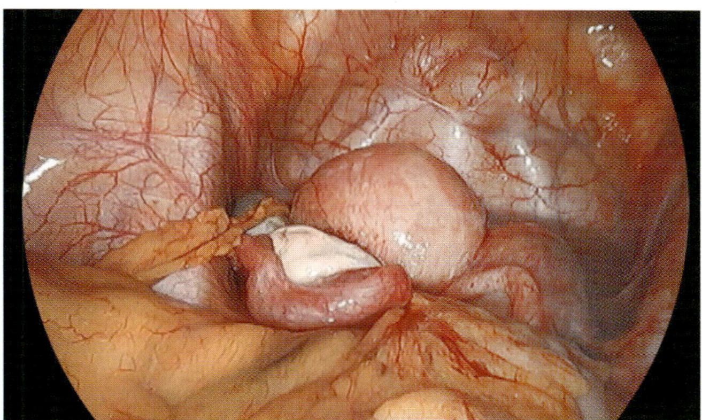

Fig. 7A: Initial appearance of pelvis in a case of recurrent endometriosis.

previous surgery. A complete check of whole abdomen is carried out and then the 10 mm port entry is optimized under direct vision. If it is a case of previous surgery, a note is made of adhesions and visually guided entry is made by 10 mm telescope avoiding adhesions. So it becomes tailor made according to the pathology, adhesions, and the patient type. Like if we are operating on a large pelvic mass, the 10 mm port can be placed much higher up under direct vision of the Jain point 5 mm port. After placing the 10 mm port, all other accessory ports are made according to the mandate of the case.

The Jain point then becomes the main operating port in due course of the surgery. Out long experience and that of our endoscopy colleagues spread in various parts of the world have all welcomed the novel idea and the methodology of Jain point entry in previous surgery cases.

Use of Jain point port as main working port in the case of previous surgery of extensive, deep infiltrating endometriosis **(Figs. 7A to L)** with adenomyotic

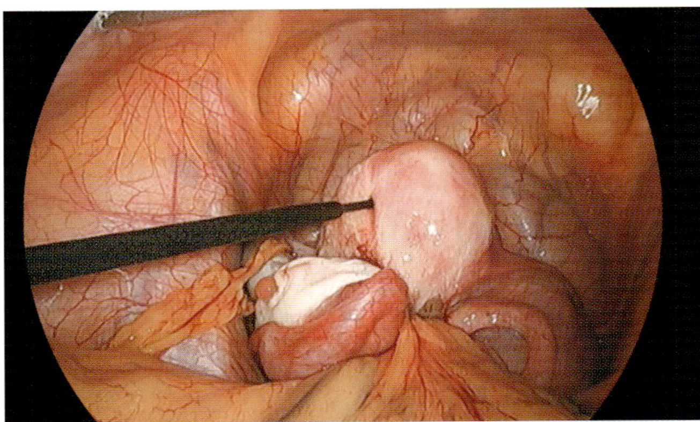

Fig. 7B: Injecting diluted vasopressin in 300 mL of saline, this helps decreasing blood loss and opens up tissue planes in dissection.

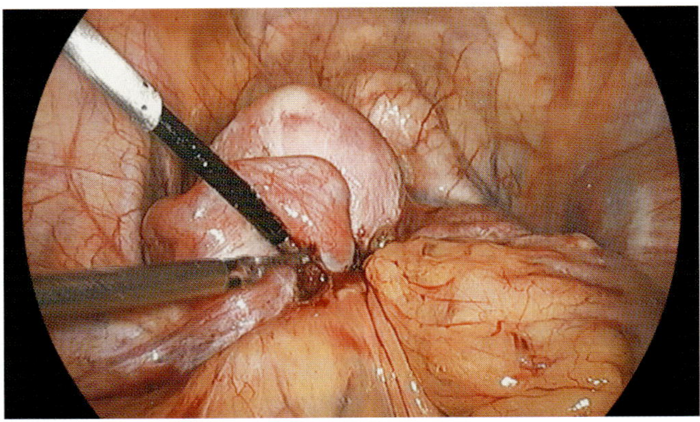

Fig. 7C: Starting dissection at left pelvic brim.

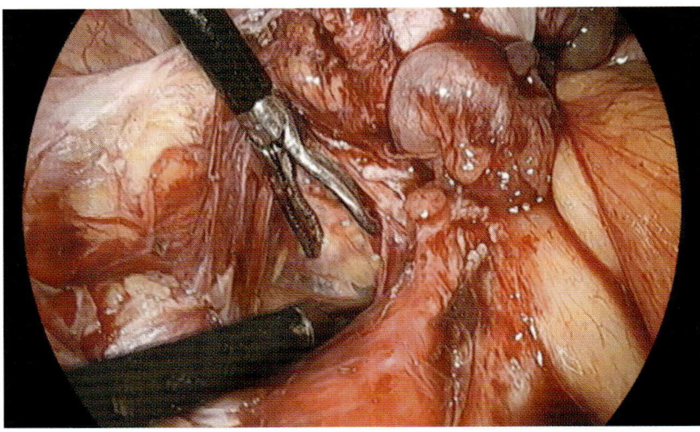

Fig. 7D: Opening up the left sided medial pararectal space.

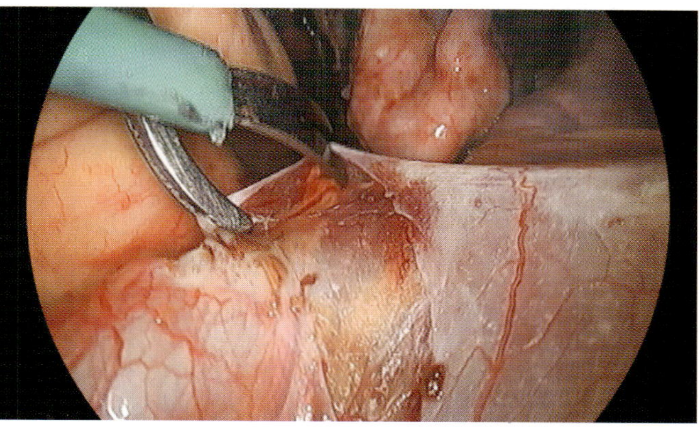

Fig. 7E: Opening the peritoneum to expose the ureter on right side of pelvis.

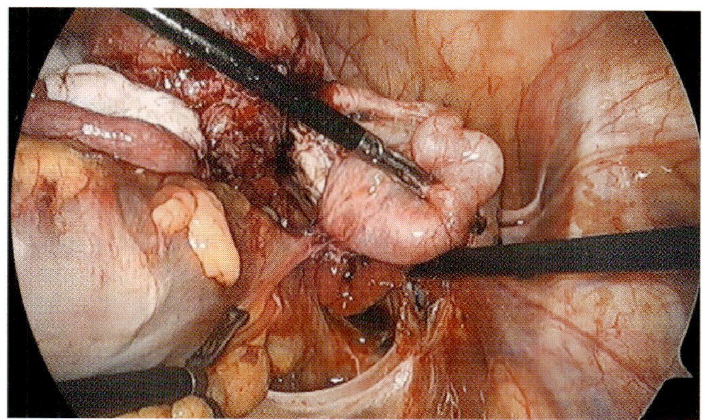

Fig. 7F: Starting dissection at right pelvic brim.

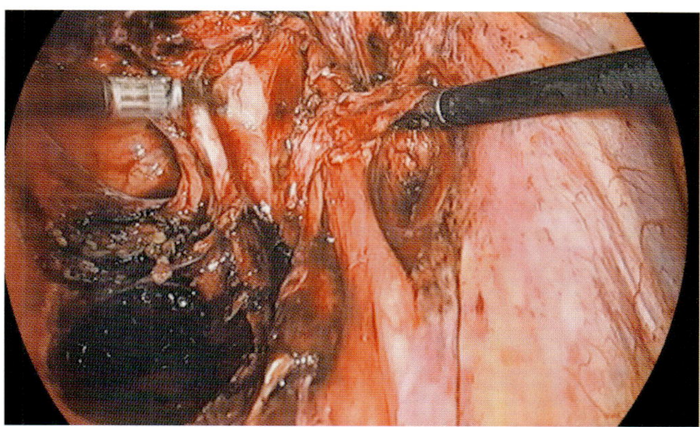

Fig. 7G: Dissection continued, right ureter exposed till rectovaginal space, both medial and lateral pararectal spaces identified and cleared.

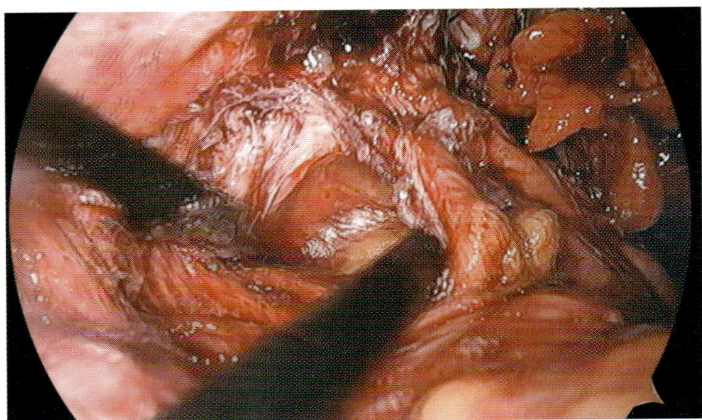

Fig. 7H: Rectovaginal space identified and entered.

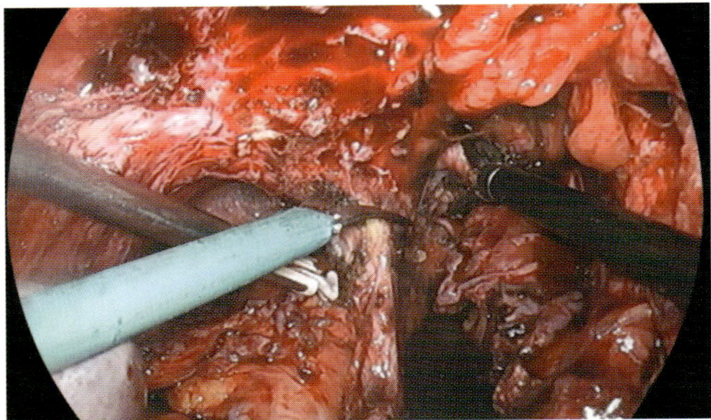

Fig. 7I: Starting excising the rectovaginal nodule, involving the uterosacral ligament, ureter much lateralized.

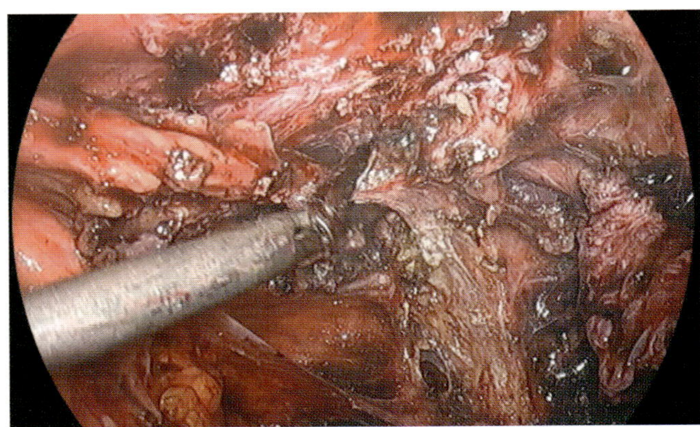

Fig. 7J: Rectovaginal nodule excised.

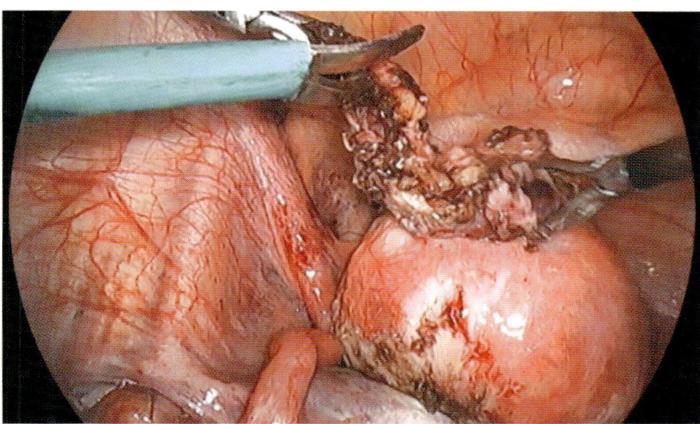

Fig. 7K: Rectovaginal nodule being removed from abdomen.

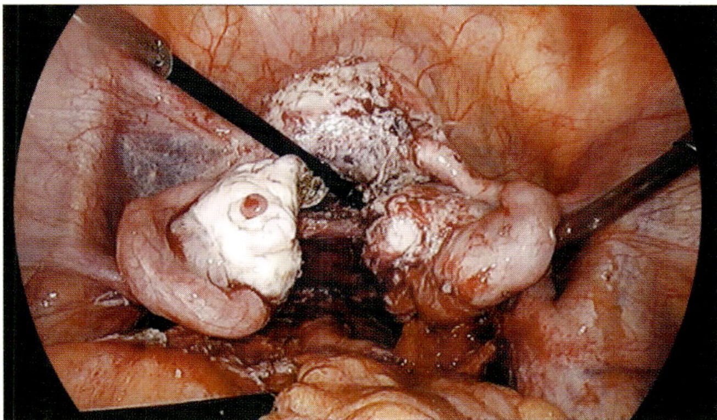

Fig. 7L: Good last picture.

uterus. Patient presented with pain and infertility. The steps of the surgery are shown by several snapshots from surgery.

▮ LEARNING POINTS

- Nonumbilical entry is suggested to avoid adhesions around umbilicus in cases of previous surgeries.
- It is applicable in all types of scars in upper abdomen as it is lower down at level of umbilicus.
- It is very safe to be used in midline vertical or paramedian scars as it is outside the umbilicus minimum 10–13 cm at the paraumbilical position.
- It is applicable in lower pfannenstiel incisions.
- Applicable in previous mesh hernia repair, where umbilicus cannot be used as the first blind entry port.

- Jain point entry is safe and can be used as main working port which becomes the ergonomic port in due course of surgery.
- It has clearly defined land marks namely the umbilicus and ASIS to make the surface marking precisely.

REFERENCES

1. Royal College of Obstetricians and Gynaecologists. Green-top Guideline No. 49. Preventing entry-related gynaecological laparoscopic injuries. London: RCOG; 2008.
2. Toro A, Mannino M, Cappello G, et al. Comparison of two entry methods for laparoscopic port entry: Technical point of view. Diagnostic and Therapeutic Endoscopy. 2012.
3. Palmer R. Safety in laparoscopy. J Reprod Med. 1974;13:1-5.
4. Lee CL, Huang KG, Jain S, et al. A new portal for gynecologic Laparoscopy. J Am Assoc Gynecol Laparosc. 2001;8(1):147-50.
5. Agarwala N, Liu CY. Safe entry techniques during laparoscopy: left upper quadrant entry using the ninth intercostal space—a review of 918 procedures. J Minim Invasive Gynecol. 2005;12(1):55-61.
6. Hasson HM. A modified instrument and method for laparoscopy. Am J Obstet Gynecol.1971;110:886-7.
7. Tu FF, Lamvu GM, Hartmann KE, Steege JF. Preoperative ultrasound to predict infraumbilical adhesions: a study of diagnostic accuracy. Am J Obstet Gynecol. 2005;192:74-9.
8. Nezhat C, Cho J, Morozov V, Yeung P. Preoperative periumbilical ultrasound-guided saline infusion (PUGSI) as a tool in predicting obliterating subumbilical adhesions in laparoscopy. Fertil Steril. 2009;91(6):2714-9.
9. Lal P, Sharma R, Chander R, Ramteke VK. A technique of open trocar placement in laparoscopic surgery using the umbilical cicatrix tube. Surg Endosc. 2002;16: 1366-70.
10. Lal P, Vindal A, Sharma R, Chander J, Ramteke VK. Safety of open technique for first trocar placement in laparoscopic surgery: a series of 6000 cases. Surg Endosc. 2012;26(1):182-8.
11. Tarnay CM, Glass KB, Munro MG. Entry force and intraabdominal pressure associated with six laparoscopic trocar cannula systems: a randomized comparison. Obstet Gynecol. 1999;94:83-8.
12. Leibl BJ, Schmedt CG, Schwarz J, et al. Laparoscopic surgery complications associated with trocar tip design: review of literature and own results. J Laparosc Adv Surg Tech A. 1999;9(2):135-40.
13. Hurd WW, Diamond MP. There's a hole in my bucket, the cost of disposable instruments. Fertil Steril. 1997;67:13-5.
14. Chan ACW, Koehler A, Crisp B, et al. Is it safe to reuse disposable laparoscopic trocars. Surg Endosc. 2000;14:1042-4.
15. Corson SL, Batzer FR, Gocial B, et al. Measurement of the force necessary for laparoscopy trocar entry. J Reprod Med. 1989;34:282-4.
16. Hurd WW, Wang L, Schemmel MT. A comparison of the relative risk of vessel injury with conical versus pyramidal laparoscopic trocars in a rabbit model. Am J Obstet Gynecol. 1995;173:1731-3.
17. Soderstrom RM. Injuries to major blood vessels during endoscopy. J Am Assoc Gynecol Laparosc. 1997;4:395-8.

18. Hashizume M, Sugimachi K. Needle and trocar injury during laparoscopic surgery in Japan. Study group of endoscopic surgery in Kyushu, Japan. Surg Endosc. 1997;11:1198-201.

19. Yuzpe AA. Pneumoperitoneum needle and trocar injuries in laparoscopy. A survey on possible contributing factors and prevention. J Reprod Med. 1990;35:485-90.

20. Krishnakumar S, Tambe P. Entry complications in laparoscopic surgery. J Gynecol Endosc Surg.2009;1(1):4-11.

21. Jain N, Mann S, Jain V. To study the safety of Jain point as an alternate to standard Palmer's point in patients with previous surgeries. J Minim Invasive Gynecol. 2014.

22. Jain N, Jain V, Kanawa S. Standard technique of port placement by new laparoscopic entry port (The Jain point). Comprehensive Video Atlas of Laparoscopic Surgery in Infertility and Gynecology. 2016; pp. 33-7.

23. Jain N, Sareen S, Kanawa S, et al. Jain point: a new safe portal for laparoscopic entry in previous surgery cases. J Hum Reprod Sci. 2016;9:9-17.

24. Jain et al. presented lecture on "Jain point: a new safe portal for laparoscopic entry in previous surgery cases" at 26th Annual ESGE Congress in Antalya, Turkey on 18th to 21st October 2017.

25. Vilos GA. The ABCs of a safer laparoscopic entry. J Minim Invasive Gynecol. 2006;13:249-51.

Jain Point in Thin Patients

Kiran Kumari Mandal, Anadeep Chandi, Nutan Jain

◼ INTRODUCTION

Safe laparoscopic entry is pivotal for completing a laparoscopic procedure. If this first hurdle is not accomplished safely, the intended operation may need to be abandoned because of an unintended complication which is associated with morbidity and sometimes mortality. Although complications associated with laparoscopic surgery are rare, a significant proportion of these occur at the time of laparoscopic entry. Women who are extremely thin, obese, or known to have abdominal adhesions are at increased risk for laparoscopic entry-related injury at the umbilical entry point. In the thin patient, visceral injury and vascular injury complications are more common because of the short distance between the anterior abdominal wall and the organs below. The overall incidence of major injuries[1] at the time of entry is 1.1/1,000. Bowel injuries[1] have occurred in 0.7/1,000 laparoscopies and major vascular injuries[1] in 0.4/1,000 laparoscopies. The incidence of bowel and major vessel injuries are low, but both of these types of injuries are potentially life-threatening, especially during the initial access.

The prime concern in patients with a Body Mass Index (BMI) of < 18.5 is that the distance between the anterior abdominal wall and the abdominal organs (in particular the great vessels) is shorter than a patient with a normal BMI or one who is obese. Special considerations need to be taken in order to further reduce the risks of laparoscopic entry.

All patients should have Veress needle entry in the flat supine position; this is particularly important in thin patients. Great care should be taken to ensure that there is no rotation or Trendelenburg positioning of the patient on the operating table, as such positions can lead to alignment of the abdominal aorta or inferior vena cava with the axis of insertion of the Veress needle. Rotation of the hips and spine can bring the iliac vessels into the path of the needle.[2]

ANGLE OF NEEDLE INSERTION FOR TRANSUMBILICAL INSUFFLATION

In very thin patients, the bifurcation of the abdominal aorta may be directly below the umbilicus. Therefore, care should be exercised when considering the angle at which the Veress needle is inserted. The needle should be inserted firstly in a vertical axis, but when the fascia has been breached any further advance of the needle should be toward the sacral promontory at a 45° angle.[3] Alternative insufflation sites should be considered (e.g. Palmer's point). Open laparoscopic entry should be considered to allow direct visualization of trocar insertion in cases of where BMI is below normal.

Palmer advocated that Veress needle should be inserted 3 cm below the left subcostal border in the midclavicular line in patients with previous laparotomy.[4] This technique may also be considered in both obese as well as very thin patients. The stomach should be decompressed using nasogastric tube and the needle should be introduced perpendicular to the skin. Patients with previous splenic or gastric surgery, portal hypertension or significant gastropancreatic masses should be excluded for Palmer's point entry.

The main concept in an open technique is to create a very small incision, incise the abdominal wall layers directly, cut the peritoneum, and enter the abdomen. As gas can easily escape around the incision, an olive should be placed over the end of the trocar so that the incision is occluded and sutures are placed on the abdominal fascia and attached to the cannula. Advantages of the open technique are avoidance of blind puncture with a needle, higher certainty of establishing a pneumoperitoneum, and better anatomical repair of the abdominal wall incision. Hasson[5] presented his review of 5,284 women who had open laparoscopies and developed complications related to primary access. Twenty one had minor wound infections, four had minor hematomas, one developed an umbilical hernia that required surgery and one had an inadvertent injury to the small bowel that was repaired intraoperatively without adverse outcome. Access to the abdominal cavity was generally secured within 3–10 minutes. Extensive use of this technique has been confined to women with previous surgery, pregnant women, very thin women where little space exists between the abdominal wall and the spine, and children. Some reasons for limited use of the open technique include difficulty with the technique, obese patients, greater time needed for performance, and difficulty in maintaining pneumoperitoneum.

Taking into account the limitations with the existing technique and points of entry for low BMI (<18.5) patients we see that a nonumbilical entry, *the Jain point* does well. Even Palmer's point is contraindicated in upper abdominal scars and upper abdominal masses, but Jain point has no contraindication and is very safe for entry in thin patients. As in thin patients, the biggest hazard is injury to major retroperitoneal vessels; in Jain point entry we made a non-umbilical entry.

TECHNIQUE OF JAIN POINT ENTRY

Jain point is located in the left paraumbilical region on the left side. These injuries are more common in extreme of BMI. In our overall experience of 30 years in operative laparoscopy, we found left side nonumbilical entry safe while standing on the left side of the patient. An article in UpToDate by HT Sharp[6] proposed Jain point as an alternative site in the sense that it is lower and more lateral in position compared with Palmer's point and may, therefore, be more easily used as the Veress needle entry and then main operating port throughout the surgery. Jain point lies on a vertical line drawn 2.5 cm medial to anterior superior iliac spine (ASIS) at the level of umbilicus in the left paraumbilical region. It is roughly 10–13 cm lateral to the umbilicus, depending on the patient's body type. Describing the technique of Jain point entry, for creating pneumoperitoneum, the preoperative preparation comprised of low residual diet for 48 hours prior to surgery. The stomach emptied of secretions and air by the use of orogastric tube by anesthetist, after endotracheal intubation. The operating table is laid in horizontal position. We made a very small 1–2 mm nick just enough for Veress needle entry. Veress needle is then inserted perpendicular to the abdominal wall, in a vertical direction irrespective of patient being obese, average weight or thin **(Figs. 1 to 12)**. The abdominal wall is not lifted and no change in direction of Veress needle makes it an easy insertion in extreme of low BMI. We put a finger as a guard on the Veress needle according to the patient's thin abdominal wall. This is a

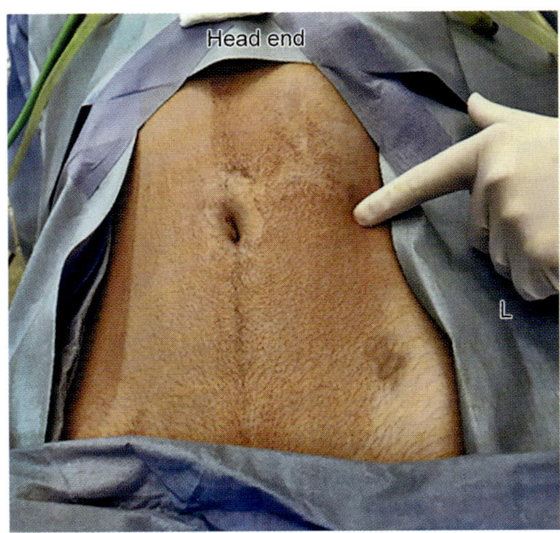

Fig. 1: It is a case of primary infertility with positive mantoux test with USG showing bilateral tubo-ovarian mass with BMI of 18.2. A index finger pointing at Jain point.

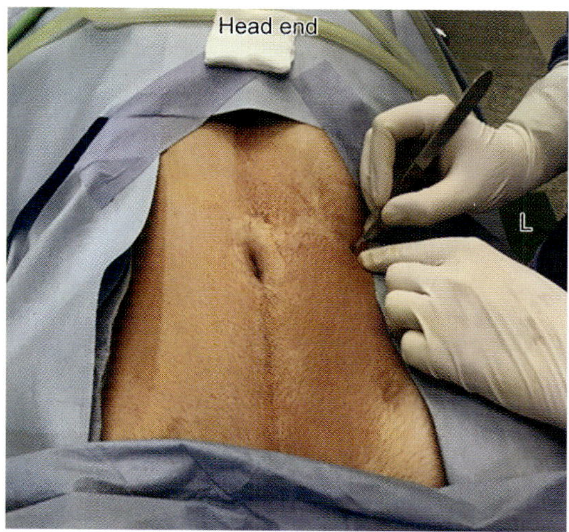

Fig. 2: Giving a 1–2 mm stab incision at Jain point with stretched skin.

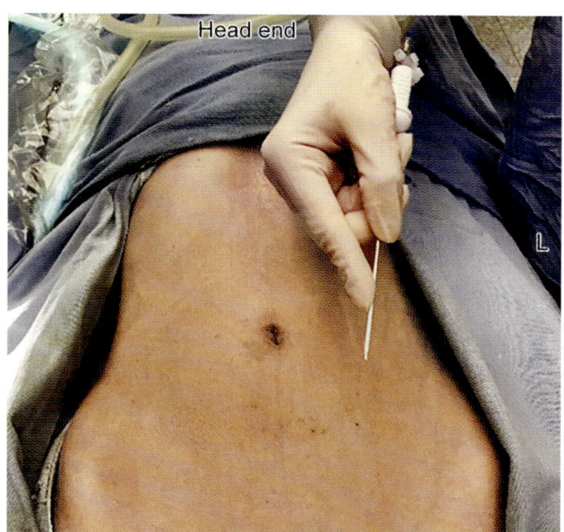

Fig. 3: Holding of a Veress needle with finger guide.

very important safety feature. In very thin patients, this entry site is a boon as the risk of retroperitoneal vessel injury is negated and the layer-by-layer entry is very well-defined due to good muscle tone.[7-9] and all the limitations, which are faced in entry in all other methods explained above, are easily minimized. After insertion of Veress needle, the 5 mm port is inserted and abdomen is inspected from all quadrants and then the 10 mm port is inserted under direct visual guidance. After insertion of telescope though the umbilicus, the Jain point port becomes the upper working port and the surgery continues in an ergonomic stress free manner.

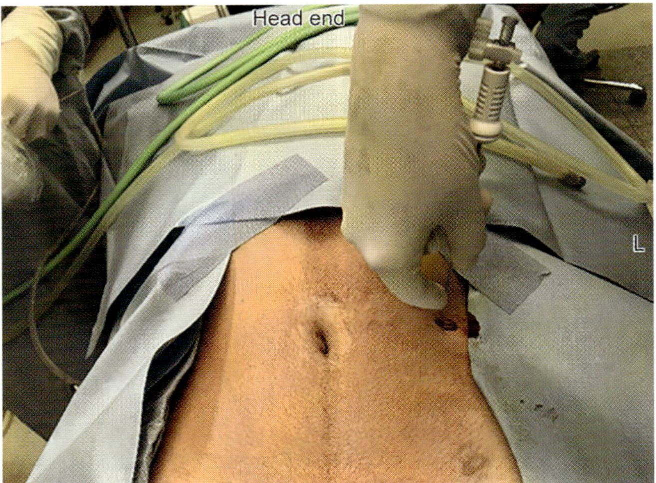

Fig. 4: Inserting the needle at 90° without lifting abdominal wall.

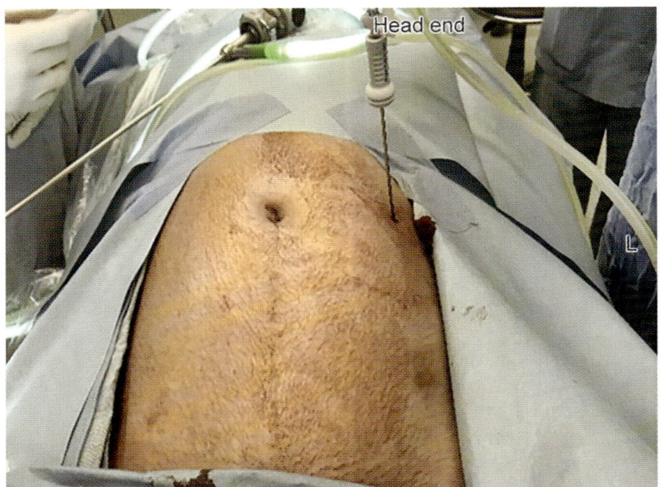

Fig. 5: Attachment with gas inflow after saline drop test.

LEARNING POINTS

- In thin patients, highest risk of major retroperitoneal vessel injury due to short distance of vessels from umbilicus.
- Catastrophic complications of Veress injury can be avoided by using the nonumbilical Jain point.
- In thin patient, muscle tone is very well-developed so hearing the pops during insertion becomes easily discernible.
- Jain point entry makes a safe nonumbilical entry.

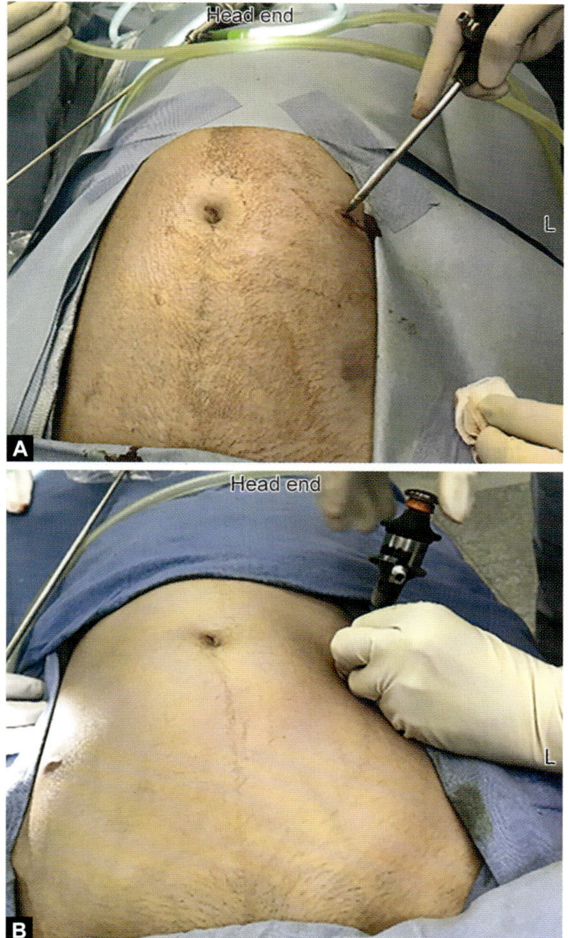

Figs. 6A and B: Insertion of 5 mm trocar holding with finger guard after pneumocreation.

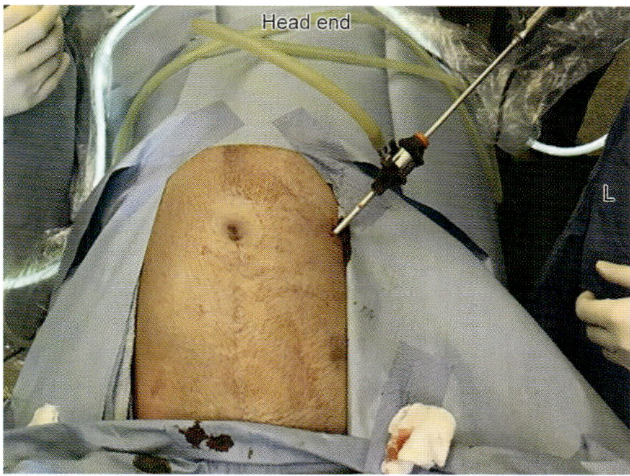

Fig. 7: Insertion of 5 mm telescope at Jain point.

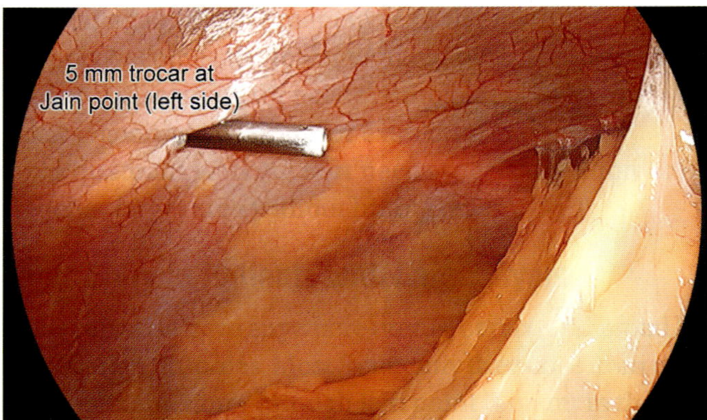

Fig. 8: Jain point inside picture that is free of adhesion.

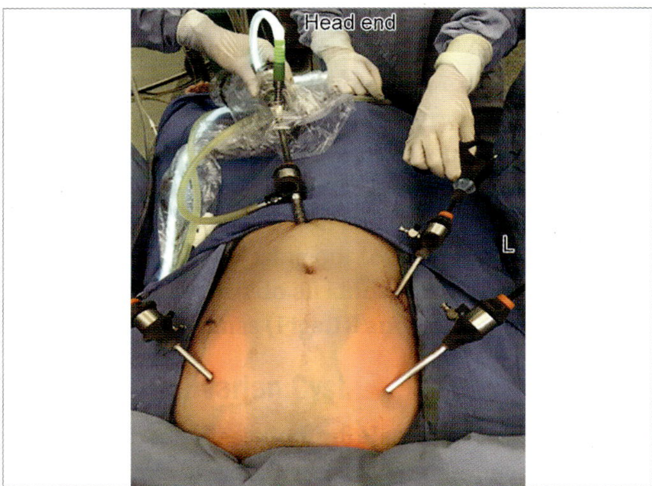

Fig. 9: Jain point as the main working port along with other accessory ports and 10 mm telescope port.

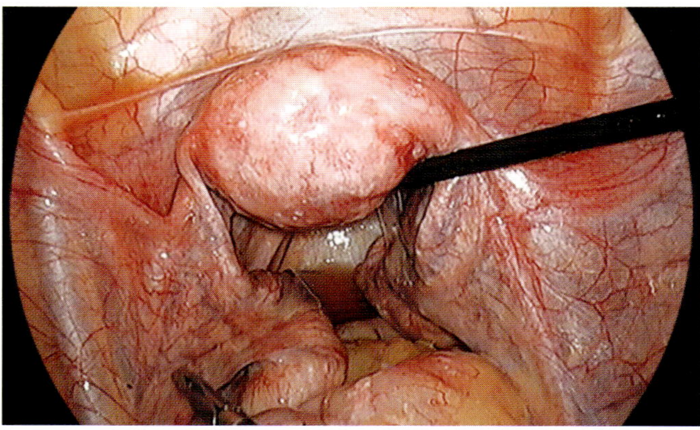

Fig.10: Initial view on telescope showing bilateral tubomass with vesicles at surface of uterus.

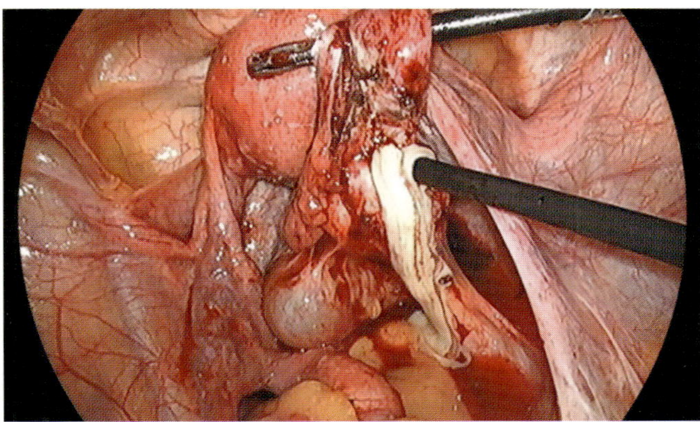

Fig.11: Frank pus seen draining from tubo-ovarian mass.

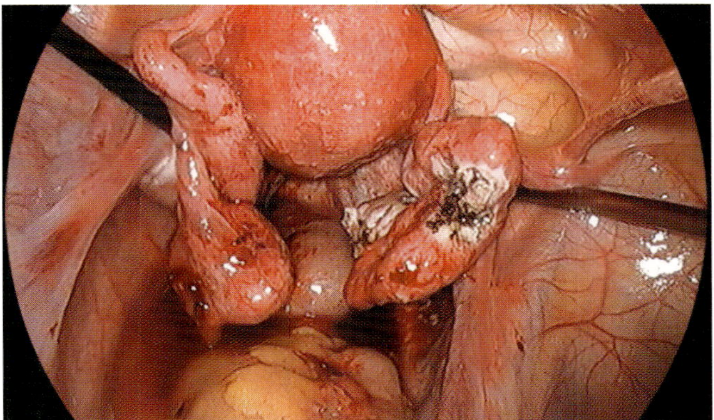

Fig.12: End pictures after drainage of pus and thorough suction and evacuation.

SUMMARY

One of the challenges of laparoscopy is access into the abdomen, particularly the insertion of surgical instruments through small incisions. All the limitations that are encountered during entry via umbilical, open technique or Palmer's technique are seen to be overcome by our technique. In our long years of practice we have not experienced major vessels injury during entry through Jain point at extremes of BMI (even <18 BMI). So, we consider it as safe entry technique.

REFERENCES

1. Krishnakumar S, Tambe P. Entry complications in laparoscopic surgery. J Gynec Endosc Surg. 2009;1(1):4-11.
2. Isaacson K. Complications of Gynecologic Endoscopic Surgery. Philadelphia: Saunders Elsevier; 2006.

3. Ahmad G, O'Flynn H, Duffy JM, et al. Laparoscopic entry techniques. Cochrane Database Syst Rev. 2012;(2):CD006583.
4. Palmer R. Safety in laparoscopy. J Reprod Med. 1974;13:1-5.
5. Hasson HM. Open laparoscopy as a method of access in laparoscopic surgery. 1999;8(6):353-62.
6. Sharp HT. (2019). Overview of gynecologic laparoscopic surgery and non-umbilical entry sites. [online] Available from https://www.uptodate.com/contents/overview-of-gynecologic-laparoscopic-surgery-and-non-umbilical-entry-sites. [Last accessed January, 2020].
7. Hurd WH, Bude RO, DeLancey JO, et al. Abdominal wall characterization with magnetic resonance imaging and computed tomography. The effect of obesity on the laparoscopic approach. J Reprod Med. 1991;36(7):473-6.
8. Hurd WW, Bude RO, DeLancey J, et al. The relationship of the umbilicus to the aortic bifurcation: implications for laparoscopic technique. Obstet Gynecol. 1992;80:48-51.
9. Nezhat F, Brill AI, Nezhat CH, et al. Laparoscopic appraisal of the anatomic relationship of the umbilicus to the aortic bifurcation. J Am Assoc Gynecol Laparosc. 1998;5:135-40.

16

Jain Point in Obese Patients

Kiran Kumari Mandal, Anadeep Chandi, Nutan Jain

■ INTRODUCTION

Obesity is becoming more prevalent in society, in both affluent as well as developing countries. About 90 million adults in the United States are estimated to be either obese [body mass index (BMI) >30 kg/m^2] or overweight (BMI 25–29.9 kg/m^2).[1] The prevalence of obese people is increasing each decade at the rate of 10% approximately.[2] According to ICMR–INDIAB study 2015, prevalence rate of obesity varies from 11.8% to 31.3%.[3] Therefore, if the current expansion of obesity continues, a majority of surgical patients will be obese soon.

Obesity is defined as having a BMI (calculated as weight in kilogram divided by height in meters squared) of 30 or greater.[4] It is further subdivided as Class I obesity as BMI 30–35; Class II obesity as BMI 35–40; and Class III obesity as BMI 40 or greater.[5,6] A prospective, multi-institutional, risk-adjusted cohort study of 1,18,707 patients who underwent nonbariatric general surgery examined mortality risk and found the highest rates in the underweight and morbidly obese and lowest rates in the overweight and moderately obese.[7] Wound complications, surgical site infections, and venous thromboembolism remain a major source of morbidity in obese patients undergoing abdominal surgery and additional risks are higher rates of atelectasis, thromboembolism, and cardiovascular dysfunction. In Cochrane review of studies on hysterectomy, risk of wound complication and surgical site infection is less when done through vaginal or laparoscopy approach as compared to open route.[8] Laparoscopy can be more complicated in the obese patients and risk of conversion to laparotomy is higher but it decreases with surgical experience.[9] Eltabbakh et al.[10] prospectively studied a cohort of 42 obese women, with BMIs between 28 kg/m^2 and 60 kg/m^2, who underwent laparoscopic hysterectomy, bilateral salpingo-oophorectomy, and lymph node dissection for stage I endometrial carcinoma. Only 7.5% of the patients were converted to laparotomy in their study. The remaining 88.1% (37/42 patients) underwent laparoscopic surgery.

When this group of women was compared with 40 other women who had the procedures performed by laparotomy, the laparoscopic group had shorter hospital stay (2.5 vs 5.6 days; P < 0.001), less pain (32.3 vs 124.1 mg of pain medication; P < 0.001), and earlier return to normal activity.

The best way to ensure safe and successful laparoscopy in obese patients is through extensive preoperative evaluation, patient counseling, and preparation for surgery. Preoperative evaluation should include a thorough cardiovascular and respiratory history. A detailed assessment of patient should be done with an extensive review of the medical history for the presence of smoking, hypertension, sleep apnea, peripheral vascular disease, or other obstructive pulmonary disease.[11] Appropriately sized blood pressure cuff must be used for measuring blood pressure. The patient should also be evaluated for evidence of peripheral vascular disease, skin changes, or ulcerations. The panniculus should also be lifted to identify the costovertebral edge, the xiphoid process, the ischial spines, and the bifurcation of the aorta in relation to the patient's umbilicus in supine and standing positions. Obese patients are predisposed to moist, dark, and anoxic spaces beneath folds of skin which need to be examined for evidence of fungal or bacterial infection. To optimize postoperative wound healing, treat any preexisting infections before surgery. The airway should be examined carefully, because difficulties in intubation can occur due to short neck, excessive fat around the face, or limited movement of the jaw and neck.

Baseline laboratory screening must include blood count, serum electrolytes and glucose concentrations, and renal function tests.[11] An electrocardiogram, chest X-ray, and arterial blood gas level are also recommended in the assessment of the patient's cardiopulmonary status. The electrocardiogram may show signs of arrhythmias, ischemia, strain, and ventricular hypertrophy. The chest X-ray is done to evaluate cardiac size or any pulmonary abnormalities.[11] Extensive patients counseling is very important in morbidly obese patients as they need to understand the technical and practical difficulties that may be encountered by the anesthetist and surgeons during laparoscopy (like intravenous access and need for central lines, panniculus repositioning, and conversion to laparotomy). Patients must also understand that their recovery depends on early ambulation and avoidance of the supine position. Proper evaluation of the patient's panniculus and body type is crucial for determining intravenous access, trocar placement, and positioning during laparoscopy. The distribution of the weight of patient should be properly evaluated (i.e. increased hip circumference vs increased waist circumference). Patients with large adipose tissue centered on their waist are likely to be more technically challenging than patients whose adipose tissue is centered on the hips. Trocar placement may be difficult in patients with large panniculi due to increased thickness and lack of mobility. If the panniculus is soft and mobile, it can be repositioned easily with the use of traction with tape or weights.

During preparation for surgery, the anesthesia teams and operating room staff must be advised of the patient's weight. Often extrasheets, blankets, padding, and lifting devices are used for appropriate positioning of obese patients. Operating rooms should be equipped with appropriate sized blood pressure cuff and monitoring devices, large compression lower extremity stockings and pneumatic boots. Facility for central vascular access should be available for patients in whom peripheral intravenous access fails.

POSITION THE PATIENT FOR OPTIMAL ACCESS

This issue in obese laparoscopy patients is explored by only 1 recent publication. Lamvu et al.[12] advocate the arms-tucked by side "military position", low lithotomy position, with liberal padding on the legs and arms and a gel pad under the lower back. Additionally, they recommend stationary shoulder blocks to help maintain positioning in the Trendelenburg position. They also use gauze, clamps, tape, and weights to maintain the panniculus in caudal position.

The success or failure of most laparoscopic surgeries is determined in the initial minutes during placement of the operative ports. Obesity increases the distance between skin and fascia, and can increase the distance between fascia and peritoneum. The difficulty of inserting the Veress needle or trocar into the peritoneal cavity increases with this distance. Preperitoneal insufflation of gas exacerbates the problem. In addition, dissection to the level of the fascia for an open (Hasson) approach sometimes requires incision extension and increases the risk of postoperative wound infection. Obesity also changes the relationship of the umbilicus to the aortic bifurcation. Utilizing computed tomography, Hurd et al.[13] demonstrated that the umbilicus migrates caudally in relation to the aortic bifurcation as the BMI increases. In nonobese patients (BMI < 25), the umbilicus had a median location 0.4 cm caudal to the bifurcation, but in 33% of patients, the umbilicus was actually cephalad to the aortic bifurcation. In overweight (BMI 25–30) and obese (BMI > 30) patients, the umbilicus had a median location 2.4 and 2.9 cm caudal to the aortic bifurcation, respectively. The same group of researchers, again using computed tomography, demonstrated that the distance between the umbilicus and peritoneum at a 45° angle from the umbilicus into the pelvis, in both nonobese and overweight patients, was only 2 cm. In obese patients, this distance increased to a median of 12 cm. Hurd et al.[14] also noted that the distance between the umbilicus and the underlying vessels was only 6 cm at a 90° angle in nonobese patients, but it averaged 13 cm in obese patients. Hurd et al. recommend a 45°angle from the umbilicus toward the pelvis in nonobese patients and a 90° approach in obese patients to optimize intraperitoneal Veress needle and trocar placement while minimizing risk to the underlying vascular structures. In overweight patients, however, the approach should range between 45°and 90°.

TECHNIQUE OF JAIN POINT ENTRY

At our institution, we routinely use Jain point **(Figs. 1 to 3)**, where there is no requirement in change in direction of Veress needle during entry. In entry, we mostly use long Veress needle in obese patients which facilitates and increases the success rate of entry in all classes of obesity.

We use a long Veress needle and hold the needle perpendicular to the patient's body. Patient is kept in horizontal position. The Veress is entered and as we go layer by layer, we hear for two pops and the third or give of peritoneum as the needle passes through the peritoneum after the fat layer. We found this entry method with long Veress needle easier as we do not need to change

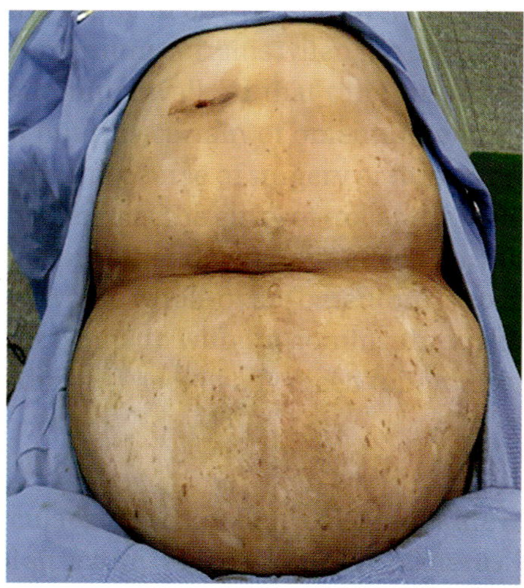

Fig. 1: It is case of morbidly obese patients (BMI > 40).

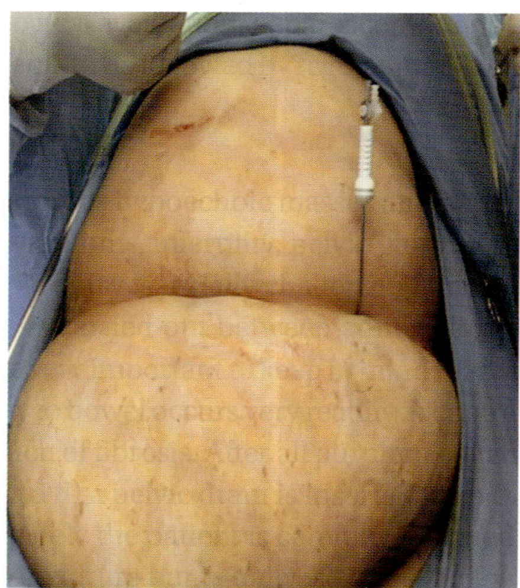

Fig. 2: Veress needle insertion at Jain point.

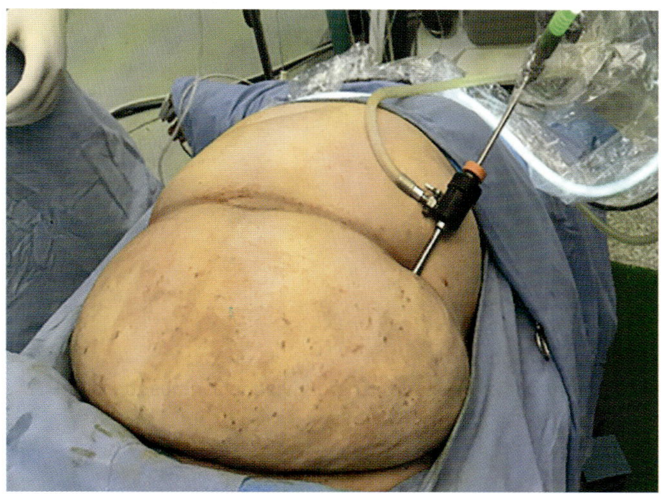

Fig. 3: First blind 5 mm trocar with 5 mm telescope.

direction or the angle of insertion. Also no risk of major retroperitoneal vessel injury, while going vertically with long Veress needle.

We perform a standard technique of entry through Jain point at a 90° in any class of obesity. There is no requirement of lifting or repositioning of abdominal wall during entry in our technique. We have concluded it as safe entry technique through long years of practice in large number of patients.

After Achieving Pneumoperitoneum

The routine safety check of drop test and low initial Veress intraperitoneal pressure (LIVIP) test are done and then CO_2 insufflation started. Once 3 liters of CO_2 has created a good pneumoperitoneum and abdomen duly tented with insufflation pressure of 25 mm Hg, then a 5 mm pyramidal tip reusable long trocar is inserted.[15] This decreases the risk of preperitoneal trocar placement by further elevating the abdominal wall. After trocar is placed successfully, intra-abdominal pressure should be reduced to 15 mm Hg immediately to avoid excessive catecholamine release, pulmonary compromise, and subcutaneous emphysema. Once the 5 mm long trocar has been introduced, we inspect the entire abdomen, all quadrants, and confirm the entry to be smooth by checking the Jain point port. Looking for adhesions and presence of big masses, etc. then we optimize the 10 mm port. After the insertion of 10 mm telescope, the Jain point port becomes free and is utilized all though the surgery as the main working port.

■ TECHNIQUES TO ENHANCE VISUALIZATION

Excess adipose tissues in the omental, pericolic, mesenteric, and retroperitoneal spaces obscure visualization of intraperitoneal and retroperitoneal structures in obese patients **(Fig. 4)**. Preoperative mechanical bowel preparation can deflate the bowel and enhance visualization. If required, visualization can be improved by extra-ancillary trocar for placement of a bowel retractor. Showing a case of TLH in morbidly obese patient **(Figs. 5 to 16)**.

Close Port Sites at the Fascial Level

The risk of bowel herniation through a trocar site is higher in obese patients than the general population because of the greater intra-abdominal pressures. Increases in atelectasis from diminished functional residual capacity also predispose the obese patient to postoperative pulmonary complications and can lead to recurrent cough and subsequent bowel herniation. Given these

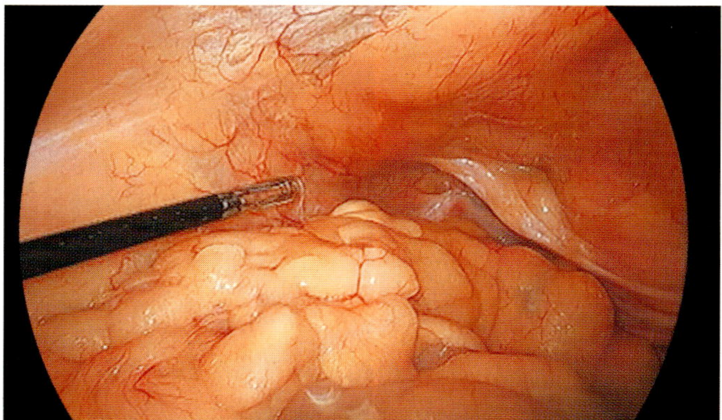

Fig. 4: Excess adipose tissue occupying pericolic, omental area obscuring uterus.

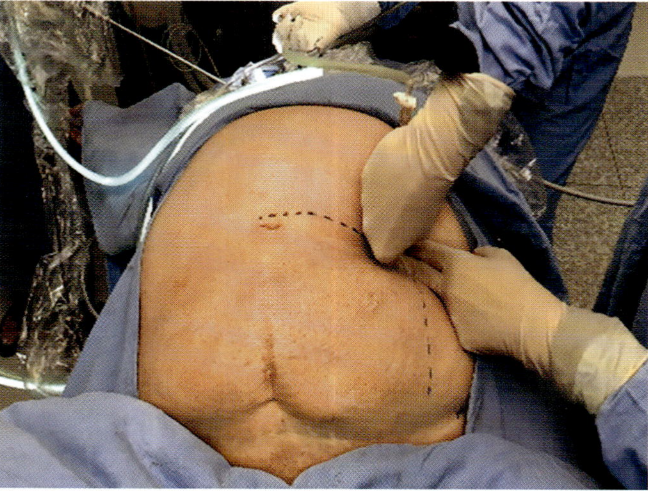

Fig. 5: A 70 years old patient with BMI of 34.85 kg/m^2 with postmenopausal bleeding undergoing TLH. Veress needle insertion through Jain point is shown.

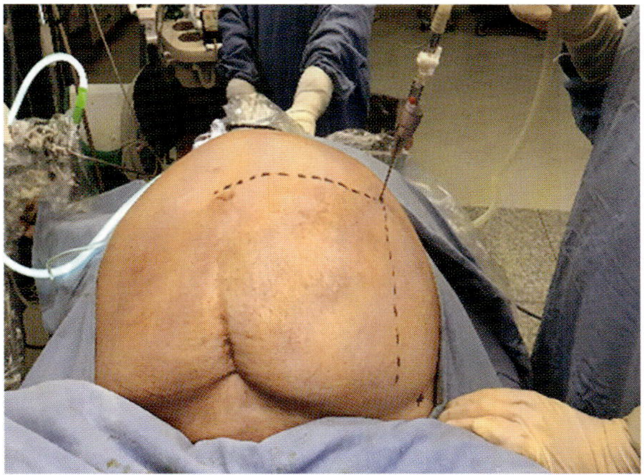

Fig. 6: Attachment of gas tubing after syringe test.

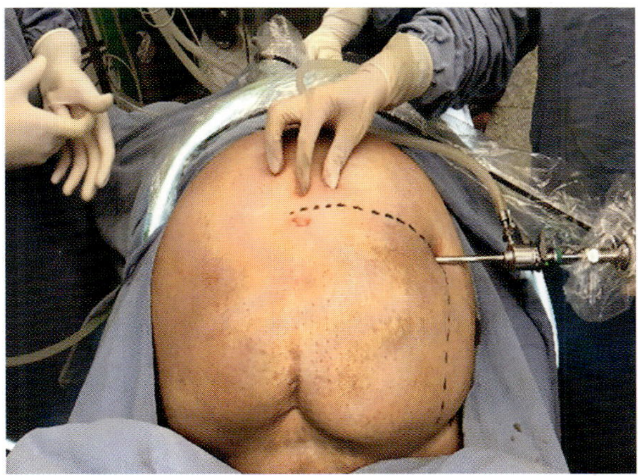

Fig. 7: A 5 mm trocar with 5 mm telescope showing site for under vision insertion of 10 mm trocar.

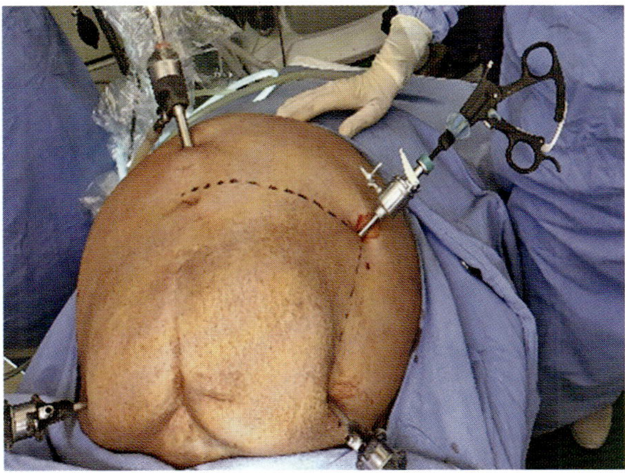

Fig. 8: All ports in situ.

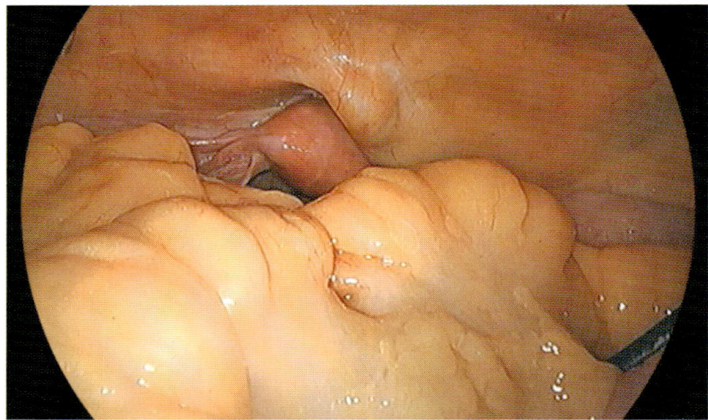

Fig. 9: Telescopic view showing initial picture of pelvic cavity.

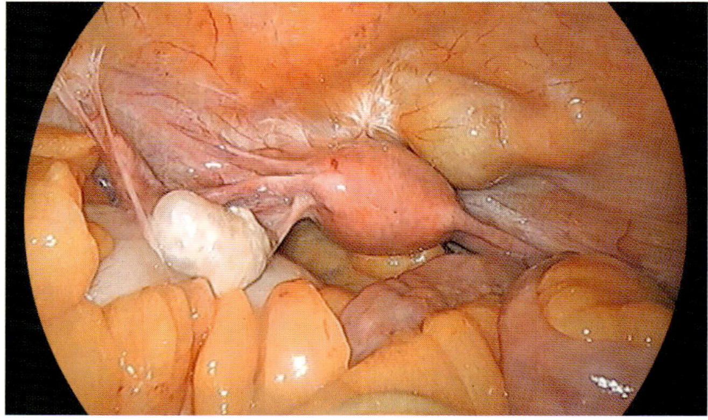

Fig. 10: Telescopic view after replacing fat.

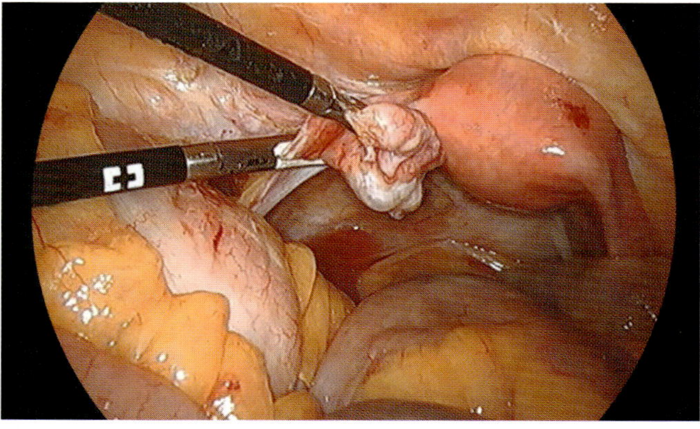

Fig. 11A

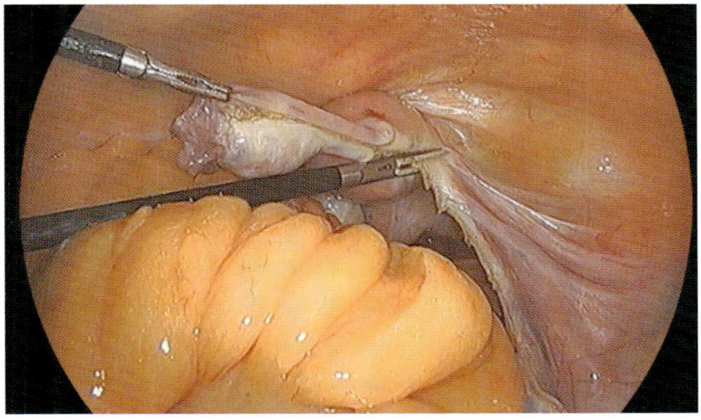

Fig. 11B
Figs. 11A and B: Bilateral infundibulopelvic ligament cut with ligasure.

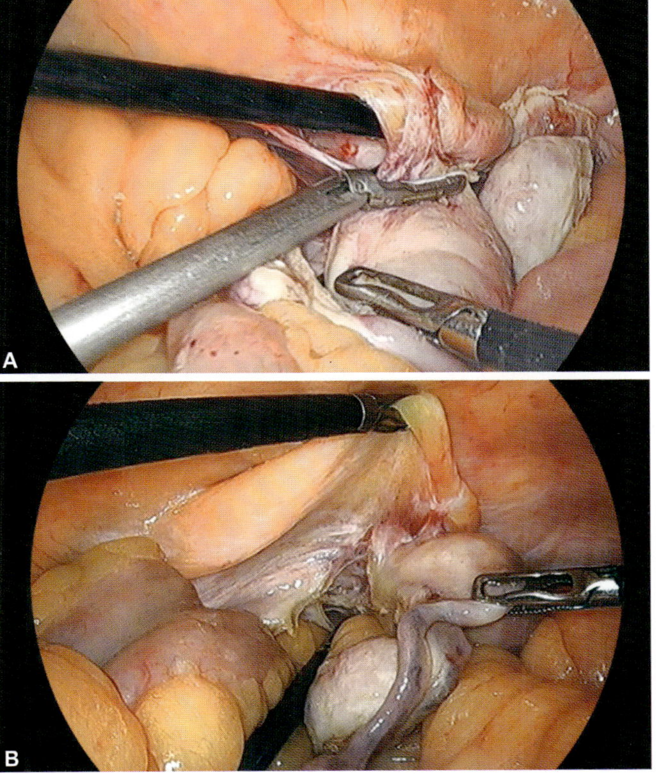

Figs. 12A and B: Bladder dissection with harmonic.

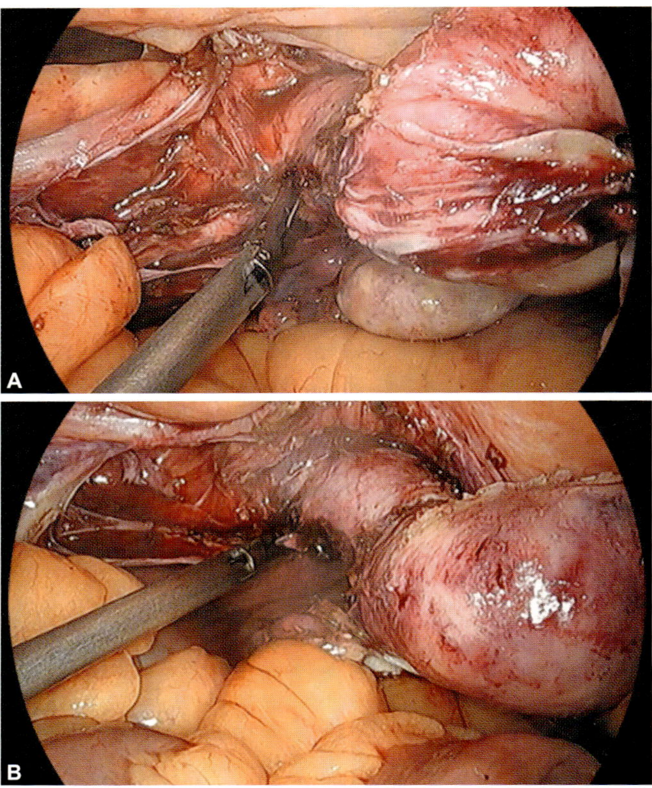

Figs. 13A and B: Bilateral uterine artery coagulation and cut done with harmonic.

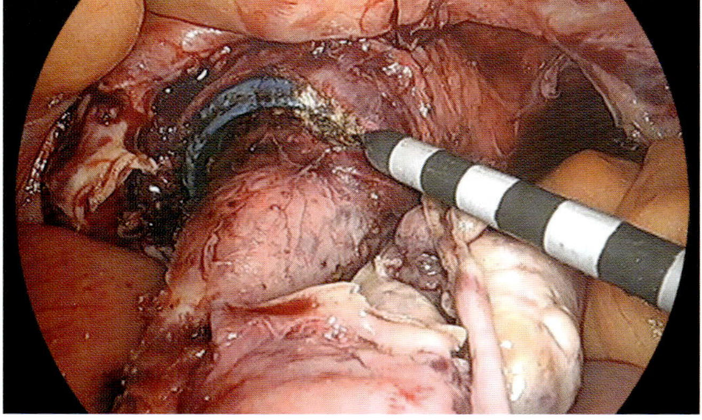

Fig. 14: Colpotomy done by monopolar hook.

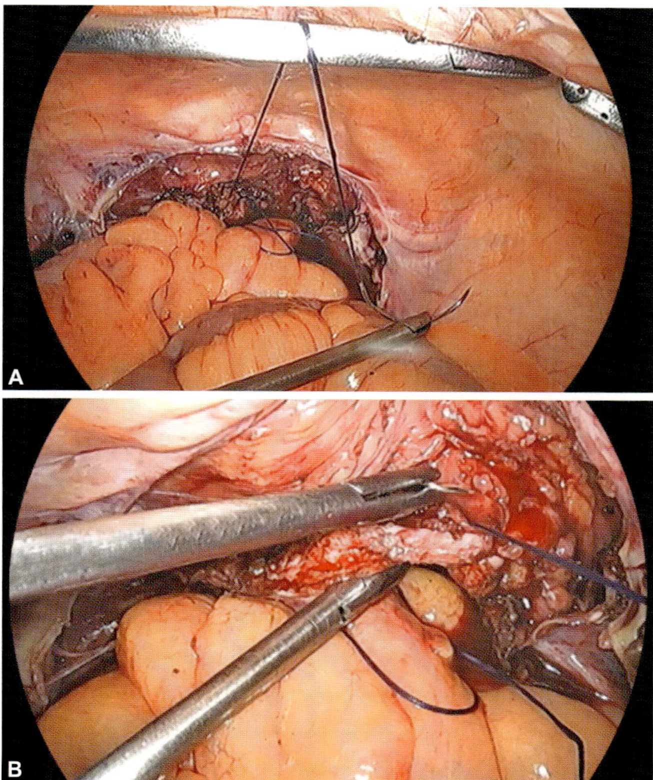

Figs. 15A and B: Suturing of vault in double layer by V-suture technique with vicryl 1-0.

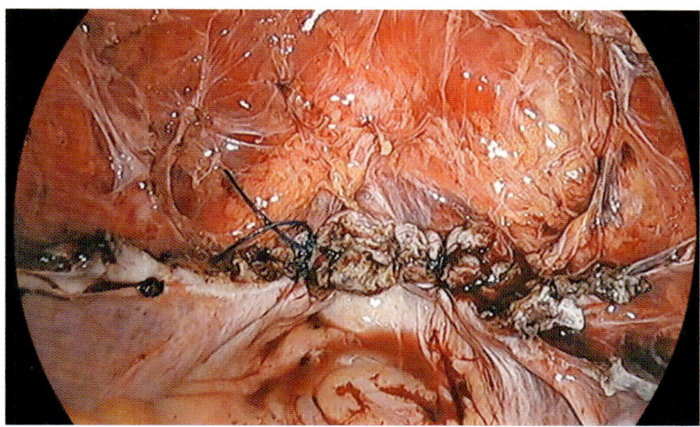

Fig. 16: Vault at the end.

risks, it is imperative that all port sites 10 mm or larger be closed at the fascial level in obese.

Encourage Early Ambulation

This requires adequate but not oversedating analgesia,[16-20] early catheter removal, and a motivated nursing staff. Early ambulation is associated with fewer episodes of deep venous thrombosis, pulmonary complications, and ileus, and also eases pain management. Continue thrombosis prophylaxis with sequential compression devices, subcutaneous heparin, or both, until the patient is spending most of her time out of bed. We routinely give injection enoxaparin to our patients in postoperative period according to risk stratification by CAPRINI SCORE for thromboprophylaxis.[21]

SUMMARY

Jain point entry has been developed over a decade of practice at our center, to avoid the complications associated with Veress needle and first blind port entry through umbilicus. It has been found to be safe entry port in obese patients. There are clinical situations, which pose a challenge and we have used Jain point in all these situations.

LEARNING POINTS

- In obese patients surface marking of other nonumbilical entry points is difficult, but as Jain point has a fixed bony reference point the ASIS it becomes easier as it is in the sterile field.
- Use a long Veress needle.
- Use a long 5 mm trocar.
- Nonumbilical entry is encouraged to avoid major vessel injury, which can happen with long Veress and long trocars from the umbilicus.
- Use the Jain point paraumbilical port to avoid retroperitoneal vessel injury.
- Challenge of obesity is overcome by a nonumbilical entry.

REFERENCES

1. NHLBI Obesity Education Initiative Expert Panel on the Identification, Evaluation, and Treatment of Obesity in Adults (US). Clinical guidelines on the identification, evaluation, and treatment of overweight and obesity in adults. Bethesda (MD): National Heart, Lung, and Blood Institute; 1998. pp. 7.
2. McTigue KM, Garrett JM, Popkin BM. The natural history of the development of obesity in a cohort of young US adults between 1981 and 1998. Ann Intern Med. 2002;136:852-64.
3. Pradeepa R, Anjana RM, Joshi SR, et al. Prevalence of generalized and abdominal obesity in urban and rural India: the ICMR—INDIAB Study (Phase-I) [ICMR-INDIAB-3]. Indian J Med Res. 2015;142(2):139-50.

4. Shields M, Carroll MD, Ogden CL. Adult obesity prevalence in Canada and the United States. NCHS Data Brief. 2011;56:1-8.

5. Flegal KM, Kit BK, Orpana H, et al. Association of all-cause mortality with overweight and obesity using standard body mass index categories: a systematic review and meta-analysis. JAMA. 2013;309:71-82.

6. Jensen MD, Ryan DH, Apovian CM, et al. 2013 AHA/ACC/TOS guideline for the management of overweight and obesity in adults: a report of the American College of Cardiology/American Heart Association Task Force on practice guidelines and The Obesity Society. J Am Coll Cardiol. 2014;63:2985-3023

7. Mullen JT, Moorman DW, Davenport DL. The obesity paradox: body mass index and outcomes in patients undergoing nonbariatric general surgery. Ann Surg. 2009;250:166-72.

8. Nieboer TE, Johnson N, Letharby A, et al. Surgical approach to hysterectomy for benign gynaecological disease. Cochrane Database Syst Rev. 2009;3:CD003677.

9. Wattiez A, Soriano D, Cohen SB, et al. The learning curve of total laparoscopic hysterectomy: comparative analysis of 1647 cases. J Am Assoc Gynecol Laparosc. 2002;9:339-45.

10. Eltabbakh GH, Shamonki MI, Moody JM, et al. Hysterectomy for obese women with endometrial cancer: laparoscopy or laparotomy? Gynecol Oncol. 2000;78:329-35.

11. Shenkman Z, Shir Y, Brodsky JB. Perioperative management of the obese patient. Br J Anaesth. 1993;70:349-59.

12. Lamvu G, Zolnoun D, Boggess J, Steege JF. Obesity: physiologic changes and challenges during laparoscopy. Am J Obstet Gynecol. 2004;191:669-74.

13. Hurd WW, Bude RO, DeLancey JO, et al. The relationship of the umbilicus to the aortic bifurcation: implications for laparoscopic technique. Obstet Gynecol. 1992;80:48-51.

14. Hurd WH, Bude RO, DeLancey JO, et al. Abdominal wall characterization with magnetic resonance imaging and computed tomography. The effect of obesity on the laparoscopic approach. J Reprod Med. 1991;36:473-6.

15. Vilos GA, Vilos AG. Safe laparoscopic entry guided by Veress needle CO_2 insufflation pressure. J Am Assoc Gynecol Laparosc. 2003;10:415-20.

16. Wilmore DW, Kehlet H. Management of patients in fast track surgery. BMJ. 2001;322:473-6.

17. Kehlet H, Wilmore DW. Multimodal strategies to improve surgical outcome. Am J Surg. 2002;183:630-41.

18. Kehlet H, Dahl JB. Anaesthesia, surgery, and challenges in postoperative recovery. Lancet. 2003;362:1921-8.

19. Arumainayagam N, McGrath J, Jefferson KP, et al. Introduction of an enhanced recovery protocol for radical cystectomy. BJU Int. 2008;101:698-701.

20. Kehlet H, Mogensen T. Hospital stay of 2 days after open sigmoidectomy with a multimodal rehabilitation programme. Br J Surg. 1999;86:227-30.

21. Laryea J, Champagne B. Venous thromboembolism prophylaxis. Clin Colon Rectal Surg. 2013;26(3):153-9.

Laparoscopic Entry in Large Pelvic Masses

Vandana Jain, Nutan Jain

"So what if they are taller? We will play big"
—**George Ireland**

INTRODUCTION

In this modern era, as technology advances, the indications for open surgery are diminishing. Laparoscopy is the chosen route not only by surgeons, even by patients. Large pelvic masses are one such indication where surgeons have now switched over to laparoscopy over conventional laparotomy, but the challenges are big. So, we, try to present few variations in entry as well as operative ports. With correct entry and port placement, one can easily operate large pelvic masses with minimum difficulty.

LARGE PELVIC MASSES

Large pelvic masses **(Figs. 1 and 2)** in the female pelvis arise from the reproductive organs (e.g. uterus, cervix, ovaries, and fallopian tubes). Majority of large masses include fibroid **(Figs. 3 to 5)**, dermoid cyst, ovarian cyst **(Figs. 6 and 7)**, ovarian cancers, and retroperitoneal tumors. However, uncommon masses such as mesothelioma, carcinosarcoma, adenocarcinoma, leiomyosarcomas, and desmoid tumors can also be seen.[1]

ENTRY IN PATIENTS WITH LARGE MASSES (FIG. 8)

About 50% of major complications occur at the time of entry.[2,3] Entry in large masses is difficult with conventional umbilical port. Most gynecologists use closed entry technique with Veress needle insertion through the umbilicus. But in patients with large fibroid or ovarian cyst, there are high chances of hitting the needle into the mass as these masses are difficult to displace and

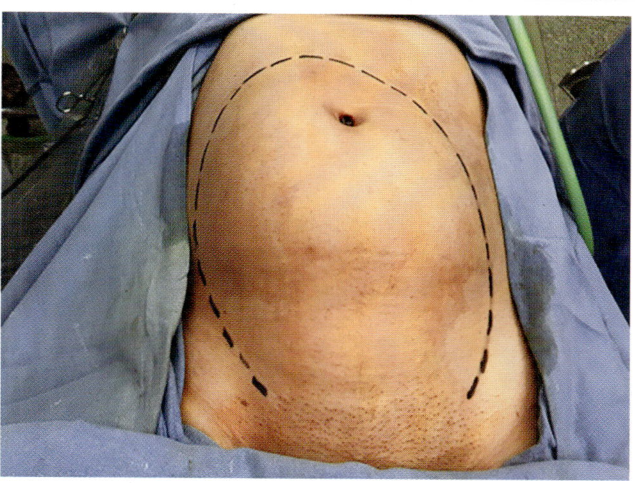

Fig. 1: Large mass (outside picture).

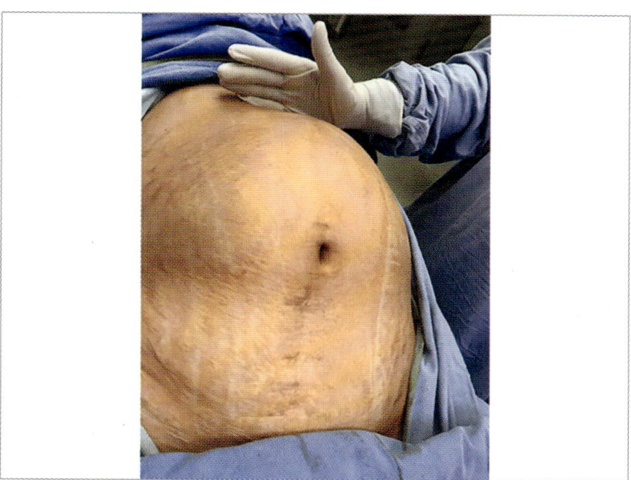

Fig. 2: Very large mass (≥30 weeks).

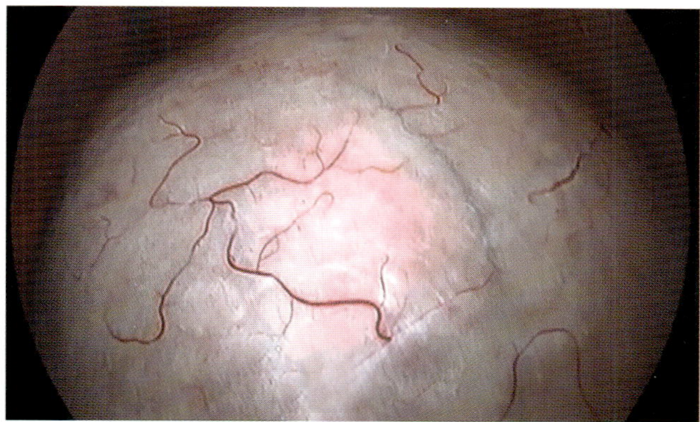

Fig. 3: Big myoma.

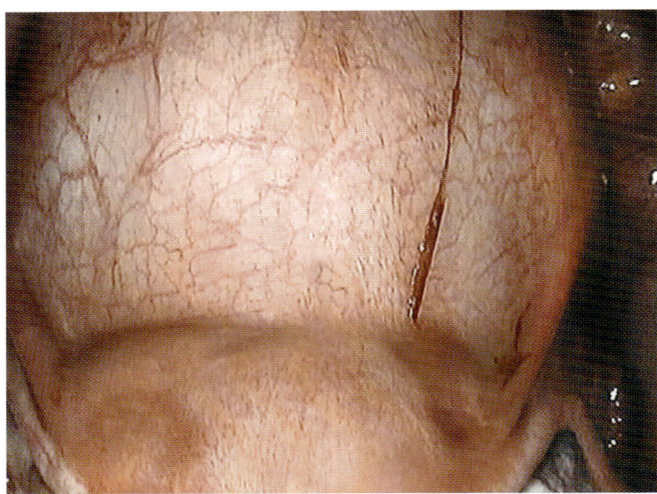

Fig. 4: Huge cervical fibroid.

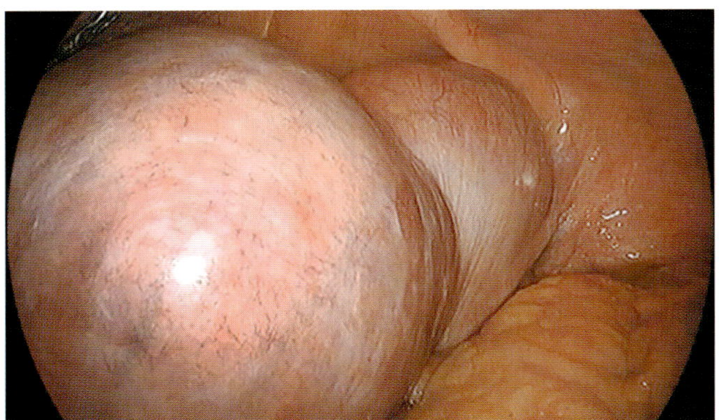

Fig. 5: Large fibroid.

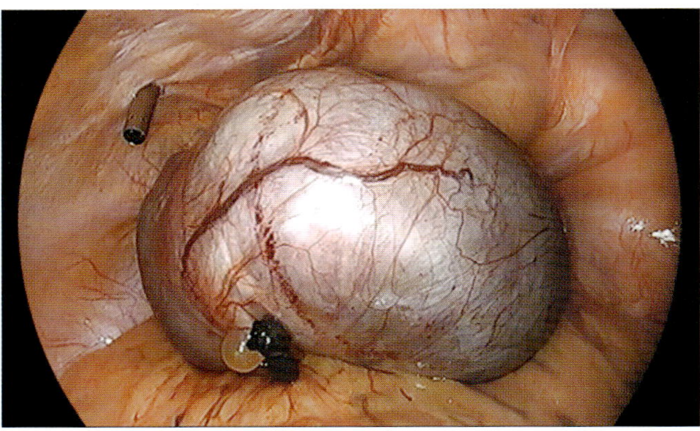

Fig. 6: Large endometriotic cyst.

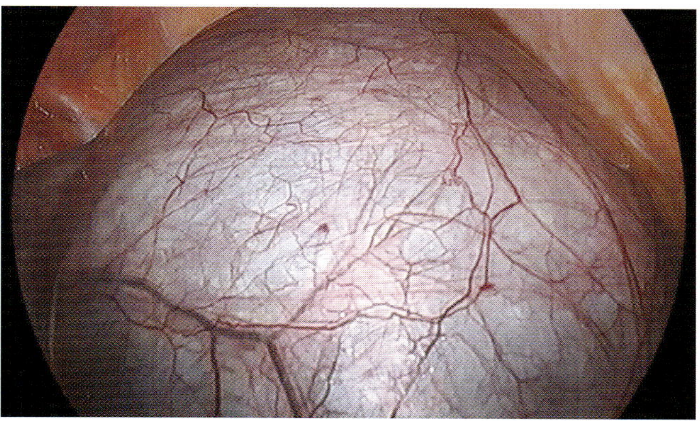

Fig. 7: Large ovarian cyst.

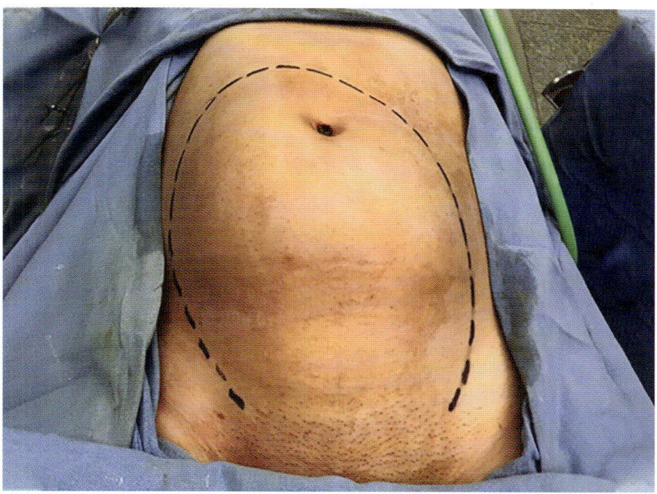

Fig. 8: Outside picture (large mass).

it is not a good idea to puncture the cyst before entry or hit the fibroids and cause bleeding.

We, at our hospital, have been using Jain point for about a decade for large pelvic masses. We report this as a safe entry point in large pelvic masses.

Jain Point

Jain point lies on a vertical line drawn 2.5 cm medial to anterior superior iliac spine (ASIS) at the level of umbilicus. It is roughly 10–13 cm lateral to the umbilicus on the left side, depending on patient's body type. It has an advantage of lateral location avoiding any entry into abdominal adhesions of the midline, median, and paramedian incision sites. Being at the level of L4, it avoids upper abdomen scar adhesions. Also no vessels (superficial or deep retroperitoneal) lie beneath it. It avoids stomach and enlarged spleen at level of T10 to L1 and kidney which is deep in retroperitoneum at T12 to L3. It is comparatively safer as no vessel or hollow viscus lie directly beneath it.

Ease of Entry

Jain point is used for Veress needle placement for creating pneumoperitoneum. Patient is laid on OT table in horizontal position. A small nick (1–2 mm) is given with scalpel at Jain's point. Incision is small, so that Veress needle is secure at that point. Veress needle inserted perpendicular to the abdominal wall in a vertical direction. Do not lift the abdominal wall. Concentrate on two pops. The first pop is entry in the aponeurosis of external oblique muscle. The second pop is the fused aponeurosis of internal oblique and transverses abdominis muscle. Feeling of give of resistance confirms the entry of needle into the peritoneal cavity. This is an important step thus requires patience and concentration to hear the pops and appreciate the loss of resistance. Then routine safety check of drop test and LIVIP (low initial Veress intraperitoneal pressure)[4] test are done.

TECHNIQUE IN LARGE MASSES (<30 WEEKS)

Primary port (5 mm) is placed through Jain point. Secondary port (10 mm) is placed higher up under vision of primary port depending upon the pathology. Another port (5 mm) is placed in left lower quadrant 2.5 cm medial to ASIS. We place another port (5 mm) for assistant in right lower quadrant and since the surgery needs more manipulation—traction we place another paraumbilical port in right side almost mirror image of Jain point.

Entry Technique Devised for Very Large Masses (≥30 weeks)

- As the mass is coming beneath Jain point, first assistant displaces it medially using his both hands.
- Usual entry through Veress needle at Jain point is made **(Fig. 9)**.
- Primary 5 mm port insertion done at Jain point **(Fig. 10)**.
- (10 mm) secondary port (camera port) is inserted under vision high up into the epigastrium, 1–2 fingers laterally on right side from midline to avoid falciform ligament. Also going lateral from midline allows better assistance with 30° camera port **(Figs. 11 to 14)**.
- Another port (5 mm) is placed in left lower quadrant **(Fig. 15)**.
- Another 5 mm port is placed on right side (assistant side) at the level of umbilicus **(Fig. 16)** *(mirror image of Jain point)*.
- On left side, upper working port comes almost at level of 10 mm port flush with the subcostal margin **(Fig. 17)**:
  - This very high placement of the upper working port allows us to reach the big mass almost straight away, without hitting the mass by the side

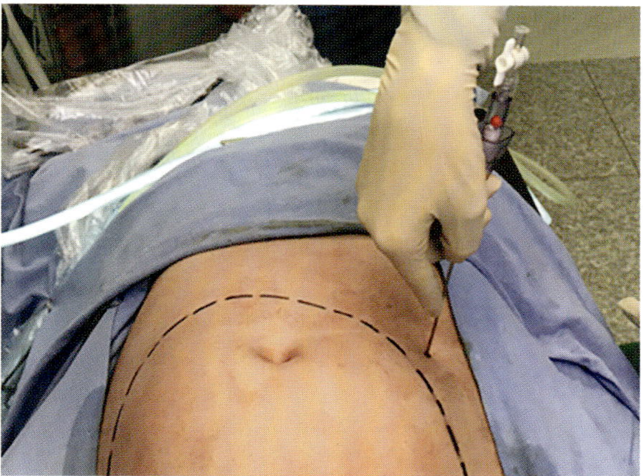

Fig. 9: Veress insertion at Jain point.

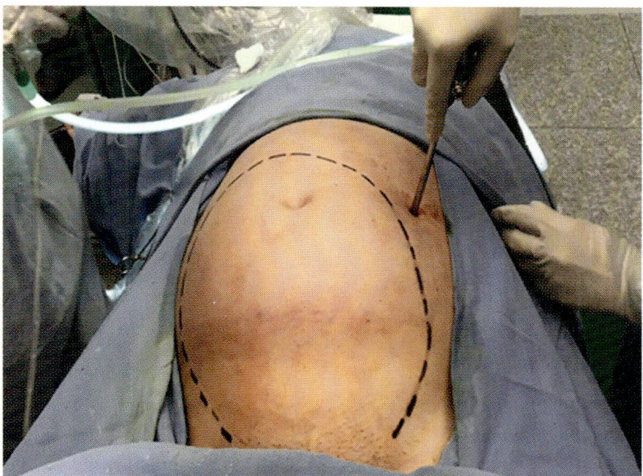

Fig. 10: Primary port (5 mm) at Jain point.

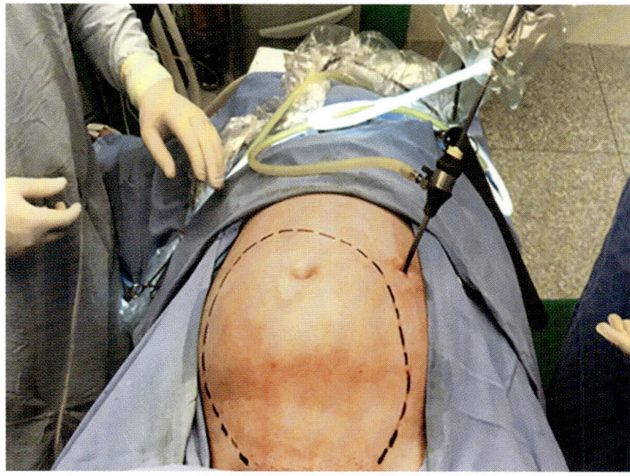

Fig. 11: 5 mm telescope in place and looking into the abdominal cavity to optimize the entry point for 10 mm port.

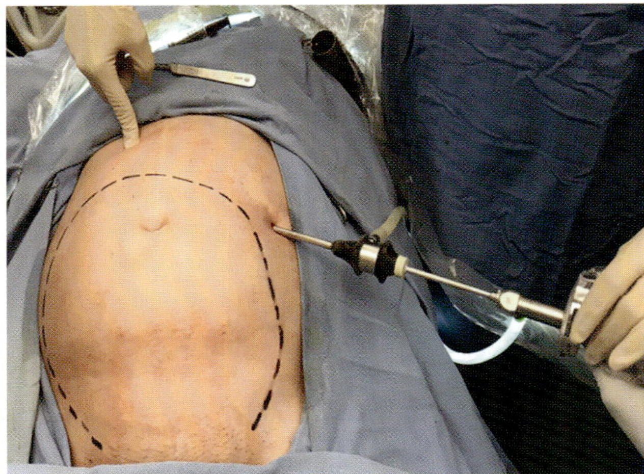

Fig. 12: Marking for 10 mm port, 1–2 cm to the right of the midline.

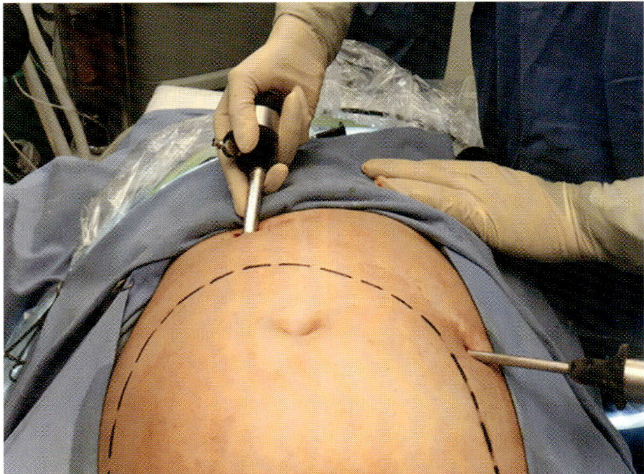

Fig. 13: Camera port (10 mm) insertion.

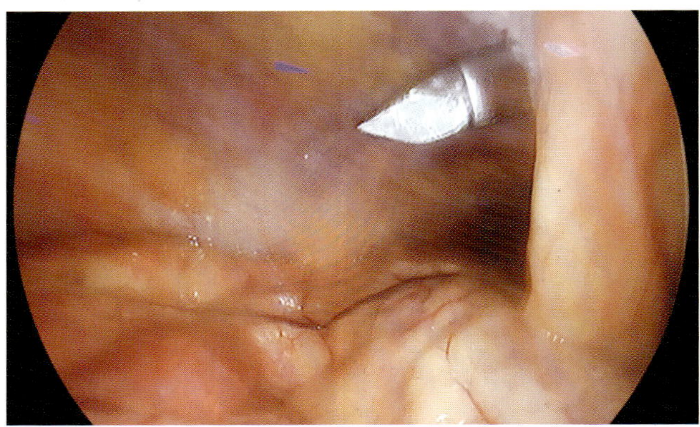

Fig. 14: Camera port inserted to avoid falciform ligament.

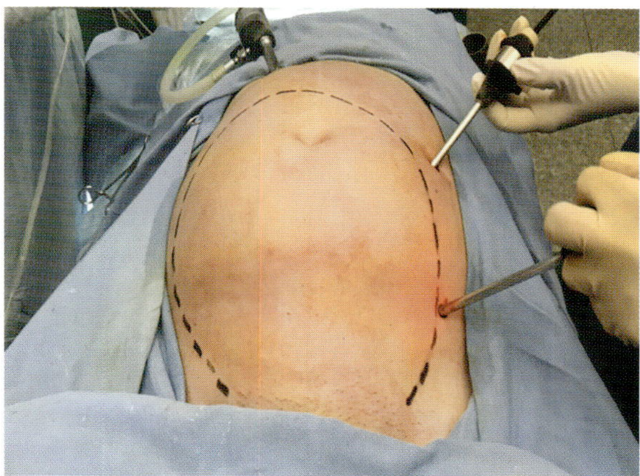

Fig. 15: Secondary port (5 mm) left lower quadrant.

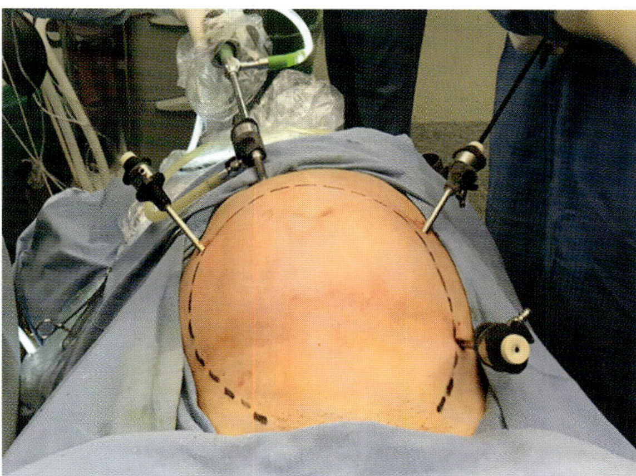

Fig. 16: 5 mm right side port paraumbilical in position for assistant surgeon.

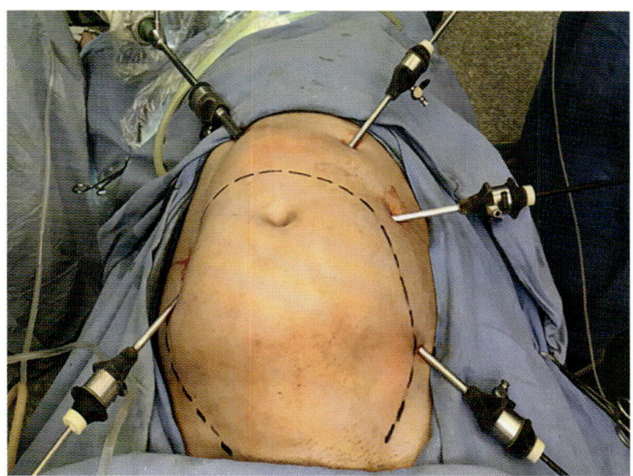

Fig. 17: Final port placement with the upper quadrant 5 mm working port on the left side becoming the upper working port and Jain point port is the lower working port.

again and again during maneuver of the instruments. This way Jain point port becomes the lower working port. This is relatively a newer way of port placement for pelvic pathologies but it works. Wonders for quicker ergonomic working for extralarge masses.

- This upper quadrant working port needs special mention as it is the one which reaches target area without hitting mass.

Laparoscopic Entry in Patients with Large Myomas

Large myomas can arise from anywhere uterus, cervix, and broad ligaments or they could be ovarian fibromas. Most frequently they arise from uterus leading to uterine enlargement. Entry through Jain point is better in these cases as we avoid hitting the myoma when we enter through a lateral point compared to umbilical one. Umbilical entry may hit the mass and initiate bleeding even before we begin the surgery. Safe entry through Jain point can be made making the myomectomy easy. Number, location, and size of myoma do not from a limitation for laparoscopic myomectomy for experienced surgeons.[5] The steps of myomectomy remain same. It is the entry and port placement, which needs to be mastered. If the ports are placed outside and above the mass, visualization becomes easy, incision can be marked accurately. Also higher port placement gives space for traction and manipulation of myoma with the screw and easier enucleation. Using our technique devised for large masses and very large masses, one can do all kinds of myomectomy without fearing the size and number of myomas **(Figs. 18 and 19)**.

Entry in Patients with Ovarian Cyst

Ovarian cysts have been classified into large if size is > 5 cm and giant/voluminous if > 15 cm. In America, 10% women need surgical procedure for ovarian cyst.[6] Large ovarian cysts are not uncommon in surgeons platter on a routine basis in today's era. Most common being endometriotic cyst,

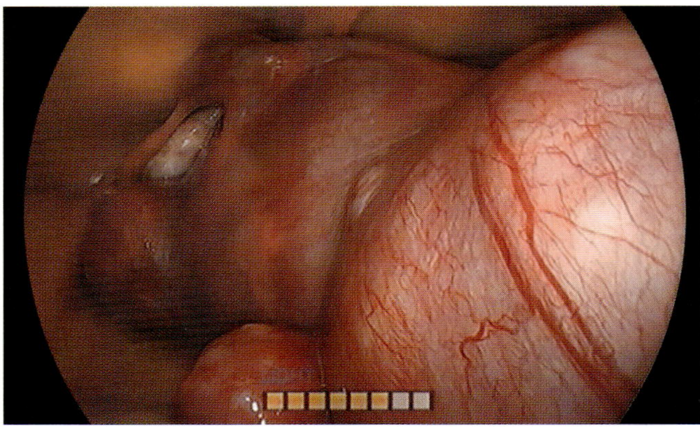

Fig. 18A: Multiple very large myomas (4 myomas of 11 × 10 cm and several other smaller ones).

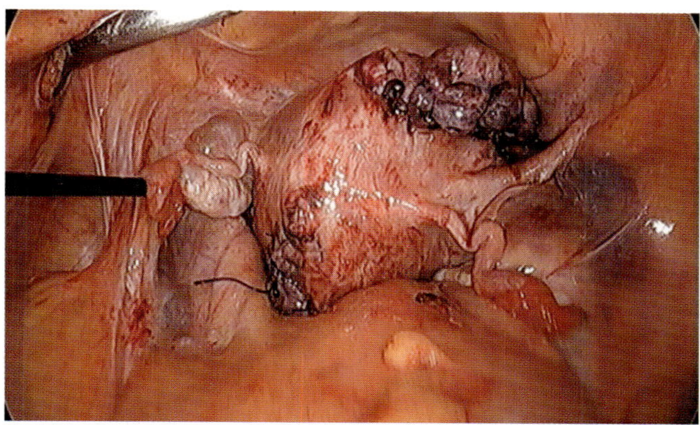

Fig. 18B: End result after removal of large masses. The suturing is carried out by the left side lower 5 mm port and Jain point port.

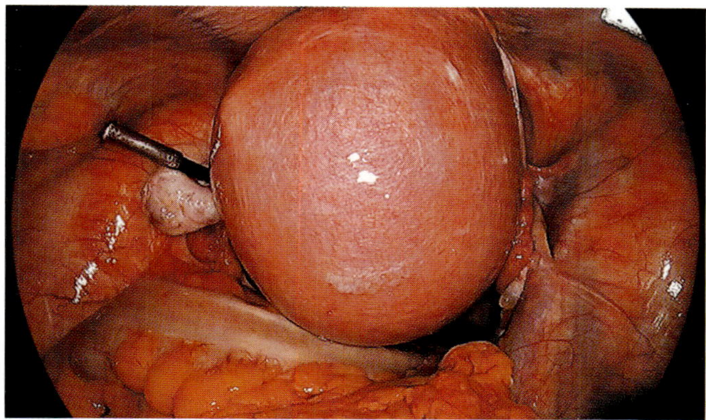

Fig. 19A: Big size fibroid uterus.

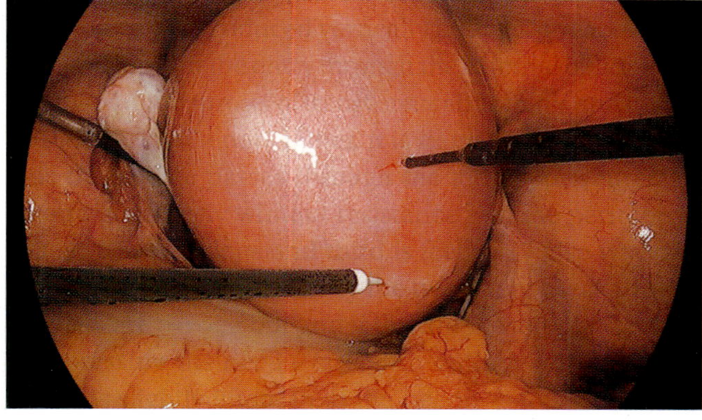

Fig. 19B: Diluted vasopressin injecting over the myoma.

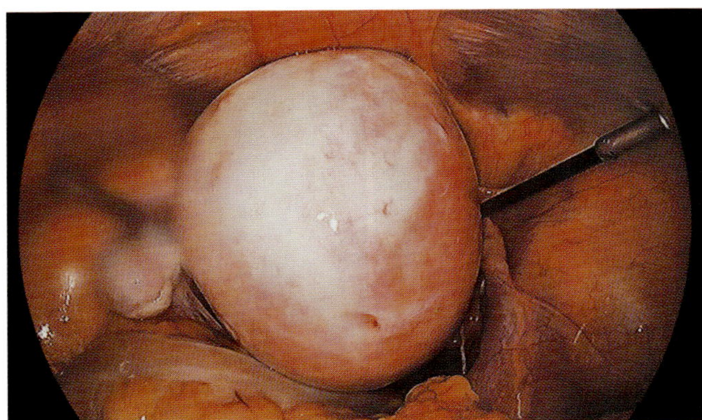

Fig. 19C: Uterus after injected diluted vasopressin.

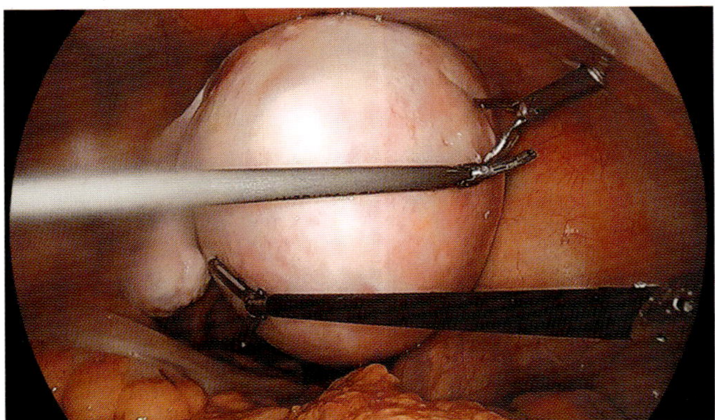

Fig. 19D: Incision over the myoma using harmonic ACE.

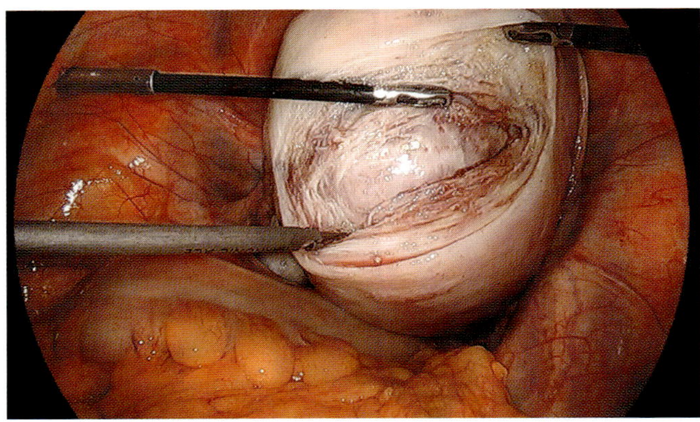

Fig. 19E: Transverse incision given.

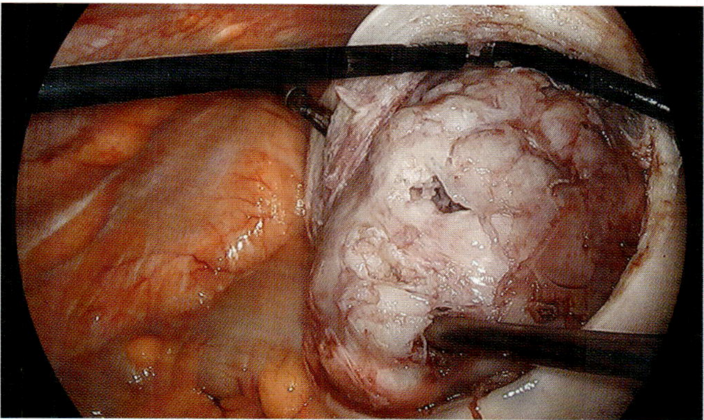

Fig. 19F: Enucleation of myoma.

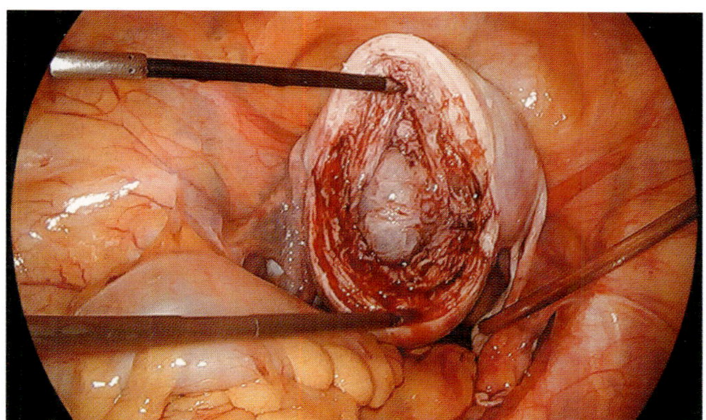

Fig. 19G: Intact cavity seen after enucleation of myoma.

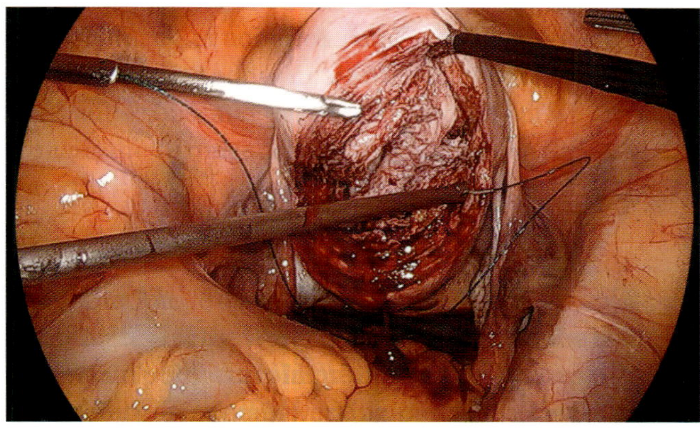

Fig. 19H: Suturing starting using V-LOC suture.

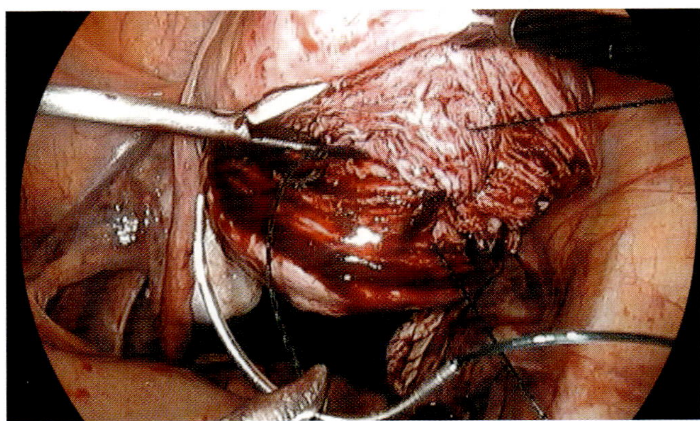

Fig. 19I: 2nd layer almost completed.

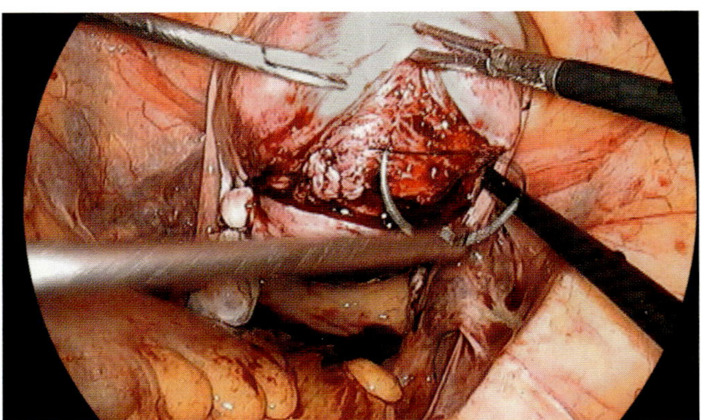

Fig. 19J: 2nd layer completed with V-LOC suture.

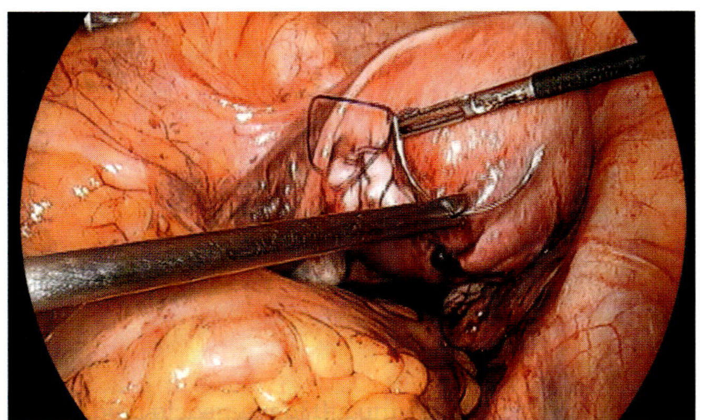

Fig. 19K: Upper layer closed with vicryl.

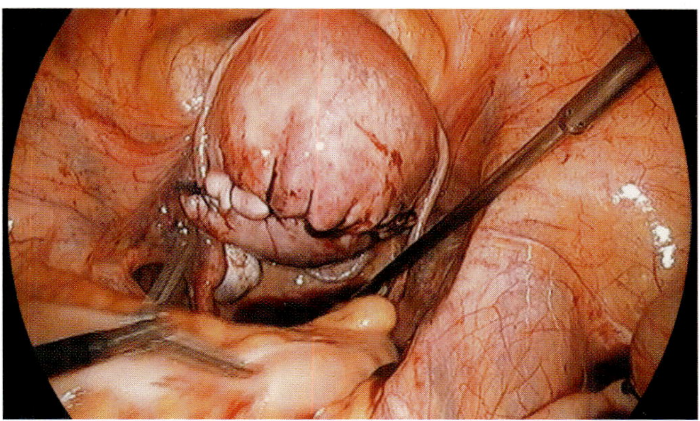

Fig. 19L: Nice appearance of myoma bed sutured.

dermoid cyst, simple cyst, paraovarian cyst, and dysgerminomas. Large cysts (all above level of umbilicus) have been managed laparoscopically without conversion to laparotomy and any complication. All cysts were benign in pathology with normal tumor marker profile and imaging. **Figures 20A to L** depict the steps of ovarian cystectomy in a large 23 cm dermoid cyst.[7]

About 90% ovarian cysts are benign. Freely mobile, smooth, and unilateral cyst with no ascites in young patients indicates benign nature of the disease.[8] Umbilical entry can lead to puncture of cyst and spillage of contents. Thus it can upgrade the tumor staging. Also initial picture cannot be appreciated if the entry itself punctured the cyst. Jain point entry avoids spillage thus it is advantageous over umbilical entry. If the cyst is left side, the first assistant can displace it sideways and safe entry can be made. Jain point is extremely helpful in cases of ovarian cyst as spillage of contents completely changes the case scenario and is the complication one wishes to avoid in such cases. With correct port placement size of cyst no more remains a limitation to laparoscopic surgeon. The ports again should be outside and above the cyst. This allows better visualization and enucleation of the cyst. For very large cyst, we can use the superior working port as described in previous page for large myomas.

Laparoscopic Entry Patients with Big Masses with Previous Surgeries

At our center, we see a lot of cases with previous one/two or multiple surgeries. Scarred abdomen is not uncommon **(Figs. 21 and 22)**. Umbilicus is found to have adhesions in 12% cases with past history of surgery (midline, paramedian, or lower abdominal).

Bowel or omentum or both could be adherent to the umbilicus.[9]

Jain point offers an adhesions free area in such cases. We commonly encounter transverse scars in lower abdomen or vertical paraumbilical scars **(Figs. 23 to 25)**. Mostly Jain point is free in such cases, also being an adhesion

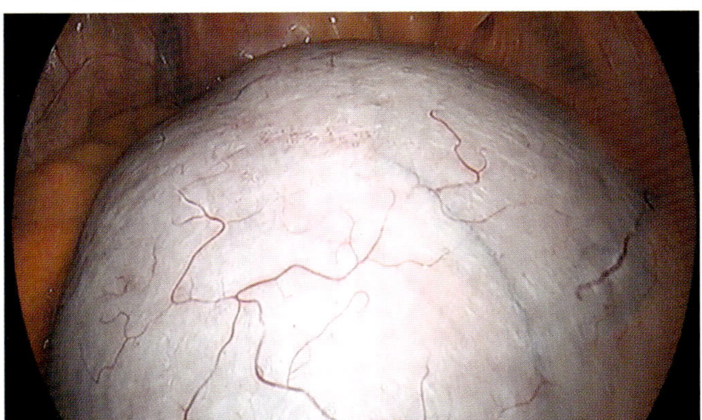

Fig. 20A: Initial appearance of 23 cm huge dermoid cyst.

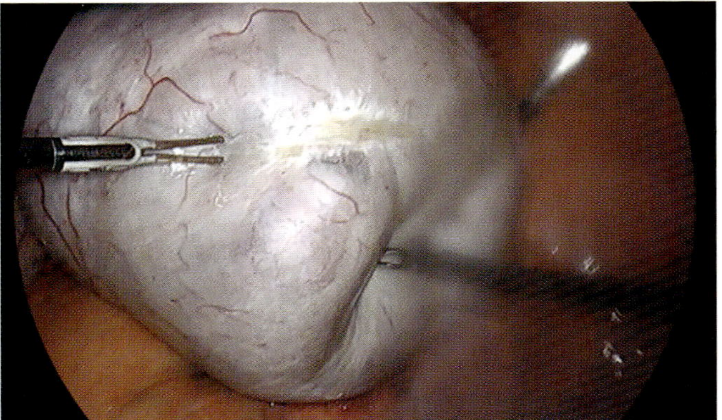

Fig. 20B: Demarcating the proposed line of incision by bipolar cautery.

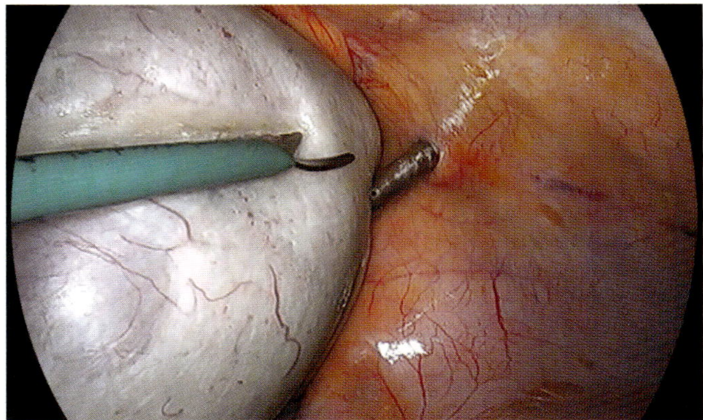

Fig. 20C: Making the initial cut to reach a good plane of cleavage.

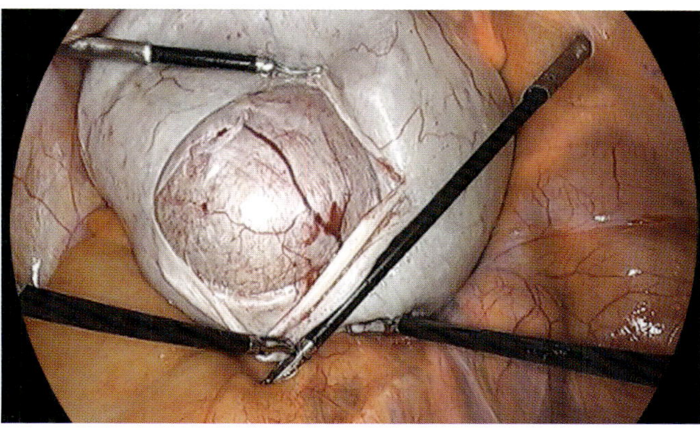

Fig. 20D: Starting enucleation.

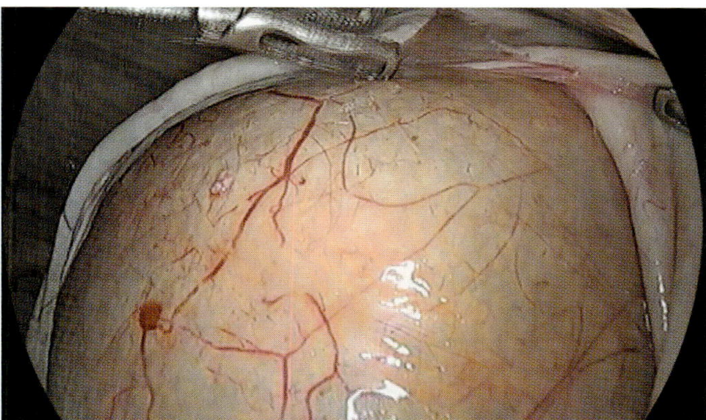

Fig. 20E: Enucleation in progress of the huge dermoid cyst avoiding spillage.

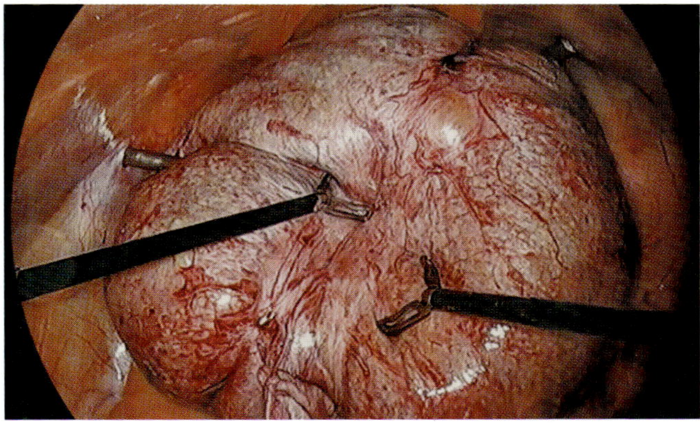

Fig. 20F: Preparing to put the enucleated cyst in endobag.

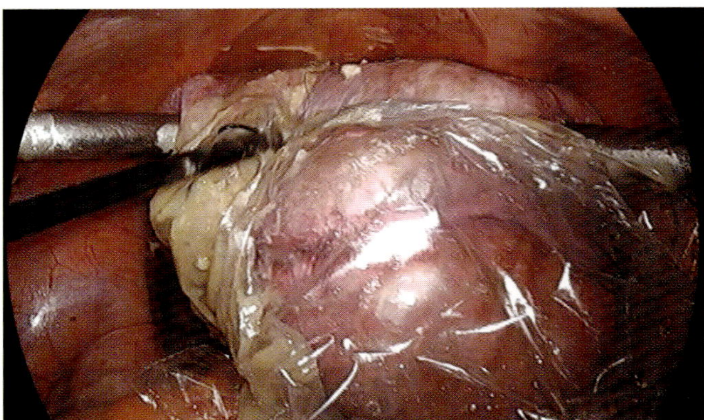

Fig. 20G: Finally putting the cyst in endobag.

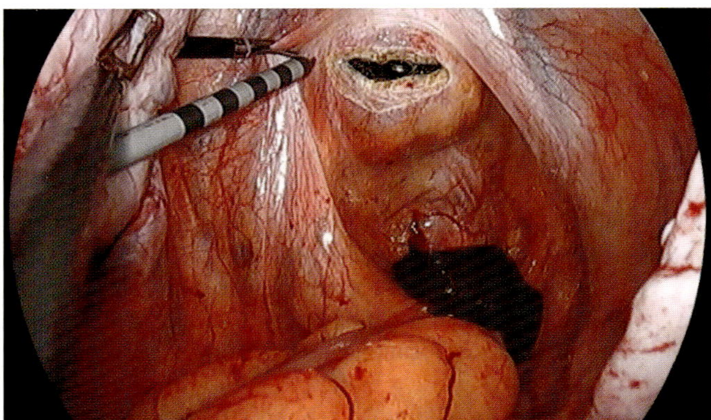

Fig. 20H: Making a colpotomy over the CCL extractor.

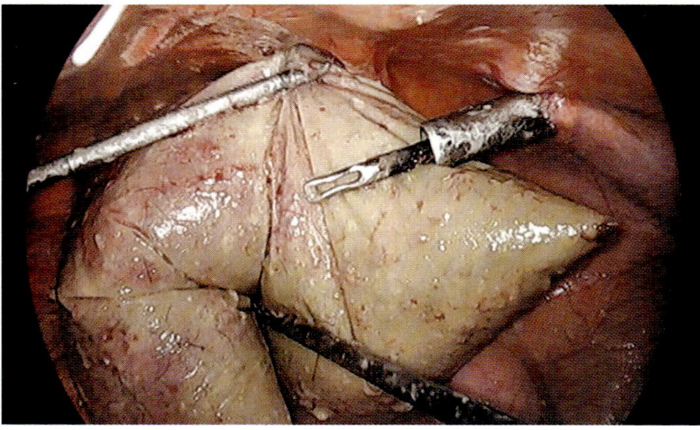

Fig. 20I: The endobag brought out of the vagina and cyst contents evacuated.

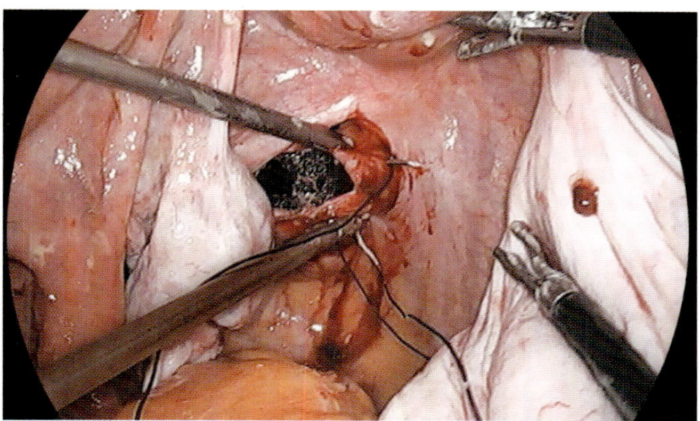

Fig. 20J: Colpotomy closure done with 1.0 vicryl.

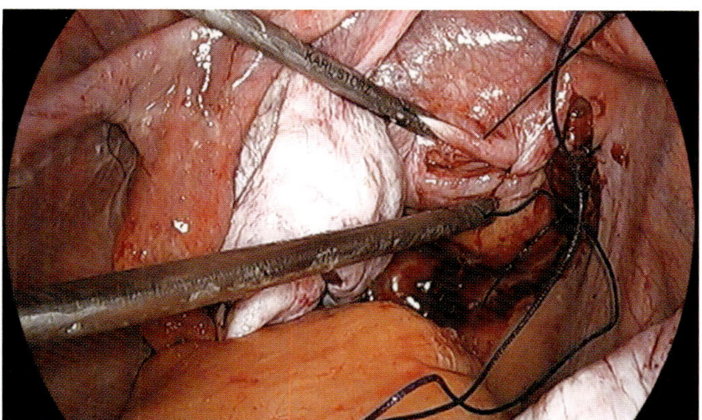

Fig. 20K: 2nd layer closure done.

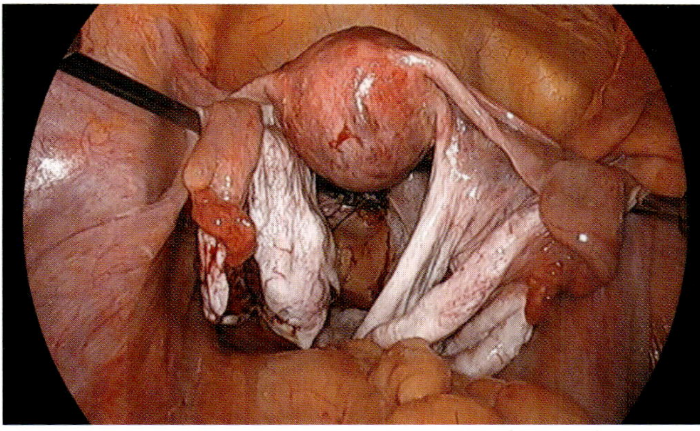

Fig. 20L: Final view at end.

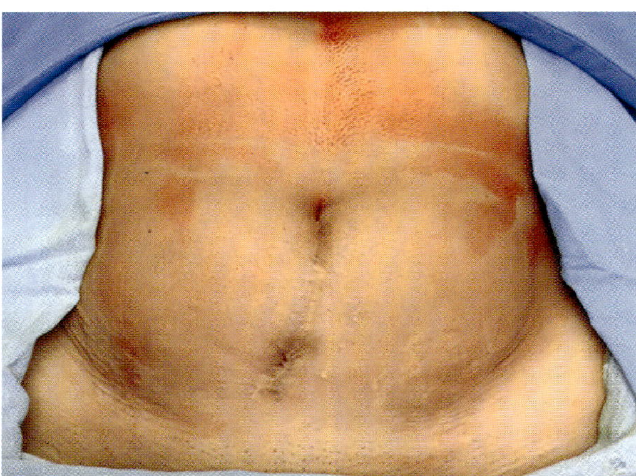

Fig. 21: Previous one surgery with large mass (vertical scar).

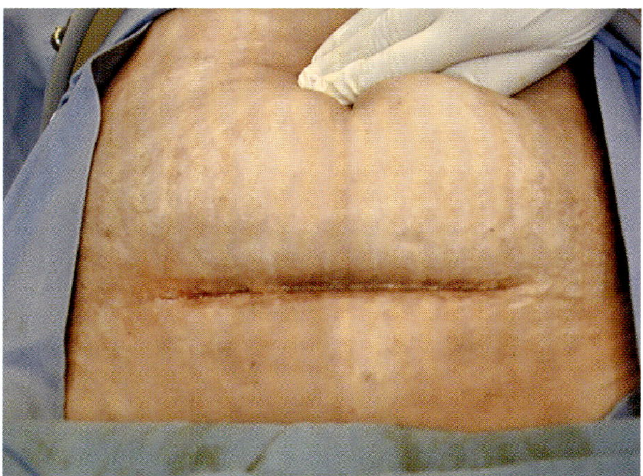

Fig. 22: Large mass with transverse scar.

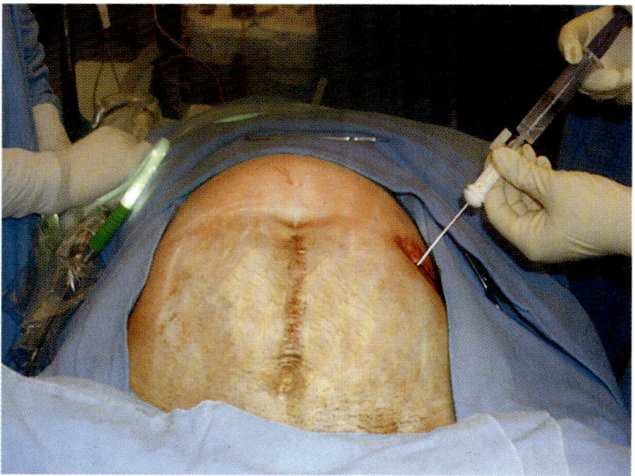

Fig. 23: Veress insertion in patient with large mass with vertical scar.

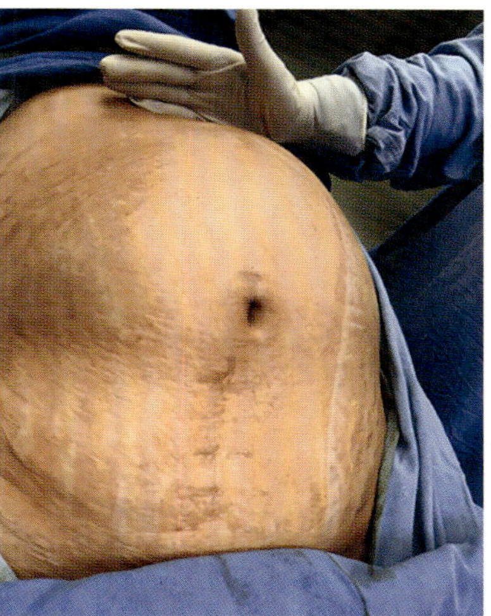

Fig. 24: Very large mass with vertical scar.

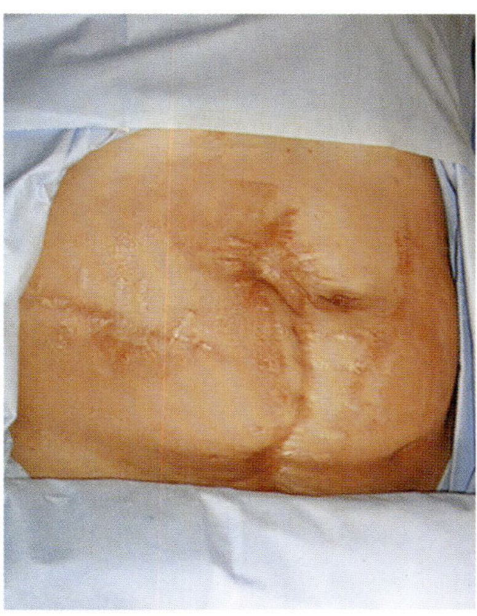

Fig. 25: Large mass in patient with multiple scars.

free area, it offers safe entry. Major complications can be prevented, if a safe entry is made in such cases **(Fig. 26)**. After inserting primary port, we insert secondary port and ensure the safety of primary port with correct placement of ports, gradual adhesiolysis can be done and these surgeries can be carried on in the same manner as patients with large pelvic masses.

Laparoscopic Entry in Patients with Large Uterine Size

Uterine enlargement due to myoma and adenomyosis is commonly seen in laparoscopic surgeries. Entry through umbilicus can directly hit the uterus and initiate bleeding. Jain point entry avoids hitting the uterus. Also, uterus can be

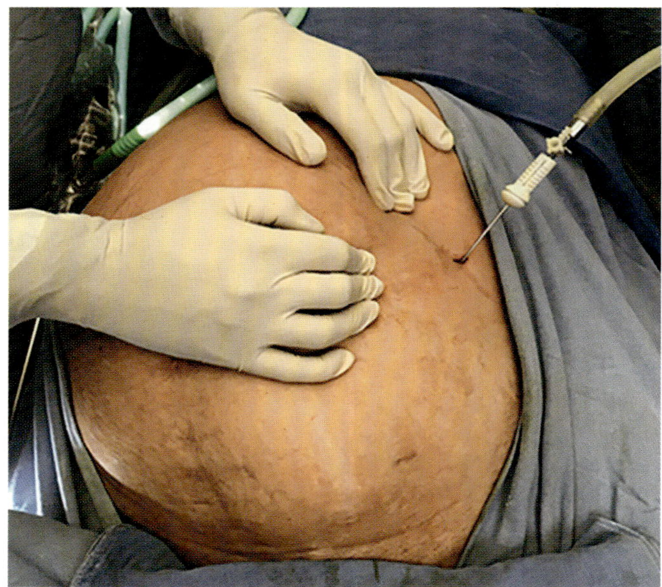

Fig. 26: Veress insertion by displacing the mass medially.

displaced sideways by assistant, and then the 10 mm port optimized to give good vision and ergonomic working through the course of a longer surgery, as it could be in large masses.

CONCLUSION

Jain point is a safe point of entry. It offers various advantages over other points of entry. Being laterally placed, there are minimum chances of hitting the mass and avoids bleeding. There are very little chances of puncturing the cyst and thus no upstaging of the tumor grade or spillage of the ovarian contents. Being ergonomically correct, it offers better working with good vision all through the surgery. It is easily duplicable by fellows, trainees, and new aspirants of laparoscopic surgery, as there are minimum risks of complications (vascular, visceral, and retroperitoneal bleeding).

Evolution of Jain point has made laparoscopic entry safe not only in routine surgery but in patients with large pelvic masses also. Size is no more a limit to minimally invasive surgery—reaching beyond the boundaries.

LEARNING POINTS

- Masses can be large (<30 weeks) or very large (>30 weeks).
- Jain point is easy entry point for both categories of large masses.
- Assistant can displace the mass with both hands if mass is on the left side.
- Minimal chances of ovarian cyst spillage with entry at Jain point.

- Minimal chances of hitting the fibroid by first blind port.
- Port placement should be above and outside the mass for easy operability of mass.
- For very large masses, camera port should go high up in epigastrium. Another secondary port could be placed above the Jain point on left side, under vision.
- Jain point is easy, duplicable and safe in patients with large/very large pelvic masses.

REFERENCES

1. Szklaruk J, Tamm EP, Choi H, et al. MR imaging of common and uncommon large pelvic masses. Radiographics. 2003;23(2):403-24.
2. Jansen FW, Kapiteyn K, Trimbos-Kemper T, et al. Complications of laparoscopy: a prospective multicentre observational study. Br J Obstet Gynaecol. 1997;104:595-600.
3. Jansen FW, Kolkman W, Bakkum EA, et al. Complications of laparoscopy: an inquiry about closed versus open-entry technique. Am J Obstet Gynecol. 2004;190:634-8.
4. Vilos GA. The ABCs of a safer laparoscopic entry. J Minim Invasive Gynecol. 2006;13:249-51.
5. Sinha R, Hegde A, Mahajan C, et al. Laparoscopic myomectomy: do size, number, and location of the myomas form limiting factors for laparoscopic myomectomy? J Minim Invasive Gynecol. 2008;15:292-300.
6. Hilger WS, Magrina JF, Magtibay PM. Laparoscopic management of the adnexal mass. Clin Obstetr Gynecol. 2006;49(3):535-48.
7. Salem HA. Laparoscopic excision of large ovarian cysts. J Obstet Gynaecol Res. 2002;28:290-4.
8. Sanfilippo JS, Rock JA. Surgery for benign diseases of the ovary. In: Rock JA, Jones HW 3rd (Eds). Te Linde's Operative Gynecology, 9th edition. Philadelphia: Lippincott Williams and Wilkins; 2003. pp. 639-59.
9. Toro A, Mannino M, Cappello G, et al. Comparison of two entry methods for laparoscopic port entry: technical point of view. Diagn Ther Endosc. 2012;2012:305428.

Jain Point in Genital Tuberculosis

Nutan Jain, Sonil Srivastava, Anshu Gupta

INTRODUCTION

Genital tuberculosis is a common problem in the developing world. Incidence of genital tuberculosis is directly related to prevalence of pulmonary tuberculosis in that region. *Mycobacterium tuberculosis* has been identified as the etiological agent of tuberculosis for many years. Genital tuberculosis is an important cause of infertility, and thereby many of these cases present for laparoscopic surgery. Laparoscopic entry in genital tuberculosis poses definite challenges. The different forms of disease pose the challenge that adhesions could be seen not only around the umbilicus but also depending upon the severity of the disease, could be involving whole of the *abdomen, upper abdomen or in the pelvis only*.

CLINICAL PRESENTATION

The problem with genital tuberculosis is that usually it remains undiagnosed in the early to moderate forms until and unless the advancing disease presents with signs and symptoms which are picked up on imaging, which could be ultrasound, or magnetic resonance imaging (MRI). Usually these patients do not complain of pain, so the diagnosis is made rather late. Most of the time, the diagnosis is made during the course of an infertility evaluation. These patients may present primarily with blocked fallopian tubes. They could present as encysted masses, slightly solid isoechoic masses, which could be because of caseous material collection which we call as caseoma. Other findings which we see could be dilated trumpet shaped, or coma-shaped hydrosalpinx, tubo-ovarian mass, and encysted collections **(Figs. 1A to E)**.

The findings on ultrasound in the uterine cavity could be jagged or irregular calcified endometrium. In more severe cases we could have pictures compatible with Asherman's syndrome. Once diagnosis of genital tuberculosis is optimized these patients are taken up for laparoscopy. Some important features to keep in mind when laparoscopy is being done.

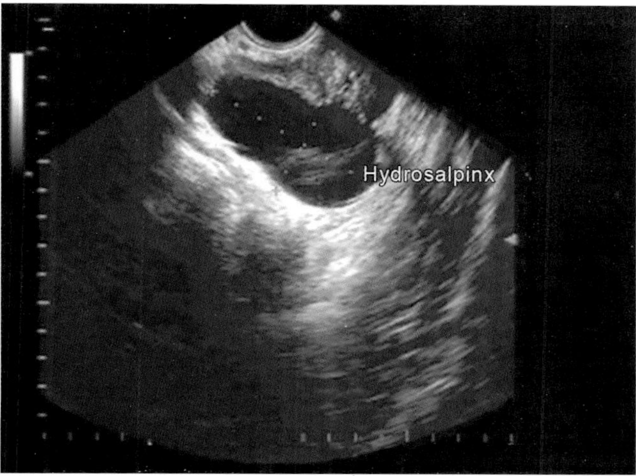

Fig. 1A: Hydrosalpinx.

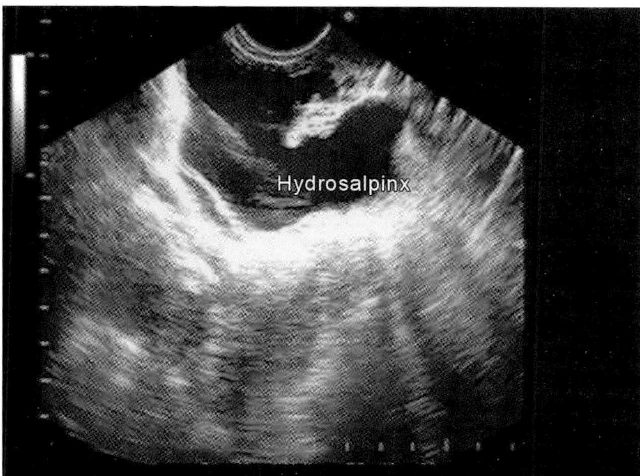

Fig. 1B: Dilated hydrosalpinx.

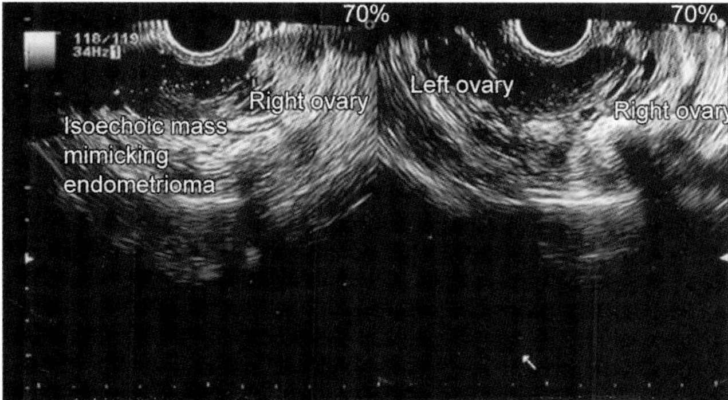

Fig. 1C: Solid isoechoic mass.

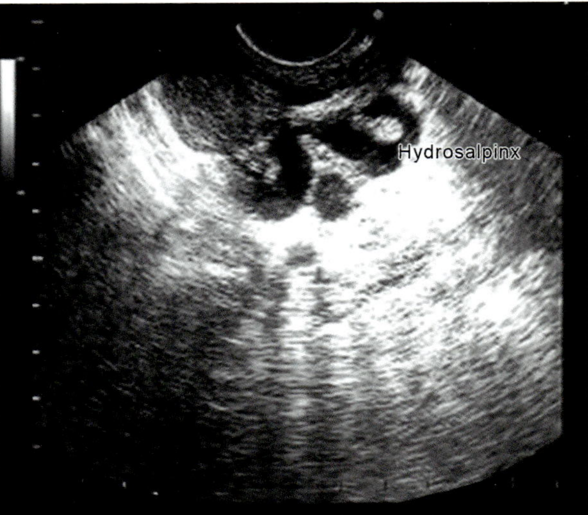

Fig. 1D: Tubo-ovarian mass.

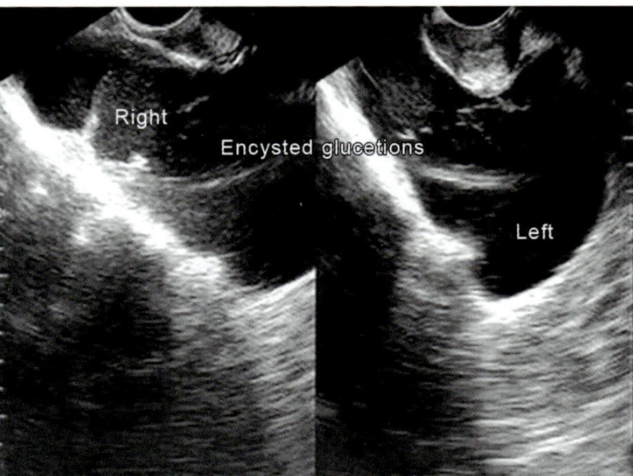

Fig. 1E: Encysted collection.

TECHNIQUE OF LAPAROSCOPIC ENTRY

In laparoscopic entry we have to keep in mind that many of these cases have had a previous surgery in childhood, in adolescence or anytime in life. If they have abdominogenital tuberculosis it may lead to intestinal obstruction. Usually the obstruction is subacute intestinal obstruction and if it leads to complete obstruction these patients might have had a complete laparotomy. In these laparotomies usually the scars are big, extending from lower abdomen going right up to the upper abdomen and they are usually long midline vertical scars **(Figs. 2A to F)**. So, the surgeon needs to be careful to optimize the port of entry where in the chances of getting into the bowel are least. As, we have

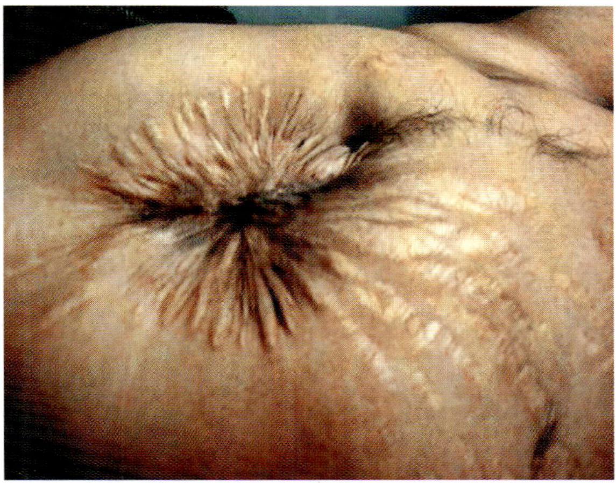

Fig. 2A: Previous surgery done for septicemia.

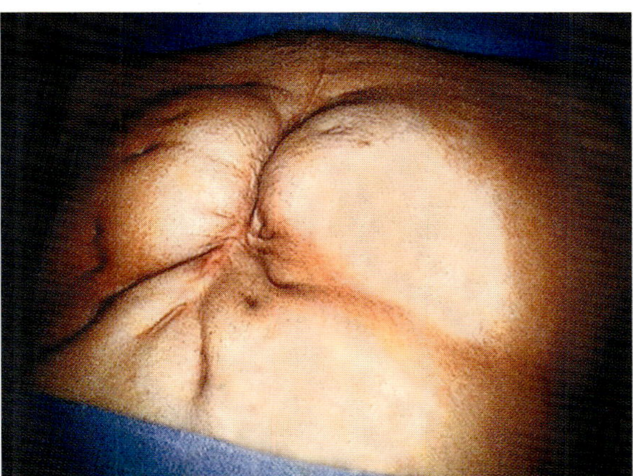

Fig. 2B: Previous surgeries for intestinal obstruction with colostomy.

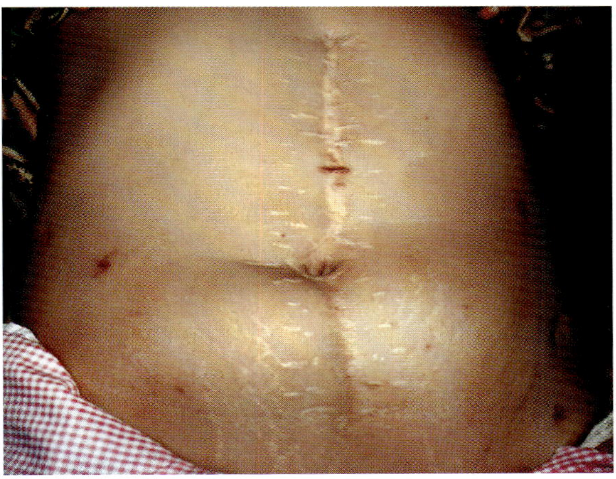

Fig. 2C: Big vertical long scar over the abdomen.

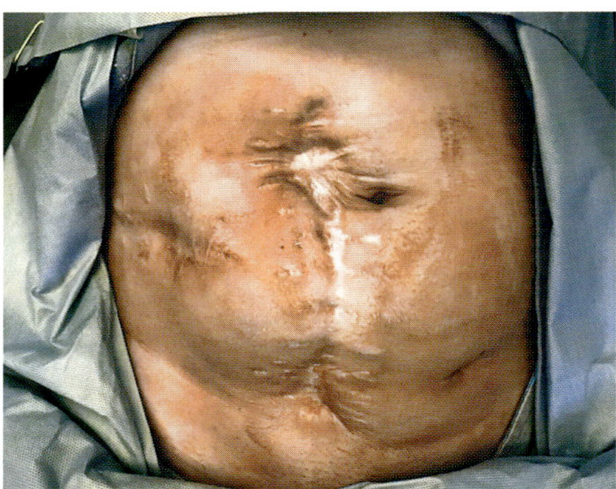

Fig. 2D: Patient had septicemia after previous laparotomy. Then multiple surgeries were done for colostomy and then colostomy closure.

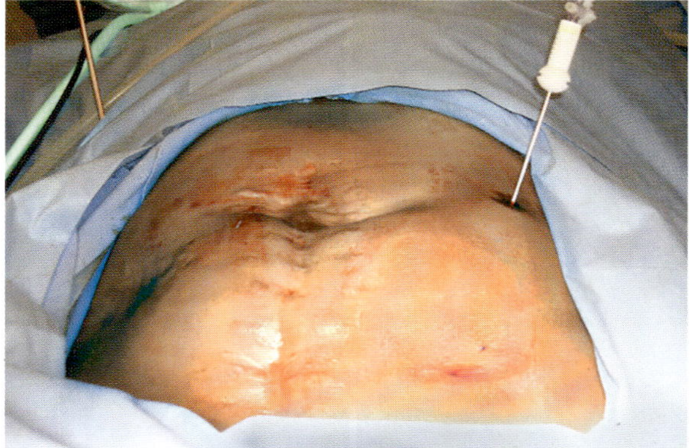

Fig. 2E: Veress needle at Jain point.

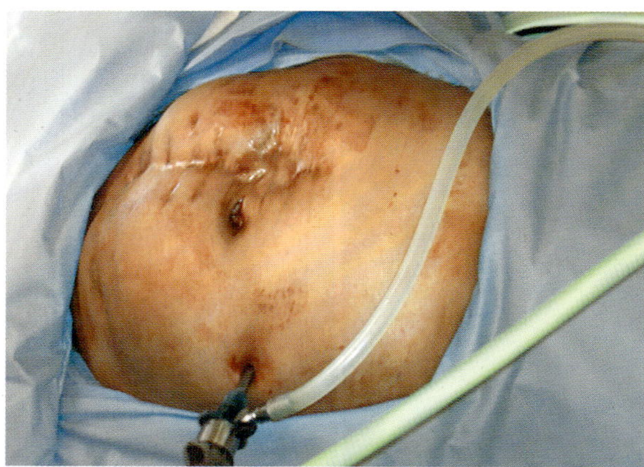

Fig. 2F: A 5 mm trocar inserted at Jain point.

a large practice of infertility patients so laparoscopic entry in such cases is quite a routine at our center. Gradually working with this subset of patients and working with Jain point entry we found that the left paraumbilical lateral port position of the Jain point favors positively while making an entry that is usually found to be free of adhesions. We have not encountered bowel entries in large number of patients who have presented with genital tuberculosis. Those patients who do not have previous surgery and have past history of tuberculosis and now need a laparoscopy, in such cases also we have to correlate the ultrasound and clinical findings with anticipated problems on laparoscopic entry.

If a patient has only dilated tubes and uterus appears to be free, this type of entry usually may not have adhesions in the mid and the upper abdomen, so the laparoscopic entry does not pose a specific challenge. The other subset of patients, who have big tubo-ovarian masses or encysted fluid collections, these patients usually have adhesions around the umbilicus and in the upper abdomen, and also over the liver which mimics the findings of a *Fitz-Hugh–Curtis syndrome.* So in these cases where in bowel loops could be plastered all over the abdominal wall or omentum is spread like a sheet over the abdominal wall, or there could be multiple loops of bowel hanging from the anterior abdominal wall **(Figs. 3A to F)**. So these are the very typical cases where in we have found repeatedly with our experience that laparoscopic entry by the Jain point port, which is much lateral and in the mid abdomen. So it avoids the adhesions which are in the pelvis and in the upper abdomen or around the umbilicus, sparing the area on the left side where we have positioned the Jain point.

To begin the laparoscopic entry we first clearly demarcate the Jain point surface anatomy. Then we make a small stab incision, first we enter with the Veress needle and then when we check that the pressure settings are normal,

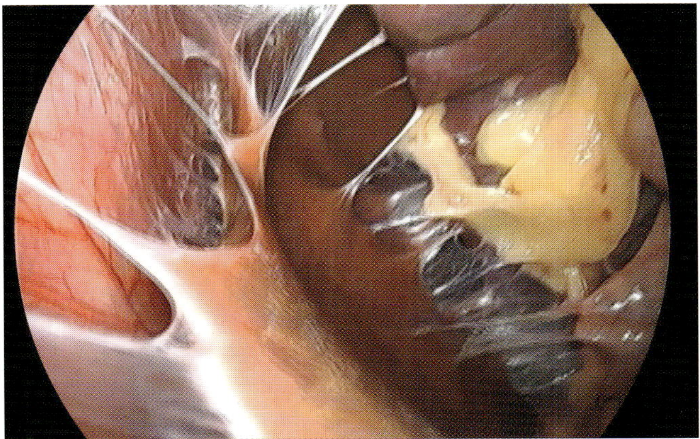

Fig. 3A: Adhesions between gallbladder and liver.

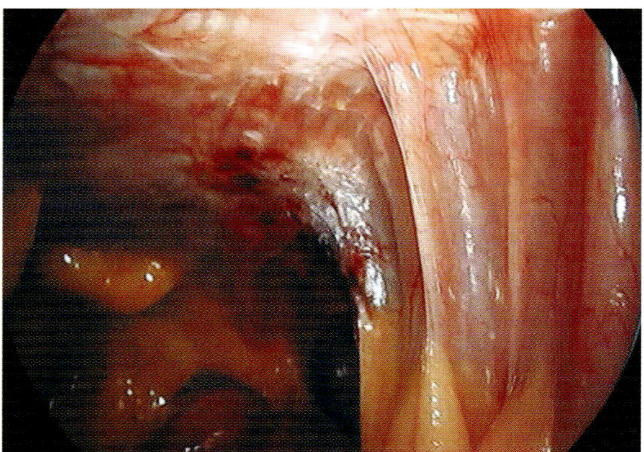

Fig. 3B: Multiple bowel loops at umbilicus.

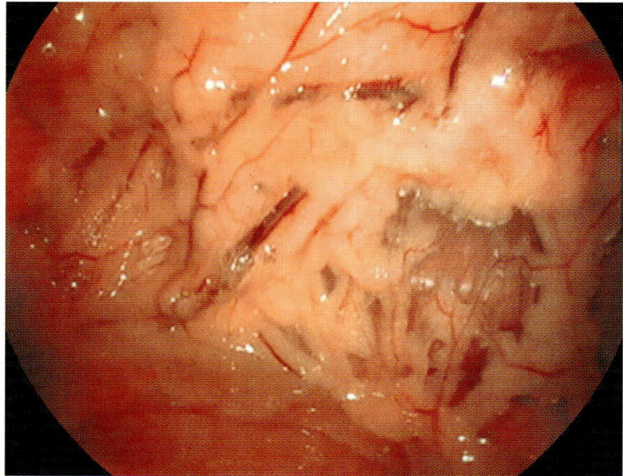

Fig. 3C: Dense omental adhesions covering the entire abdomen.

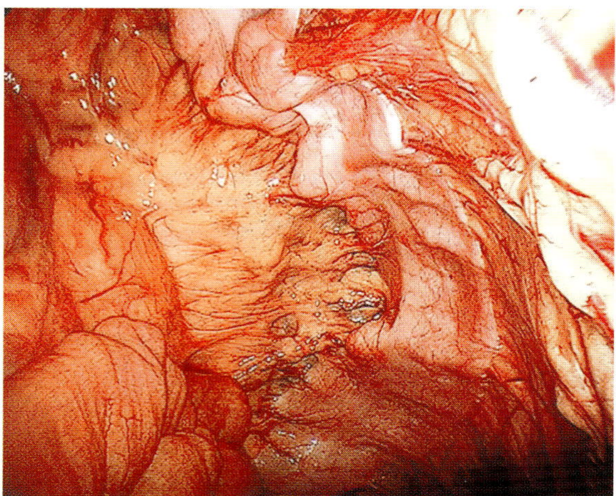

Fig. 3D: Multiple bowel loops stuck everywhere.

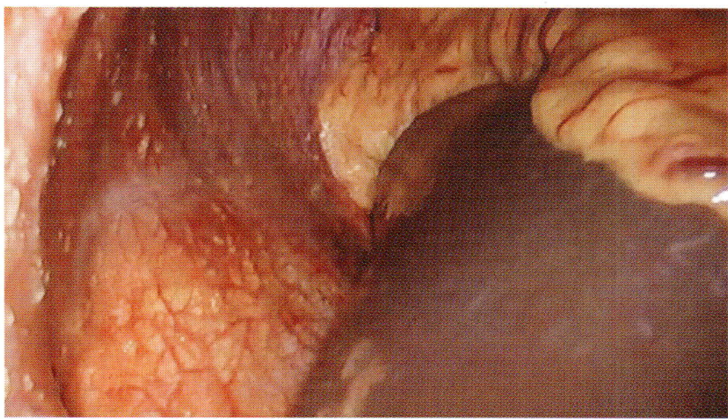

Fig. 3E: Multiple caseoma noted.

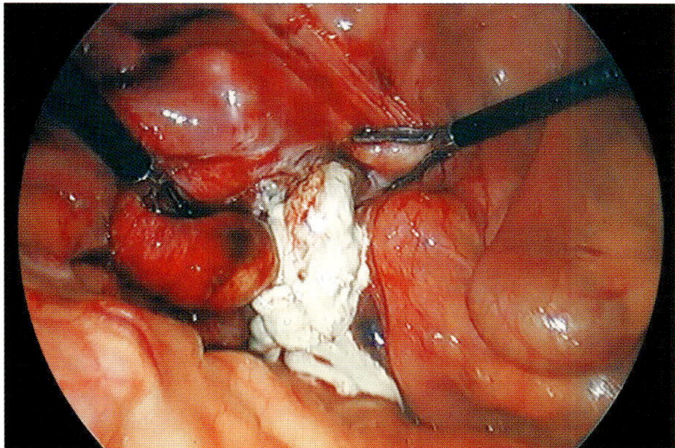

Fig. 3F: Copious amount of caseous material drained.

then we go ahead by making 5 mm trocar blind entry. It is again connected to the CO_2, and we make a complete check of the total situation inside the abdominal cavity taking into account adhesions at the mid abdomen, right side of abdomen and the upper abdomen, liver, and gallbladder. Many a times we find that the gallbladder is almost stuck to the anterior abdominal wall with the adhesions of tuberculosis. We can also find generalized tubercles all over the abdominal wall, or we find multiple caseous balls hanging from the anterior abdominal wall all over the abdomen and pelvis. So, after noting these findings we optimize the 10 mm port avoiding the bowel and omental adhesions. Many a times after making entry with the Jain point we find that it is totally frozen pelvis and no further progress can be made and that is the time when we have to abandoned the procedure and start the patient on antitubercular medicines. In this situations the telescope is very carefully removed layer by layer to reconfirm no bowel injury has been sustained.

Rationale of Jain point in genital tuberculosis lies in the fact that abdominogenital tuberculosis is usually confined at the ileocecal junction, which is on the right side, and the adhesions are primarily in the pelvis. In genital tuberculosis adhesions could be according to severity of disease and in the upper abdomen involving the liver between the liver and diaphragm. Whenever there is diffuse tuberculosis, the bowel loops and omentum are stuck around the umbilicus and anterior abdominal wall. So, umbilicus may not at all be a good point of entry in suspected case of genital tuberculosis. Our experience of these cases over a long period have consistently shown that entry in case of genital tuberculosis has been made safely by the use of Jain point as the first primary nonumbilical port. The first 10 mm port and other ports are then made at the optimum point according to the mandate of the case. It is very important to immediately check the Jain point port after putting the 10 mm port, to see that it is free of bowel. At times, the Jain point port could be coming through the omentum curtains when the omentum is totally covering the whole of the abdominal wall. At that time trocar may come through a curtain of omentum but this curtain of omentum entry does not bleed and has no sequelae during the course of surgery or during recovery and later on. We have consistently seen that the entry of trocar through omentum does not cause any bleeding or any other deleterious effect. So, this has to be borne in the mind that in cases where whole of the omentum is covering the abdominal wall, the entry cannot be made without coming through omentum, and that is quite a routine finding in cases of advanced tuberculosis.

Encysted Collections

Many a times, tubercular straw color fluid collections are noted in the pelvis in between the adnexal structures and back surface of uterus. They usually tend to be covered with rectosigmoid and bowel adhesions. Difficult adhesiolysis has to be carried out and all collections drained and tissue taken for biopsy. Fluid is subjected to cytological evaluation. Laparoscopy is an ideal route of surgical correlation and patients to be followed by regular medical treatment for Koch's.

Tubercular Cold Abscess

Presents on sonography as hypoechoic masses and patients present with low grade fever, vague symptoms, infertility, pelvic pain or intestinal obstruction. Patient's laparoscopic entry is usually challenging. In the surgical procedure careful adhesiolysis is carried out between adnexa, rectosigmoid, and back surface of uterus. It is very important to keep in mind that adhesiolysis in Koch's is very tricky as injury to bowel occurs very readily in contrast to endometriosis, where there is so much of fibrosis. After all purulent collection of cold abscess is drained **(Figs. 4A to F)** a pelvic drain is inserted from the left lower port for 24 hours. Postoperatively the patient is carefully followed for return of bowel sound. Pus is sent for culture but usually is sterile. Follow-up of patient with anti-Koch's treatment is mandatory.

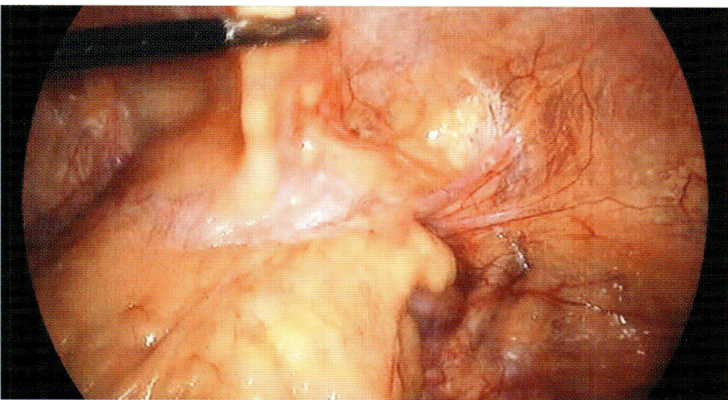

Fig. 4A: Initial appearance of pelvis, uterus tubes and ovaries not visualized.

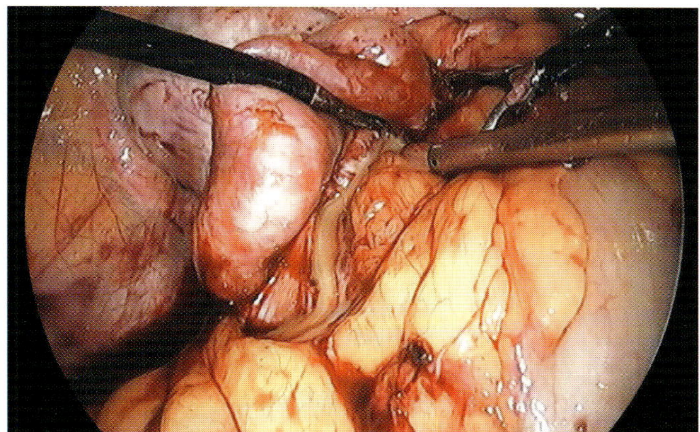

Fig. 4B: Pus coming out on adhesiolysis.

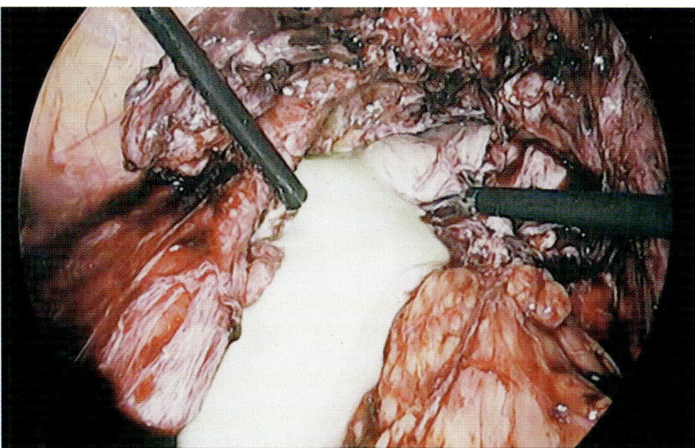

Fig. 4C: Copious amount of pus coming out from tubercular pyosalpinx.

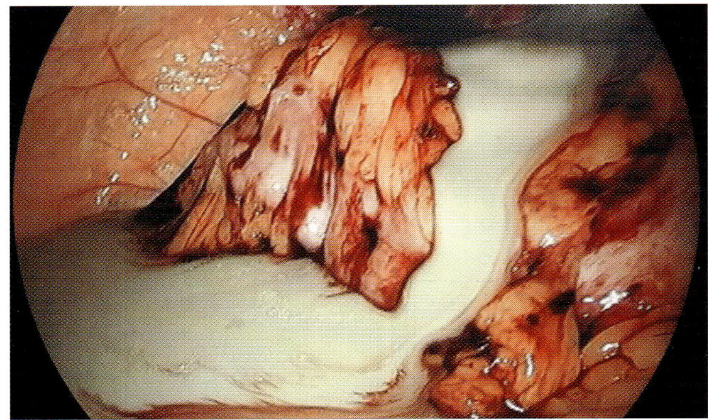

Fig. 4D: Copious amount of pus collected in pouch of Douglas.

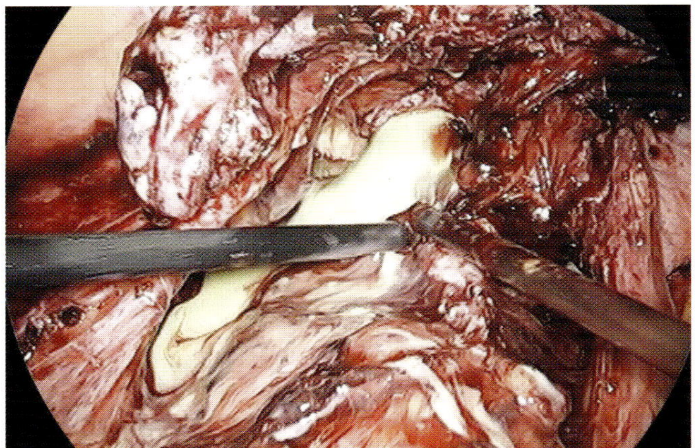

Fig. 4E: Pus drained from pouch of Douglas.

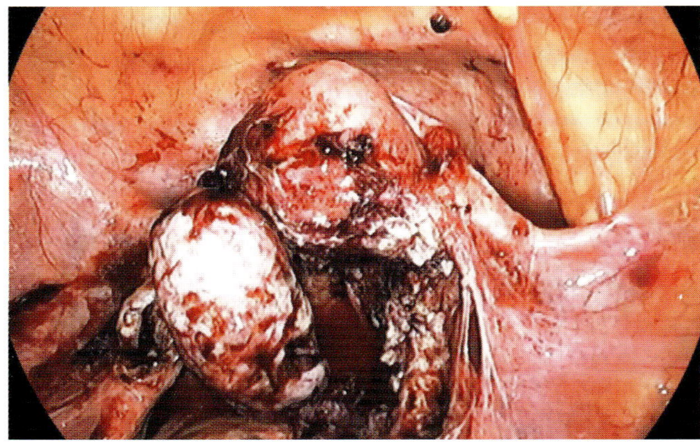

Fig. 4F: Pelvis at end.

LEARNING POINTS

- Optimize the case history with ultrasound findings.
- Thorough history of previous surgery or medical treatment for Koch's.
- Bowel preparation to be kept thorough in cases of advanced anticipated Koch's.
- Insert all ports under vision of Jain point port and also remove all ports under laparoscopic vision.
- Entry through omentum does not alter the course of surgery and postoperative recovery.
- Postoperative AKT to be charted out according to body weight, severity of disease and whether patient has already received previous AKT.

SUGGESTED READING

1. Chimote RA, Chimote A, Chipotle IN. Genital tuberculosis and infertility in Indian population. In: Studd J, Tan SL, Chervenak FA (Eds). Current Progress in Obstetrics and Gynaecology, 1st edition. Mumbai: True-Life India; 2017. pp. 205-28.
2. Goel G, Khatuja R, Radhakrishnan G, et al. Role of newer methods of diagnosing genital tuberculosis in infertile women. Indian J Pathol Microbiol. 2013;56:155-7.
3. Grace GA, Devaleenal DB, Natrajan M. Genital tuberculosis in females. Indian J Med Res. 2017;145:425-36.
4. Gupta N, Sharma JB, Mittal S, et al. Genital tuberculosis in Indian infertility patients. Int J Gynecol Obstet. 2007;97:135-8.
5. Jahromi BN, Parsanezhad ME, Ghane-Shirazi R. Female genital tuberculosis and infertility. Int J Gynaecol Obstet. 2001;75(3):269-72.
6. Mala YM, Prasad R, Singh N, et al. Role of laparoscopy in diagnosing genital tuberculosis in suspected women: A cross-sectional study from a tertiary care hospital in Northern India. Indian J Tuberc. 2018;65(1):23-9.
7. Sharma JB, Mohanraj P, Jain SK, et al. Surgical complications during laparotomy in patients with abdominopelvic tuberculosis. Int J Gynaecol Obstet. 2010;110:157-8.
8. Sharma JB, Roy KK, Pushparaj M, et al. Increased difficulties and complications encountered during hysteroscopy in women with genital tuberculosis. J Minim Invasive Gynecol. 2011;18:660-5.
9. Sharma JB, Roy KK, Pushparaj M, et al. Laparoscopic findings in female genital tuberculosis. Arch Gynecol Obstet. 2008;278:359-64.
10. Sharma JB, Sneha J, Singh UB, et al. Comparative study of laparoscopic abdominopelvic and fallopian tube findings before and after antitubercular therapy in female genital tuberculosis with infertility. J Minim Invasive Gynecol. 2016;23:215-22.

Jain Point in Upper Abdomen Scar

Chetna Agarwal, Nutan Jain, Priyanka Bansal

INTRODUCTION

In recent era, laparoscopy is being increasingly performed with great benefits for more complicated procedures with each passing day.

However, major challenge lies in entry technique. The overall incidence of major injuries at the time of entry is 1.1/1,000.[1] Bowel injuries have occurred in 0.7/1,000 laparoscopies[1] and major vascular injuries in 0.4/1,000 laparoscopies.[1] Despite considerable advances in endoscopic techniques and instrumentation, inadvertent and potentially avoidable entry injuries continue to occur.

Laparoscopic entry by left upper abdomen (i.e. Palmer's point) or the middle upper abdomen (i.e. Lee-Huang point) could be considered in patients with suspected periumbilical adhesions, history of umbilical hernia or previous three failed attempts of insufflations through umbilicus.

PALMER'S POINT (LEFT UPPER QUADRANT)

- Palmer's Point was developed by Raoul Palmer in 1974.
- It lies 3 cm below subcostal margin in midclavicular line.

Advantages

It can be used in:
- Previous laparotomy cases
- Obese patients
- Very thin patients.

Disadvantages (Limitations)

- Previous splenic or gastric surgery
- Previous upper abdomen surgery

- Hepatosplenomegaly
- Portal hypertension
- Gastropancreatic mass
- Improper nasogastric tube placement.

LEE-HUANG POINT (MIDDLE UPPER ABDOMEN POINT)

Lee-Huang point lies midway between the xiphoid process and the umbilicus.

Advantages

It can be used in:
- Gynecological malignancies
- Large pelvic pathologies.

Disadvantages (Limitations)

- A previous midline vertical incision
- Hepatomegaly and splenomegaly
- Intestinal obstruction.

MODE OF ENTRY IN PREVIOUS UPPER ABDOMEN LAPAROTOMY CASES

In cases like previous gastric surgery, pancreatoduodenal mass, portal hypertension, hepatomegaly or splenomegaly, or any hepatic surgery, we can neither use Palmer's point nor ninth intercostal space and the Lee-Huang entry point because they lie in the upper quadrant of the abdomen, and, therefore, concern for upper abdomen adhesions remains. In these cases, Jain point offers benefit because of its anatomic rationale.

JAIN POINT

It lies more lateral and lower down on the left side at the level of the umbilicus in a straight line drawn vertically upward from a point 2.5 cm medial to the anterior superior iliac spine **(Fig. 1)**. Because of its more lateral location, it avoids intra-abdominal adhesions of the midline and paramedian vertical incision sites. Being lower down at level L4 avoids upper abdomen incision-related adhesions also. It totally avoids the stomach, enlarged spleen (T10–L1), and kidney, which is deep in the retroperitoneum at the T12 to L3 level **(Figs. 2A and B)**. Another important factor is that there are no superficial or retroperitoneal deep major vessels beneath the Jain point. Therefore, it becomes safe because no vessel or hollow viscus is directly beneath it. The Jain point becomes the main working port during the course of the surgery. Hence, it has a dual benefit of being the main working port as well as the entry port. It has good ergonomic

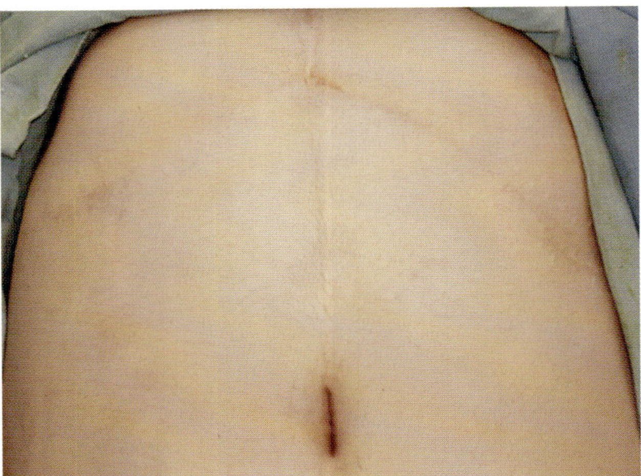

Fig. 1: Chevron incision[2] or rooftop incision for previous hepatic surgery.

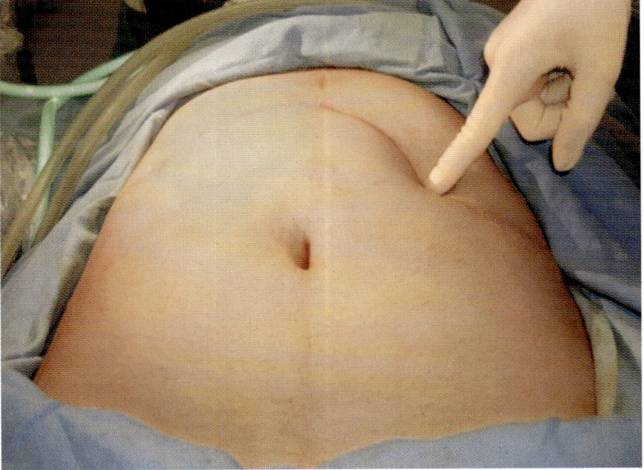

Fig. 2A: Palmer's point lying on Chevron incision.

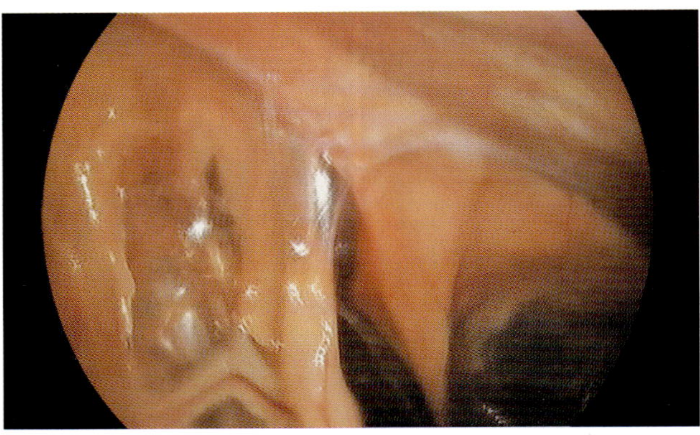

Fig. 2B: Adhesion at Palmer's point.

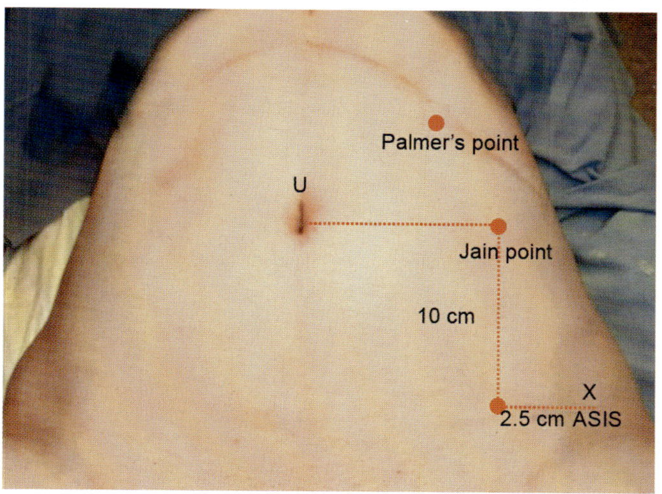

Fig. 3: Anatomic location of Jain point in previous abdomen surgery cases. (ASIS: anterior superior iliac spine).

rationale because it is placed 10–13 cm away from the lower port on the same side offering comfortable working **(Fig. 3)**.

In case with upper abdomen scars we make our entry by Jain point and has been seen that adhesions at Palmer's Point **(*see* Fig. 2B)** are usually seen as Palmer's Point falls on the incision line here we describe a case of myomectomy with chevron incision, where Jain point entry was made and adhesions noted at Palmer's Point. We then optimized the 10 mm port under the vision of 5 mm Jain point port. First thing we did after inserting the 10 mm port is to inspect the Jain point port and found it to be free of adhesions in spite of dense adhesions in upper abdomen. Patient had a posterior wall myoma. Dilute vasopressin one ampoule (20 units) in 400 mL of saline is injected over the myoma **(Figs. 4A to L)**. Transverse incision given by Harmonic ACE™ at the most bulging part of myoma. Exact plane of cleavage reached which showed the pearly white myoma. Due to large amount of vasopressin good plane of enucleation achieved and hardly any bleeding. Myoma bed was pretty large as it was a big myoma. We decided to do the suturing in four layers. The deepest myometrial layers were taken with barb sutures, the V-LOC, as it gives good approximation of the myoma bed and keeps equal tension throughout. Hemostasis is achieved only by suturing and cautery is used very sparingly. The upper muscular and serosal layer are taken by 1-0 vicryl, this is done to bury the barb sutures beneath the layers stitched by vicryl, as there could be stray incidents of bowel getting stuck to the barb suture and cause intestinal obstruction.[3] Good anatomical end result is achieved. Myoma morcellated and removed. In this case of difficult entry, surgery was easily contemplated avoiding the upper adhesions of previous surgery by entering through the nonumbilical port, the Jain point.

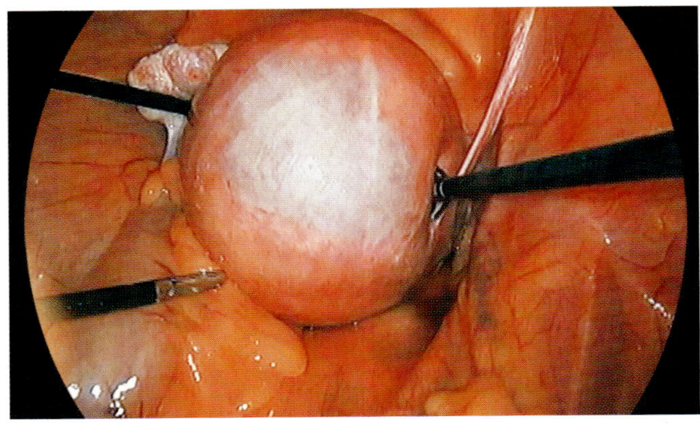

Fig. 4A: Big deep posterior wall myoma.

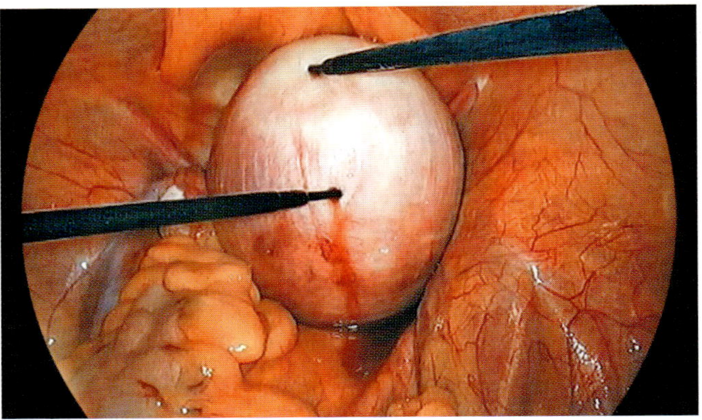

Fig. 4B: Dilute vasopressin injecting over the myoma.

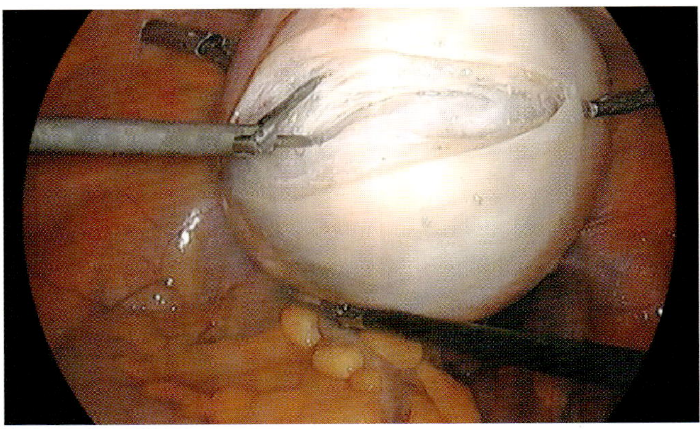

Fig. 4C: Transverse incision given using Harmonic ACE.

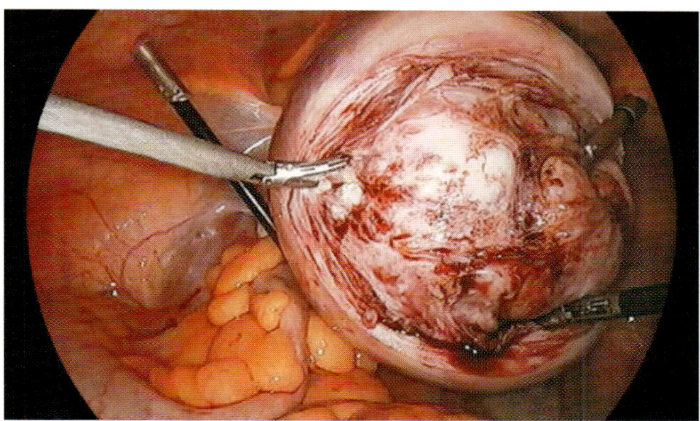

Fig. 4D: Enucleation of myoma.

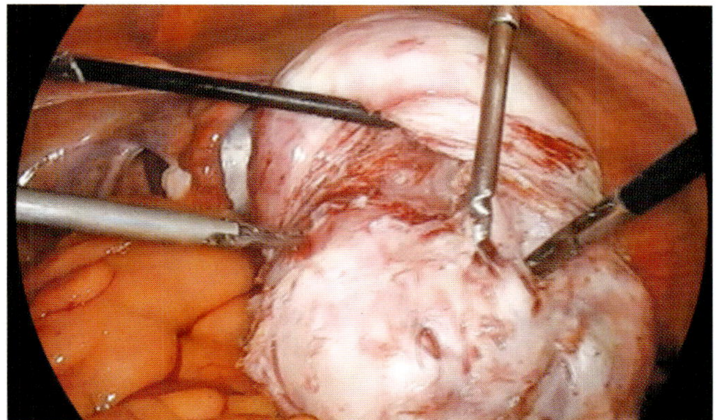

Fig. 4E: Myoma prayed out of myoma bed with a myoma screw.

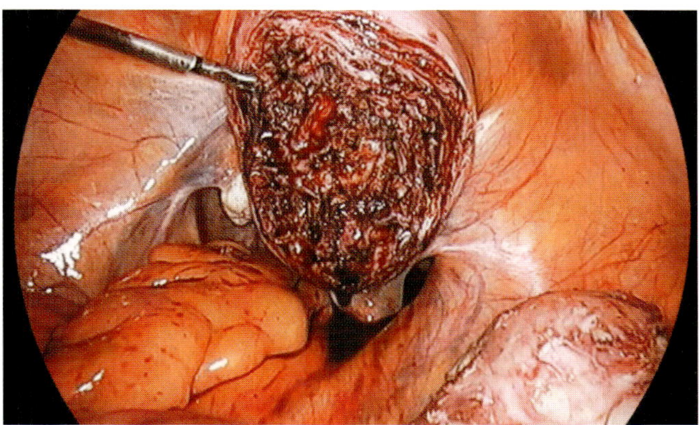

Fig. 4F: Myoma bed after myoma enucleation.

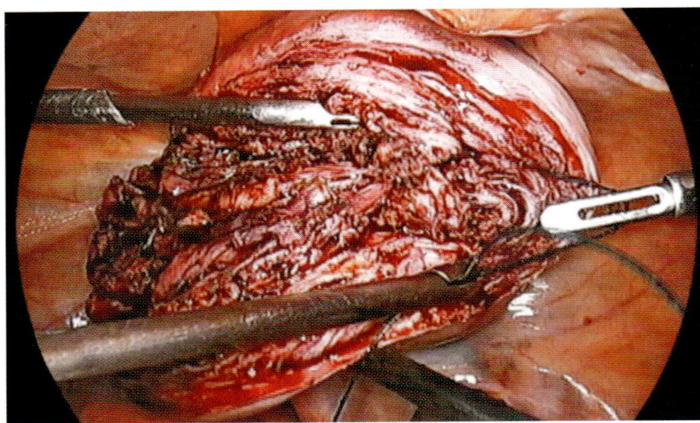

Fig. 4G: Needle passing through posterior edge with V-LOC suture.

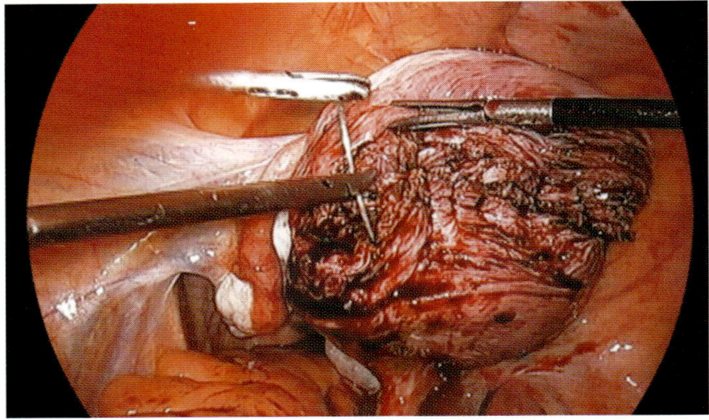

Fig. 4H: Second layer completed with V-LOC suture.

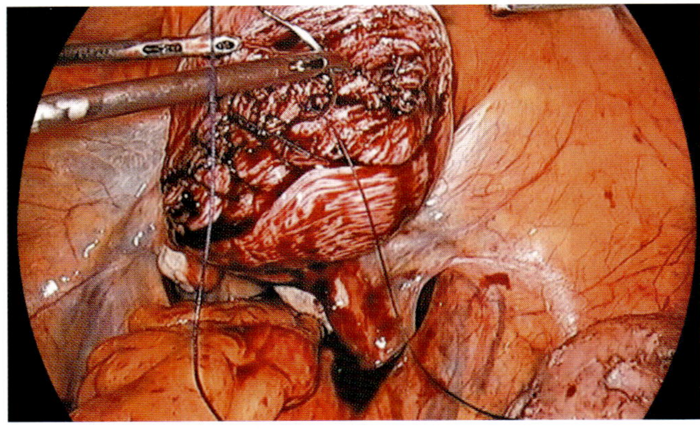

Fig. 4I: Third layer in progress.

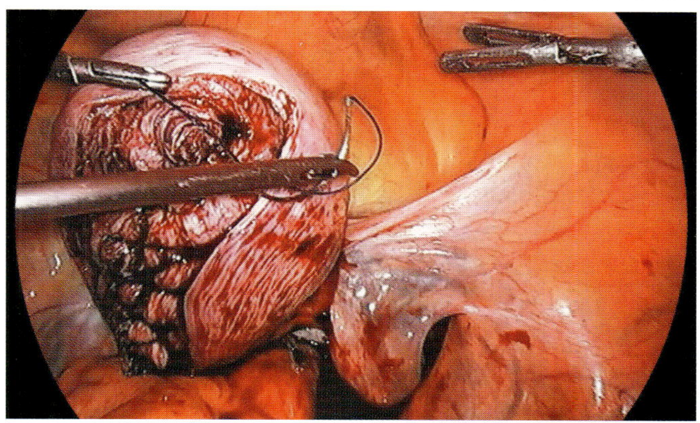

Fig. 4J: Third layer completed with 1-0 vicryl.

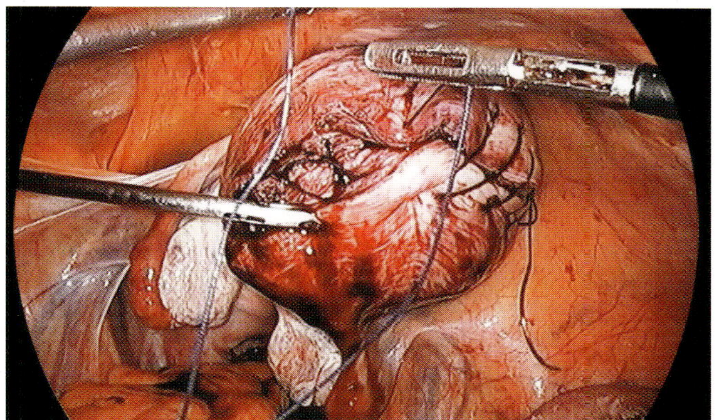

Fig. 4K: Serosal layer in progress with 1-0 vicryl.

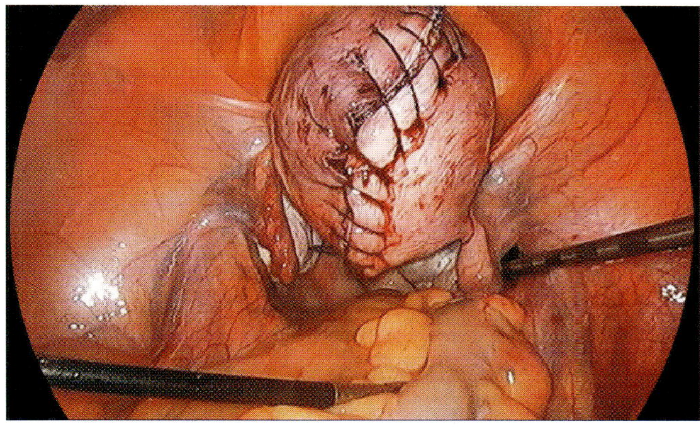

Fig. 4L: Final appearance of myoma bed sutured.

LEARNING POINTS

- Jain point avoids visceral injury.
- It avoids superficial and deep vessel injury.
- It works as both entry port and working port.
- It has good ergonomic rationale.
- It has easily located, fixed reference points for entry namely the umbilicus and ASIS.
- It is feasible in upper abdomen scars, midline vertical scars and low pfannenstiel incisions.

CONCLUSION

Jain point is feasible as first entry port in upper abdomen scars as all other three nonumbilical entry ports lie in the upper quadrant, namely the Palmer's, Lee-Huang, and 9th intercostal space. Only Jain point lies in paraumbilical position in the mid-quadrant of abdomen, hence, it can be safety used in upper abdominal scars.

REFERENCES

1. Krishnakumar S, Tambe P. Entry complications in laparoscopic surgery. J Gynecol Endosc Surg. 2009;1(1):4-11.
2. Wikipedia. Surgical incision. [online] Available from https://en.wikipedia.org/wiki/Surgical_incision [Last accessed January, 2020].
3. Lee ET, Wong FW. Small bowel obstruction from barbed suture following laparoscopic myomectomy: a case report. Int J Surg Case Rep. 2015;16:146-9.

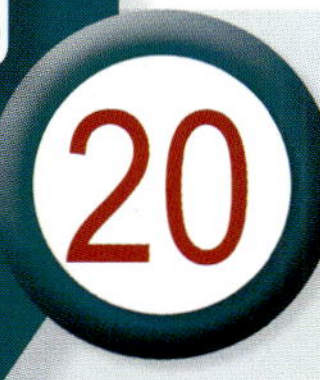

Surgeries Deep in the Pelvis using Jain Point Pelvic Floor Repair

Nutan Jain, Gunjan Saxena

INTRODUCTION

After being the first blind entry port, Jain point continues to work as the main working port, deep down in pelvis for the repair of pelvic floor defects. It is at the level of the umbilicus, so, one may feel that it is at a higher level for working deep down in pelvis and in the retropubic space of Retzius space. We have been using the left-sided ports for the last 20 years in the pelvic floor reparative surgery. We have developed a mature system to evaluate and treat various pelvic floor defects. Laparoscopy offers a feasible alternative to open laparotomy for space of Retzius repairs and paravaginal repairs for various grades of prolapse.

The anatomical supports of the uterus and cervix are the upper vertical support offered by uterosacral ligaments. The level two supports are the pubovesicocervical fascia anteriorly and rectovaginal fascia posteriorly and they attach to the arcus tendinous fascia white line laterally. Lastly, the level three support is offered by muscles of the perineum and the urogenital diaphragm.

In this chapter, we shall provide mostly a step-by-step description of surgical steps by the help of surgical snapshots. The videos of the concerned procedures will be provided separately.

BURCH COLPOSUSPENSION

The bladder is filled with about 200–300 cc of normal saline and then incision started above the highest point of bladder and entry into space of Retzius is obtained. The entry is confirmed by appearance of cotton candy space. The Cooper's ligament is identified and the dissection is done laterally up to the obturator neurovascular bundle. Two Burch sutures are applied on either side with nonabsorbable suture material between the paraurethral and paravaginal tissue and passed over to the Cooper's ligament[1] **(Figs. 1A to L)**. A loose sling

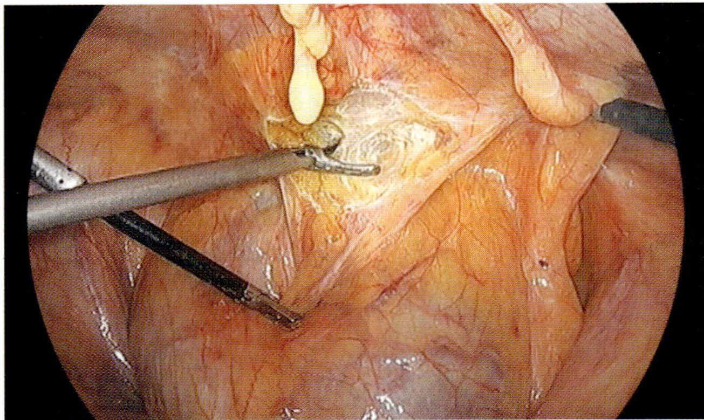

Fig. 1A: Holding the peritoneum fold to enter in space of Retzius by Harmonic ACE.

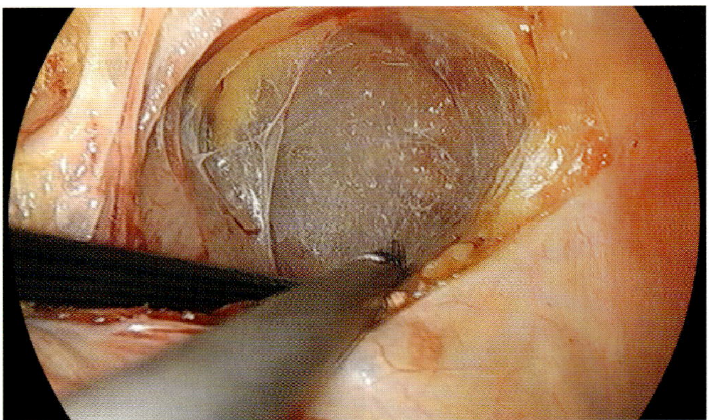

Fig. 1B: Cotton candy space to confirm space of Retzius.

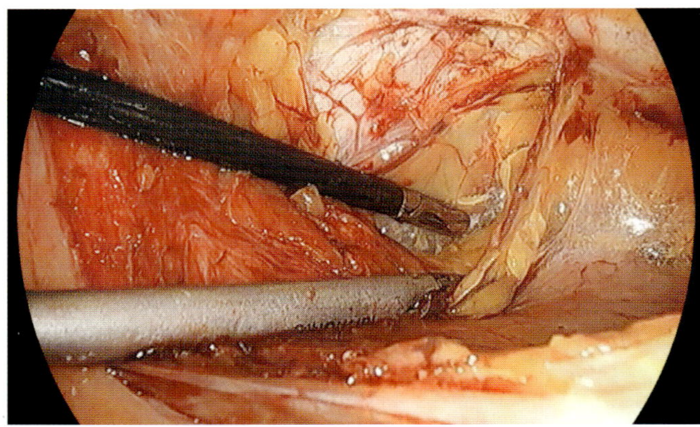

Fig. 1C: Exposure of Cooper's ligament on left side.

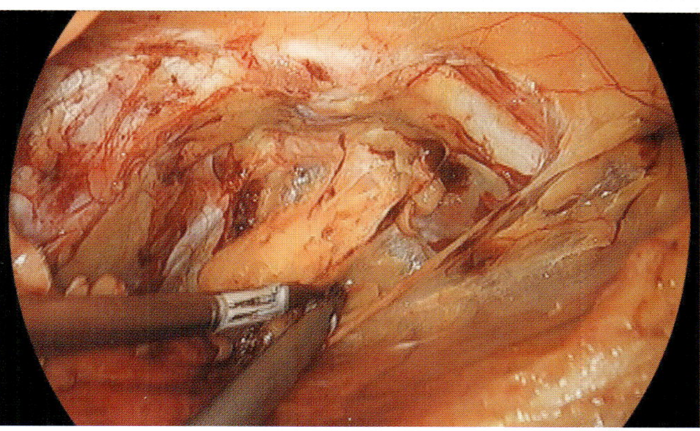

Fig. 1D: Exposing the right side arcus tendineus fascia white line.

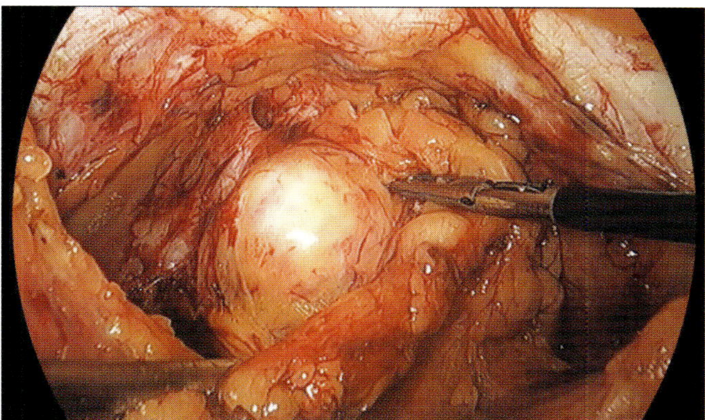

Fig. 1E: Elevating the paraurethral tissue.

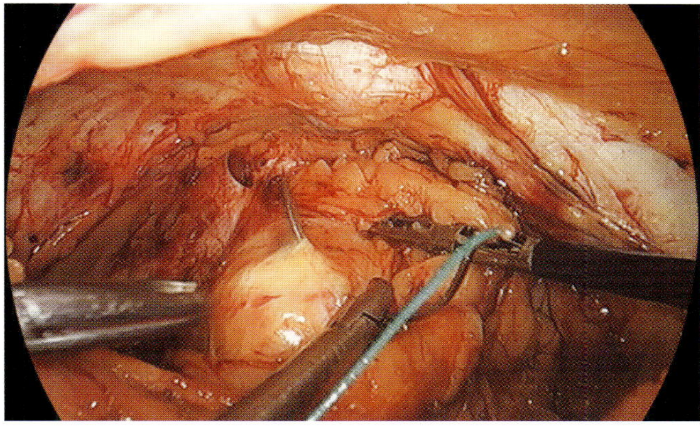

Fig. 1F: Suture taken through paravaginal tissue with no. 1 polyester suture.

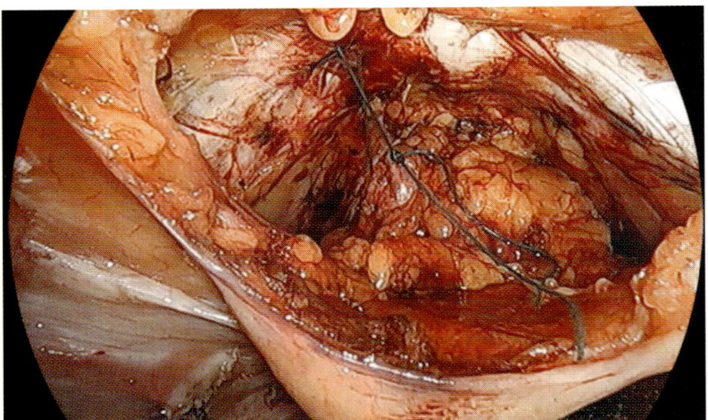

Fig. 1G: Suture passed through the Cooper's ligament and tied.

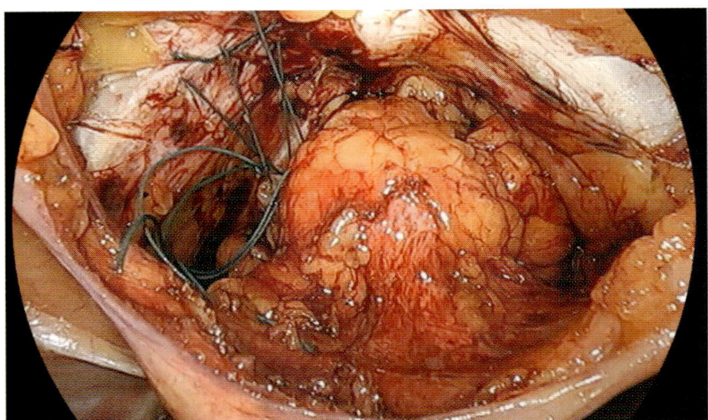

Fig. 1H: Two sutures on the left side placed.

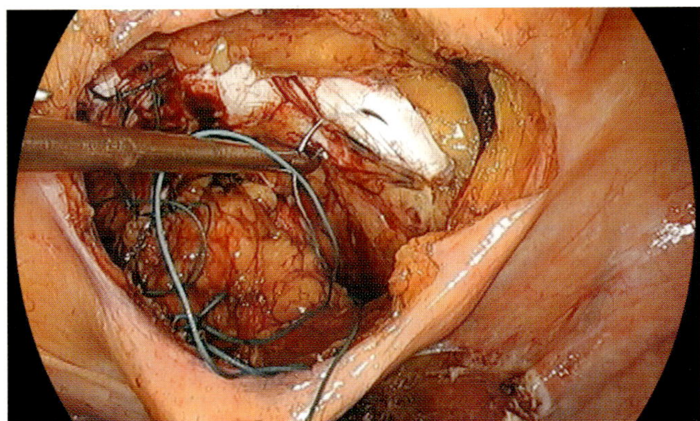

Fig. 1I: Suture passed through the Cooper's ligament on right side.

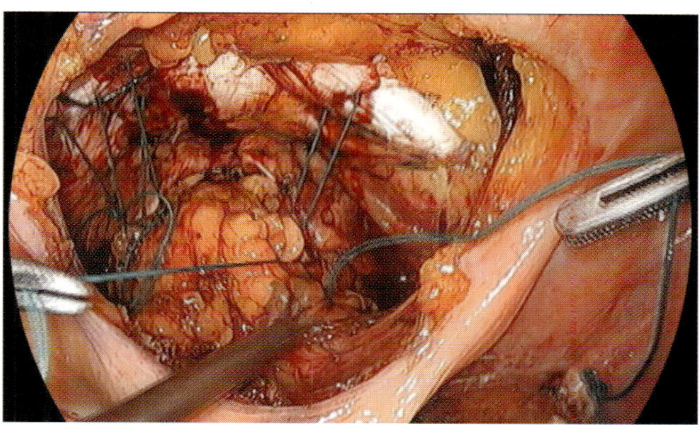

Fig. 1J: First suture completed on right side.

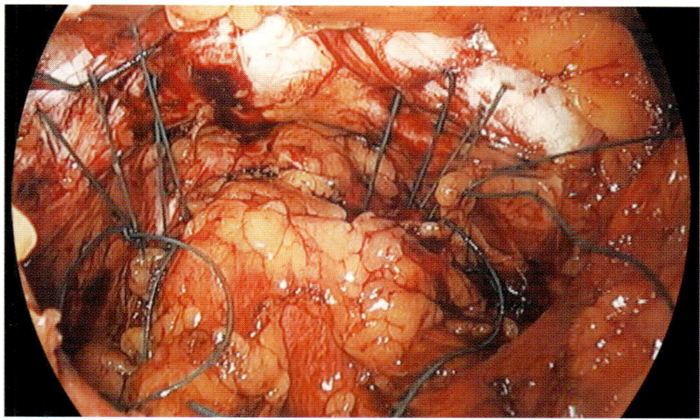

Fig. 1K: Four Burch sutures completed.

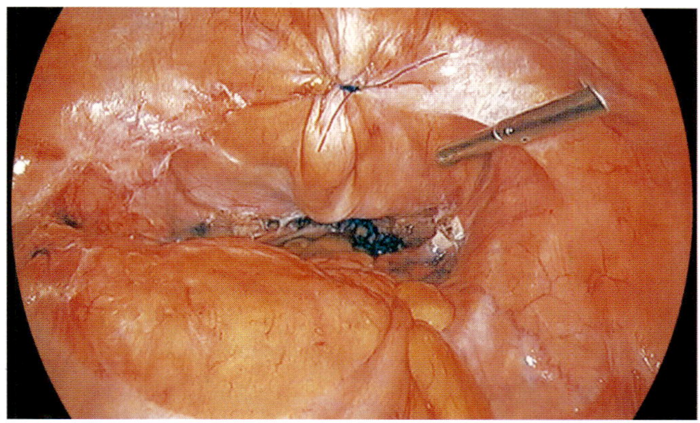

Fig. 1L: Final view of peritoneum closure.

is made and care taken not to tighten them too much, otherwise the patient can land into postoperative urinary retention.

PARAVAGINAL DEFECT REPAIR

It is a very nice procedure for central cystocele. Many times, these defects are seen as isolated defects with the cervix well supported at ischial spine and in that situation laparoscopic repair becomes an ultimate procedure. Entry into space of Retzius is gained by the method described earlier. The bladder pushed medially and Foley's bulb brought down at the level of the bladder neck. Arcus tendineus fascia white line is identified by its tough and shiny white appearance. Then paravaginal defect repair sutures are applied separately on both sides right and left starting at the level of ischial spine and working toward the pubic bone. Nonabsorbable suture material is employed. At least four sutures are applied on either side. Very nice anatomical repair is achieved. The space of Retzuis is closed by a running suture on the peritoneal defect[2] (**Figs. 2A to L**).

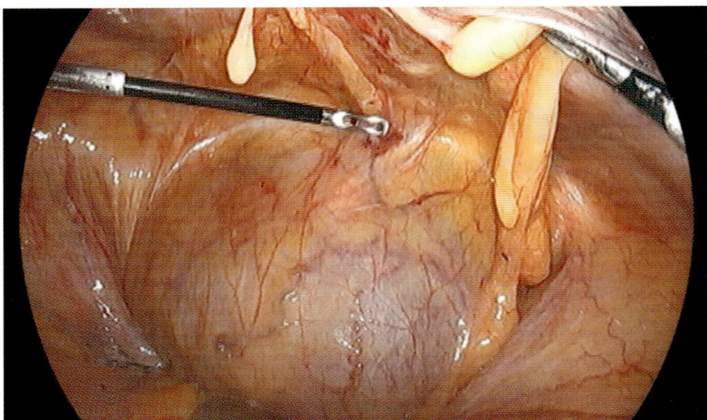

Fig. 2A: Bladder retrograde filled with 300 mL of sterile normal saline.

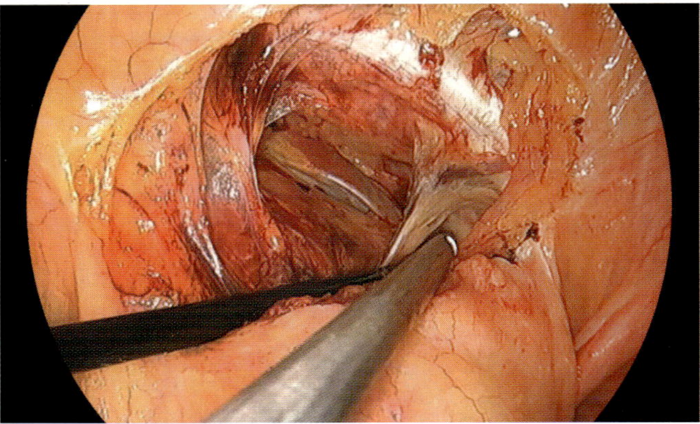

Fig. 2B: Entry into the space of Retzius.

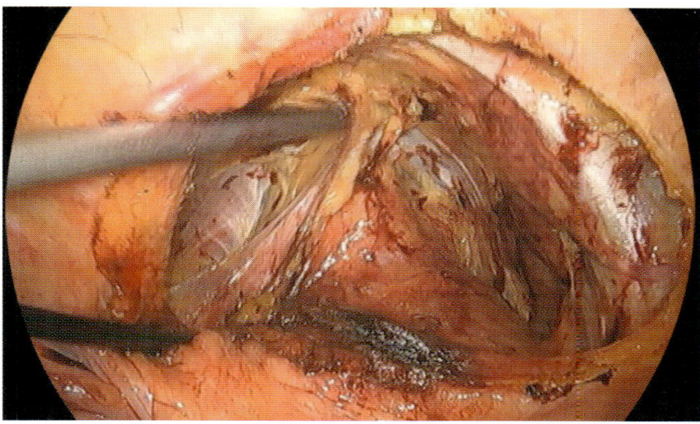

Fig. 2C: Complete exposure of space of Retzius.

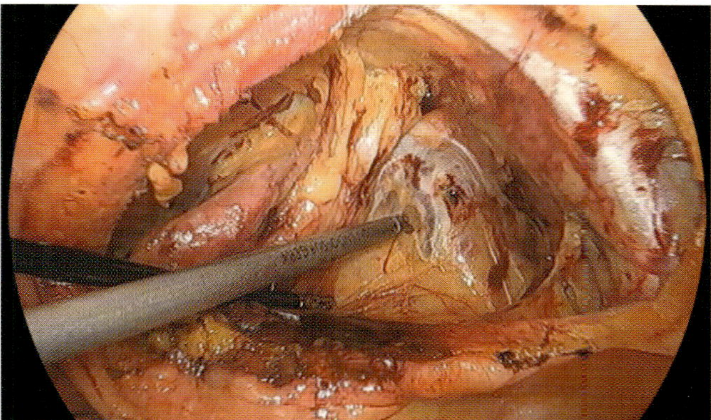

Fig. 2D: Dissection into the right side showing arcus tendineus fascia white line.

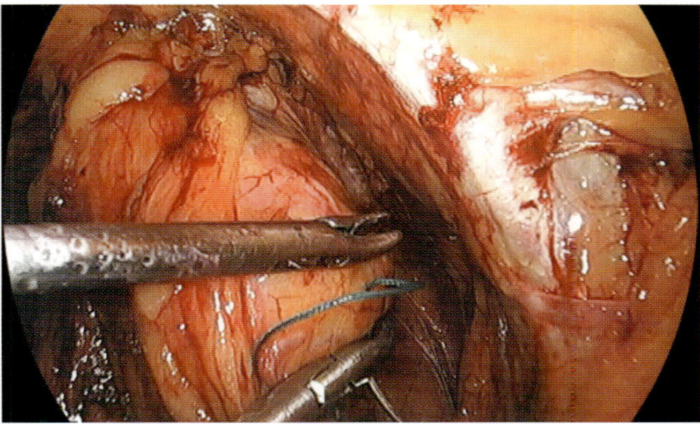

Fig. 2E: First suture passed in paravaginal tissue by Ethibond no.1 on the right side to be tied to arcus tendineus fascia.

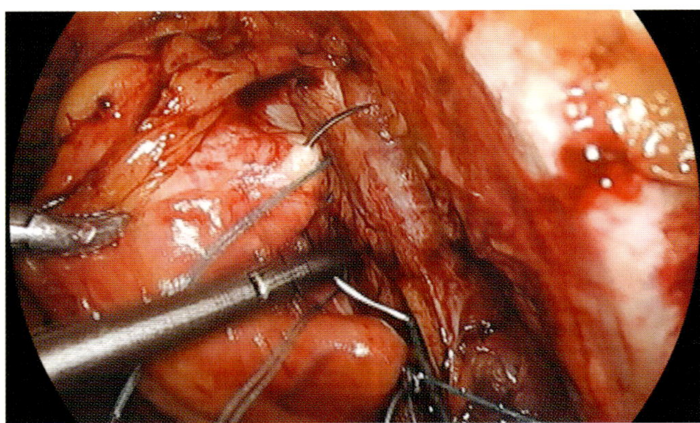

Fig. 2F: Passing another suture 1 cm apart to be tied to arcus tendineus fascia.

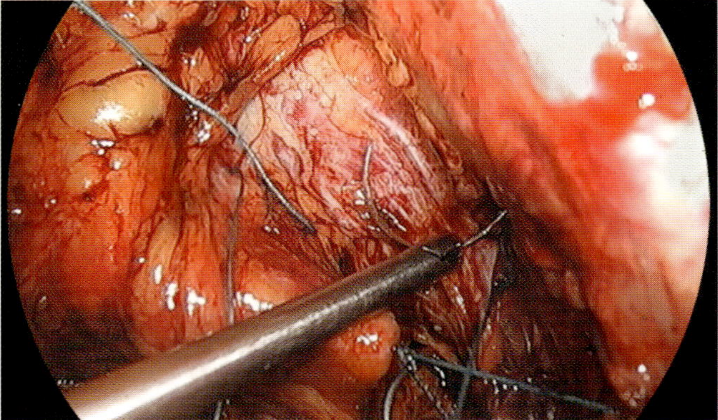

Fig. 2G: Suture passed through arcus tendineus fascia on right side.

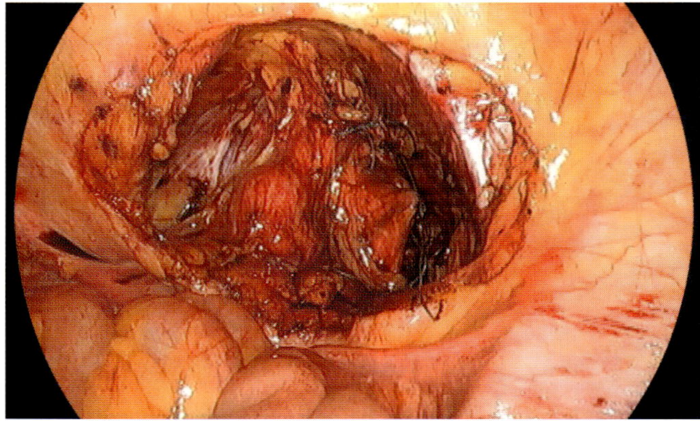

Fig. 2H: Four paravaginal suture completed on the right side.

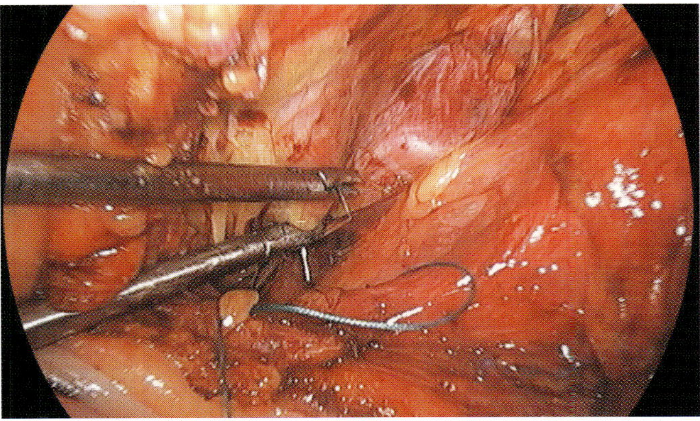

Fig. 2I: Full thickness suture passed through arcus tendineus fascia on left side.

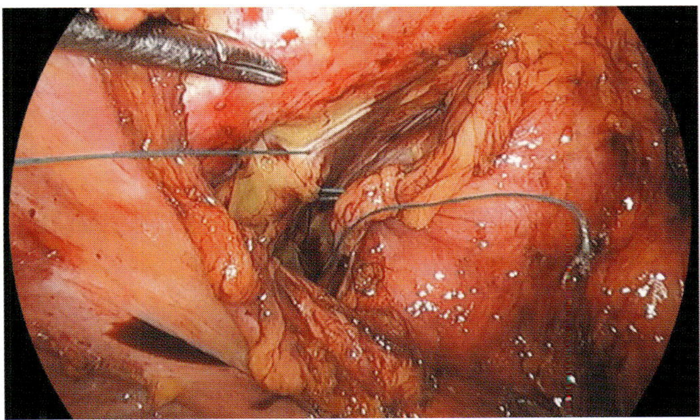

Fig. 2J: Suture passed through paravaginal tissue.

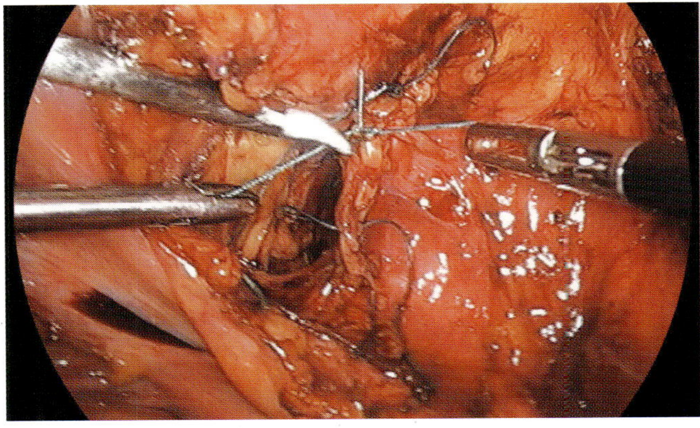

Fig. 2K: Another suture tied on left side.

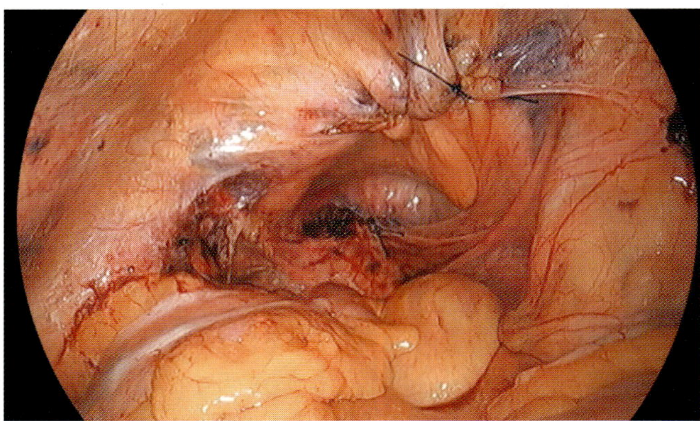

Fig. 2L: Peritoneum closure done.

■ PECTOPEXY

Pectopexy is relatively a newer procedure. It was first described by VM Joshi, et al.[3] in 1993, they did it by laparotomy as well as laparoscopy and was revived by Gunter Noe[4] as solely a laparoscopic procedure. We have done it mostly as a part of total pelvic floor procedure, combining it with other site-specific repair procedures. In our technique we push the bladder down and expose a large area of the pubovesical fascia. We pass buttressing sutures in 3–4 tiers starting just above the bladder anteriorly and going upward toward the cervix. We use nonabsorbable Ethibond 1-0 then apply a mesh over this strengthened platform. The mesh size is 3 cm in width and 15 cm in length. It is fixed in the midline with nonabsorbable sutures over the cervical isthmus. The lateral ends of the mesh strip are anchored over the iliopectineal ligaments, the posterior, prolongation of the Cooper's ligament. To expose the ileopectineal ligament we make an incision with Harmonic ACE starting by the side of the round ligament and also by feeling the bony iliopectineal ligament. The other landmarks are the external iliac vessels. About 4–5 cm segment of the ileopectineal ligament is exposed. Two suture bites are taken over this ligament and mesh fixed in place. Reperitonization is completed **(Figs. 3A to L)**. We usually combine it with a site-specific repair of the posterior compartment by plicating the uterosacral ligaments. We follow the philosophy of global repair where in both the anterior and posterior compartments are repaired and strengthened in an equal manner. In this way, when the patient becomes ambulatory and the forces of gravity fall, the posterior compartment does not sag causing an enterocele.

Likewise, if we repair only the posterior compartment by sacrocolpopexy, patient tends to develop stress incontinence by forces of gravity falling on unsupported anterior compartment. By this logic, we at our center combine the mesh repairs with site-specific repairs, attaching the broken or weak support mechanism and then anchoring the mesh.

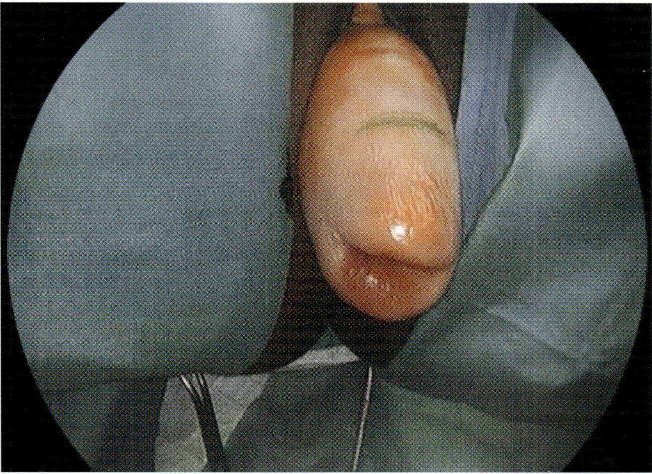

Fig. 3A: Grade IV uterovaginal prolapse.

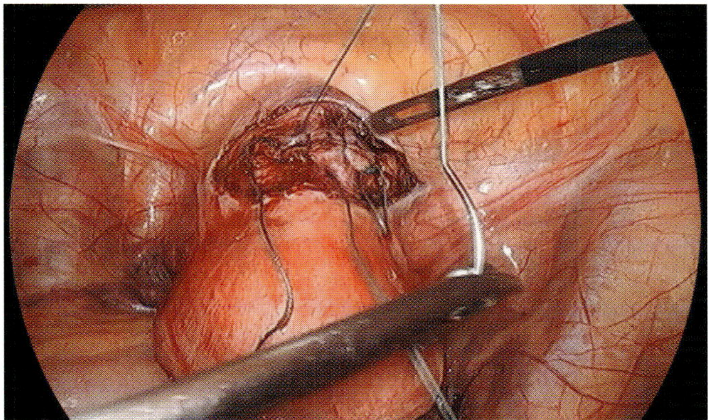

Fig. 3B: Pubovesicocervical fascia plication done using nonabsorbable suture (Ethibond).

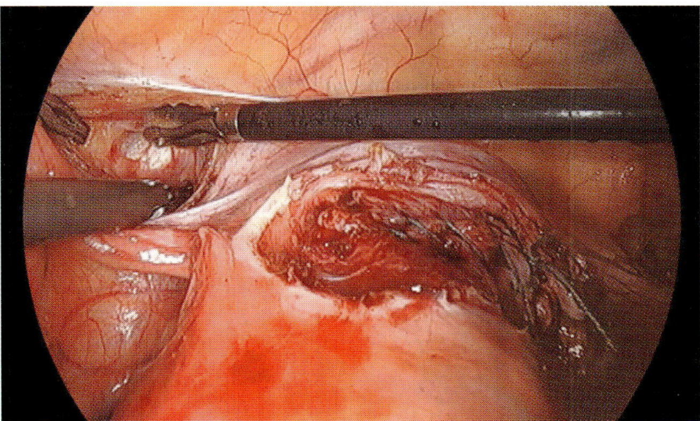

Fig. 3C: Left-sided iliopectineal ligament (Cooper ligament) exposed.

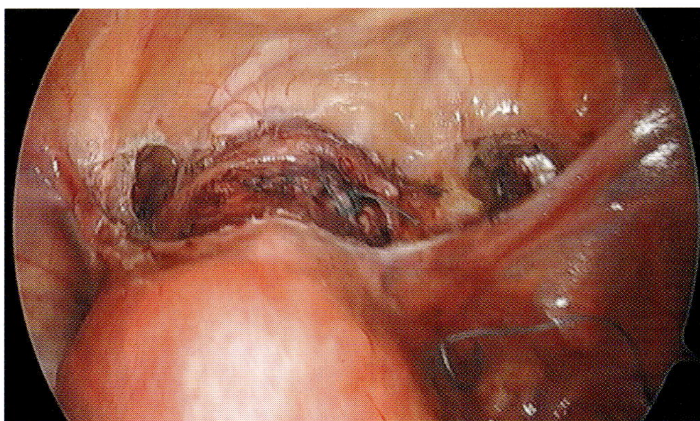

Fig. 3D: Right-sided iliopectineal ligament (Cooper ligament) exposed.

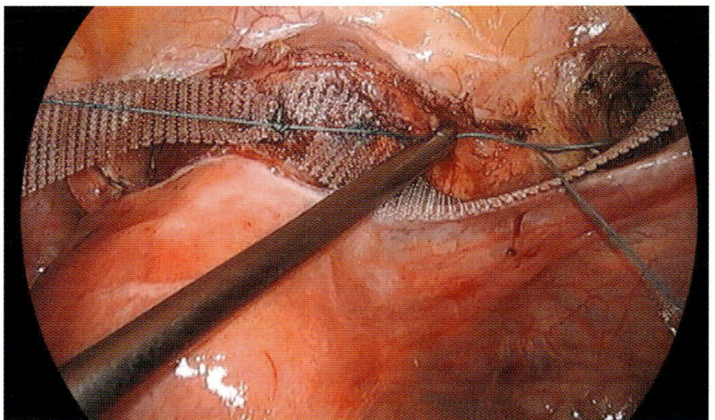

Fig. 3E: Soft mesh (size 15 × 2.5 cm) fixed at the vaginal apex.

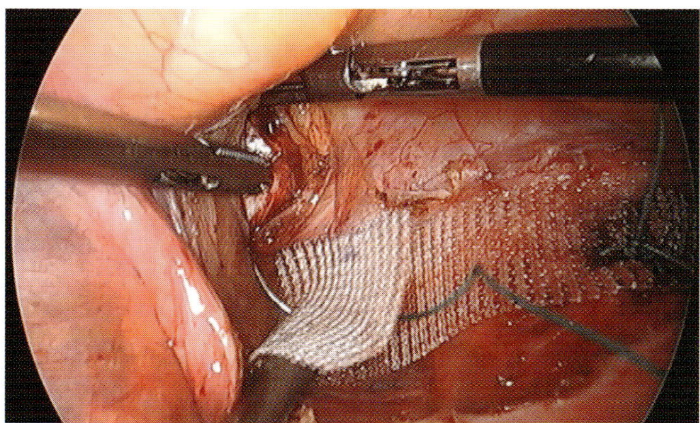

Fig. 3F: Left side suture taken through iliopectineal ligament.

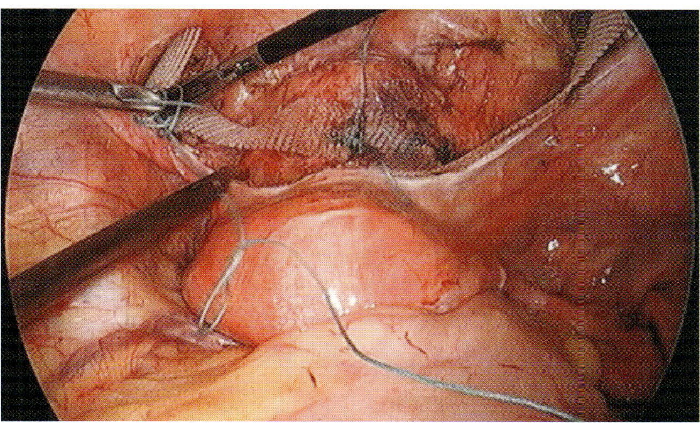

Fig. 3G: Left-sided mesh fixed to iliopectineal ligament using nonabsorbable suture.

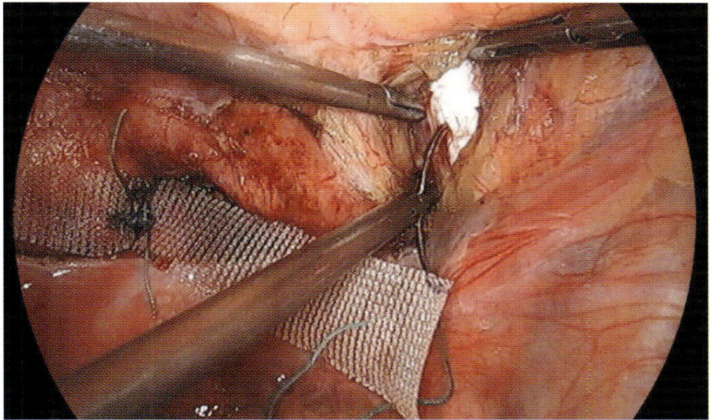

Fig. 3H: Right-sided needle passed through iliopectineal ligament.

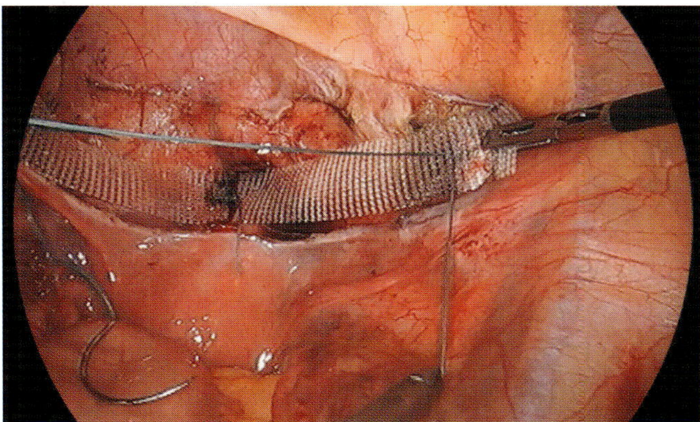

Fig. 3I: Right-sided mesh fixed to iliopectineal ligament using nonabsorbable suture.

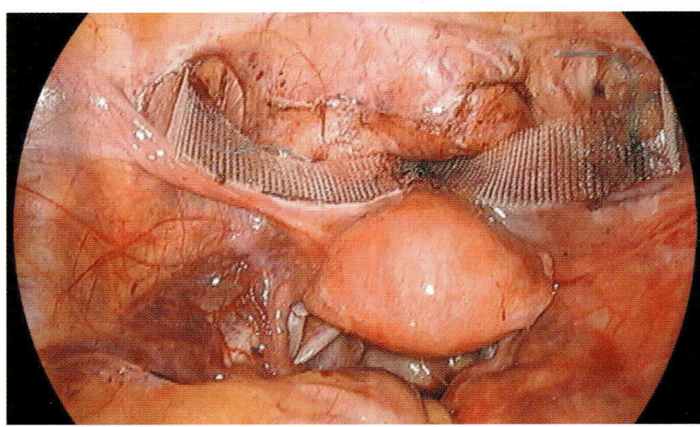

Fig. 3J: Mesh ends attached to both iliopectineal ligaments using nonabsorbable suture material (Ethibond 1.0).

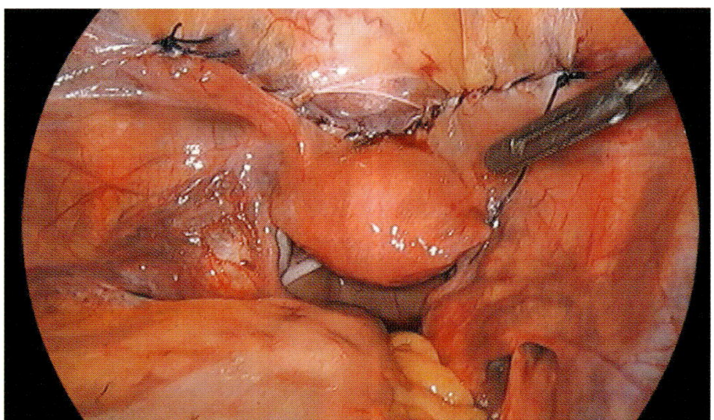

Fig. 3K: Peritoneum closure done.

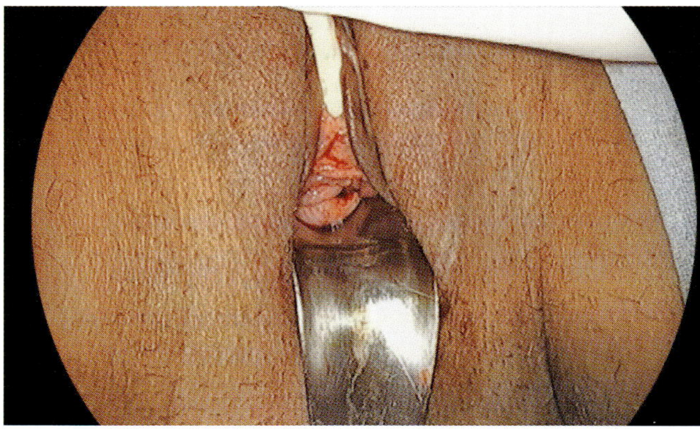

Fig. 3L: Final picture after prolapse repair.

UTEROSACRAL LIGAMENT PLICATION

This technique is offered for uterovaginal prolapse and has been advocated largely by CY Liu.[5] We do this bilaterally, on right and left side on both uterosacral ligaments, but separately. The sutures begun at the level of ischial spine 2 cm medial to it and takes a good deep bite in the fibrous portion of uterosacral ligament. We then continue with continuous sutures with nonabsorbable material till the junction of cervix and uterosacral ligament. In fact, I take a deep bite in the arcus tendinous a quadrangular area just above the insertion of both uterosacral ligaments. This gives a good attachment of uterosacral ligament to a higher fixed point and also incorporates the rectovaginal septum. Uterosacral ligament plication done bilaterally gives excellent support to the posterior compartments **(Figs. 4A to F)**. I usually combine it with other procedures to strengthen the anterior compartment

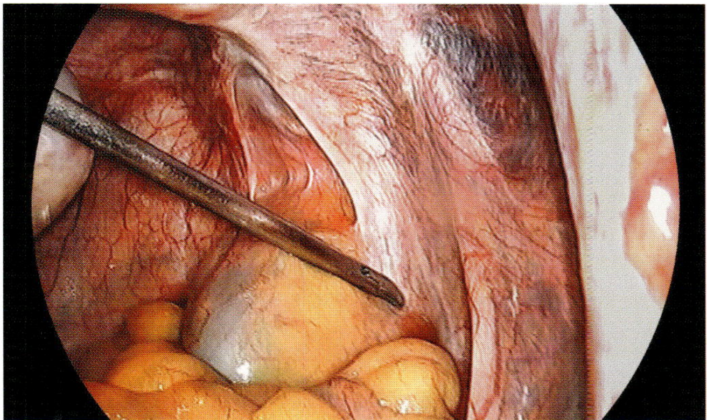

Fig. 4A: The right side uterosacral ligament.

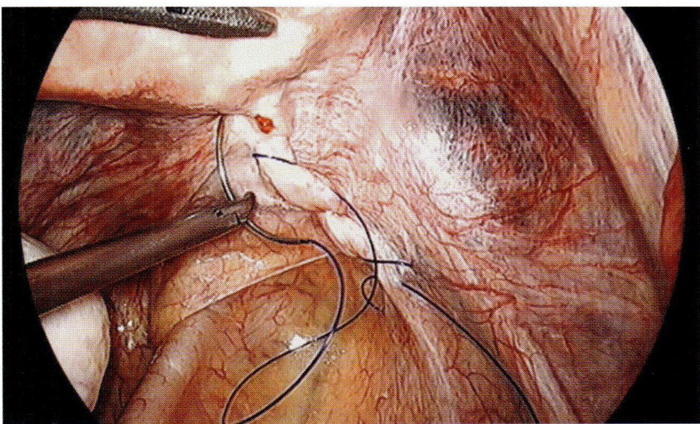

Fig. 4B: Plication of uterosacral ligament.

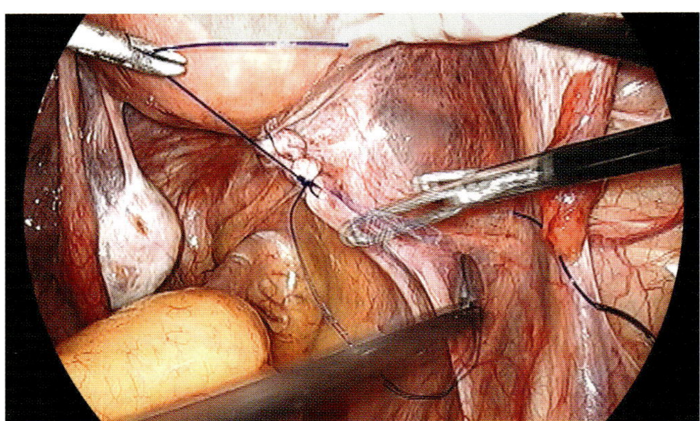

Fig. 4C: Knot tied.

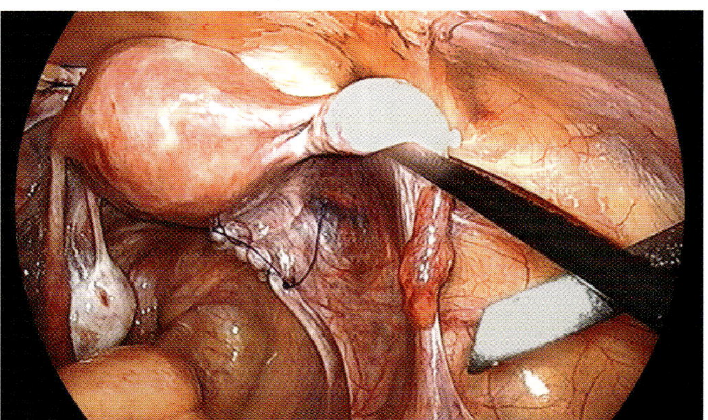

Fig. 4D: Completed picture after plication of right uterosacral ligament.

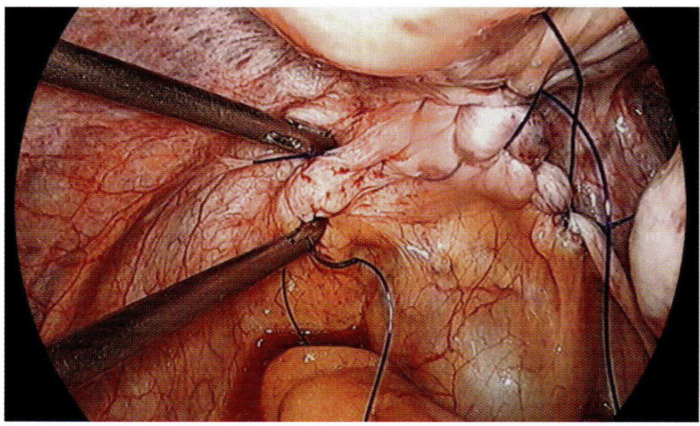

Fig. 4E: Left side uterosacral ligament plication done.

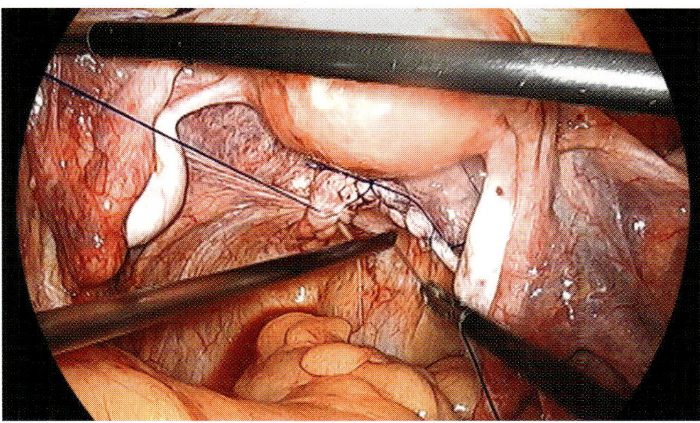

Fig. 4F: Both side uterosacral ligament plication done using Prolene suture.

like plication of pubovesical fascia and as a part of pectopexy for posterior compartment repair to give a uniform global repair.

LEARNING POINTS

- To contemplate pelvic floor repair surgeon needs to be well versed with laparoscopic suturing.
- Always assess preoperatively all defects of the anterior as well as posterior compartments and fashion out a procedure which addresses all the defects.
- It is always good to combine site-specific repair to strengthen the support structures like the pubovesicocervical fascia, rectovaginal fascia, and uterosacral ligaments.
- Mesh augmented repair to be considered according to patient's age, the strength of supporting muscles and fascia, and the extent of prolapse.
- No single procedure addresses all defects. So, it is good to be conversant with many procedures and tailor make a combination of repair technique for each individual patient.

REFERENCES

1. Moore RD, Miklos JR, Kohli N. Laparoscopic paravaginal repair and Burch urethropexy. Laparoscopic management of prolapse and stress urinary incontinence. 2008;12:96-107.
2. Miklos JR, Kohli N. Laparoscopic paravaginal repair plus Burch colposuspension. Urology. 2000;56:(suppl 6A)64-9.
3. Joshi VM. A new technique of vault suspension to the pectineal ligaments in the management of uterovaginal prolapse. Obstet Gynecol. 1993;81:790-3.
4. Noé KG, Schiermeier S, Alkatout I, et al. Laparoscopic pectopexy: a prospective, randomized, comparative clinical trial of standard laparoscopic sacral colpocervicopexy with the new laparoscopic pectopexy-postoperative results and intermediate-term follow-up in a pilot study. J Endourol. 2015;29:210-15.
5. Jenkins TR, Liu CY. Laparoscopic uterosacral uterine suspension (LUSUS). Laparoscopic management of prolapse and stress urinary incontinence. 2008;20:184-92.

Jain Point: Fellow's Experience

Anadeep Chandi, Kiran Kumari Mandal

"Surgery is all about learning and practicing new skills."

INTRODUCTION

The introduction and evolution of laparoscopic surgeries has changed the face of modern practice and has nearly replaced open surgical procedures. It's been a while, since we joined fellowship in gynecological endoscopy under Dr Nutan Jain at Vardhman Trauma & Laparoscopy Centre Private Limited, India. It was this place where we were introduced with a newer blind entry point, i.e. Jain point. In our past experiences, umbilical entry port was the preferred way of entering into the abdominal cavity. However, its known risks and complications make most of the new laparoscopic surgeons, nervous and scared during its application. Thus we would like to share our learning about Jain point entry through this write up, in a hope that this would help most of the budding endoscopic surgeon to understand and apply this technique of blind entry in an easier and safer way without fearing any complications.

Jain point is situated on the left lateral part of the abdomen, i.e. left lumbar quadrant. To be precise, it lies on a vertical line drawn 2.5 cm medial to anterior superior iliac spine at the level of upper border of umbilicus **(Fig. 1)**. Beneath this point, there is no major vessel and viscera. Spleen and kidney are above at T10–L1 level, descending colon is retroperitoneal, and sigmoid colon is adherent at the level of pelvic brim. So, there is a nascent area in the left middle quadrant where there is no major structure to fear of. Only small gut and greater omentum are the structures usually encountered beneath the Jain point and these are mobile. Thus, Veress needle insertion is quite safe through this point.

The anterior abdominal wall at the level of Jain point consists of four main layers[1] (outside to inside) **(Fig. 2)**:

- First layer is made up of skin and subcutaneous tissue.
- Second layer is superficial fascia (adipose and membranous tissues).

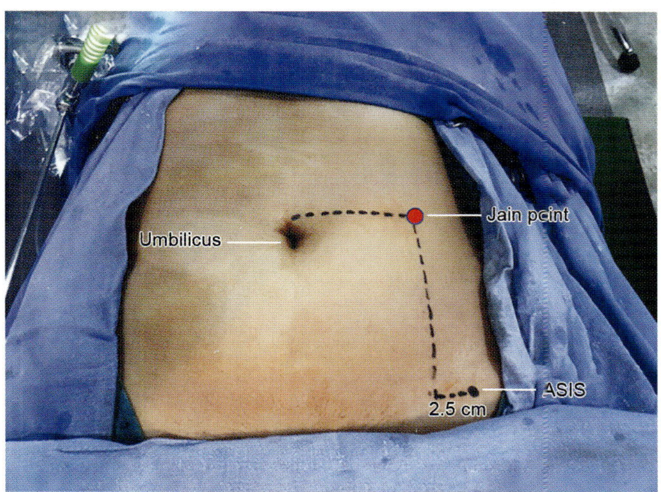

Fig. 1: Surface marking of Jain point in relation to anterior superior iliac spine (ASIS) and umbilicus.

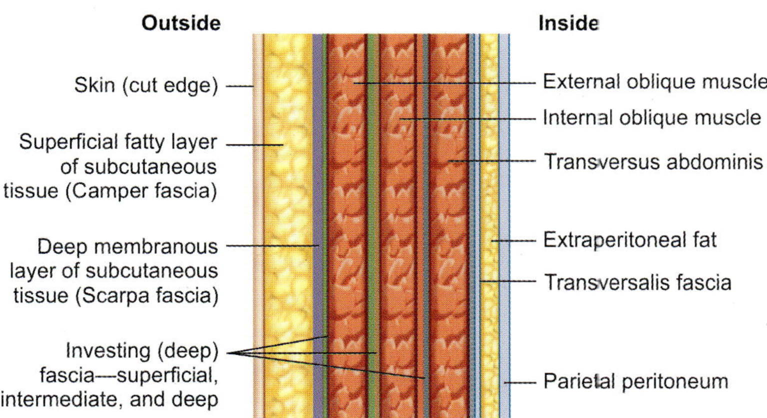

Fig. 2: Layers of anterior abdominal wall.

- Third layer is deep fascia, muscles (external oblique, internal oblique and transverses abdominis muscle), and underlying fascia (transversalis fascia).
- Fourth layer is parietal peritoneum.

Also, one needs to notice that, as we move laterally over the abdomen, the plane of the abdominal wall changes from being flat to convex edges **(Fig. 3)**. It is very important to understand the anatomy of abdominal wall, as this will guide our Veress needle insertion through the abdominal wall into the peritoneal cavity.

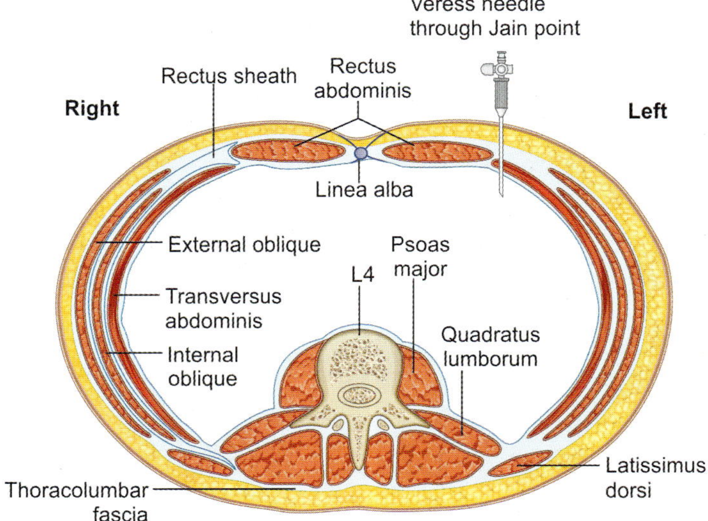

Fig. 3: Transverse section of anterior abdominal wall at the level of umbilicus.

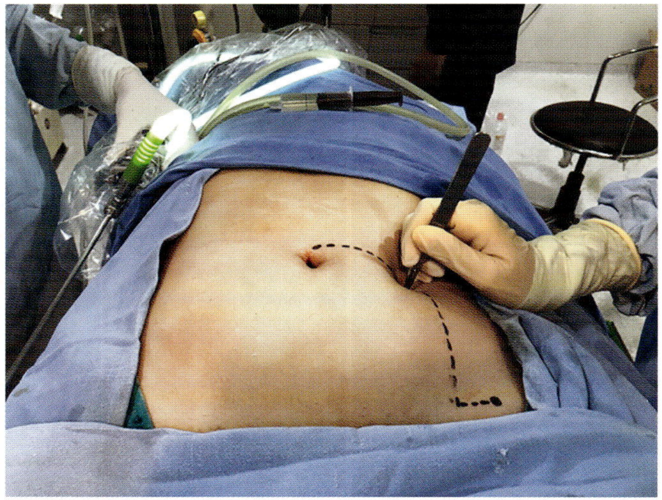

Fig. 4: Stab incision made by blade number 15 at Jain point.

STEPS OF VERESS NEEDLE INSERTION AND TROCAR PLACEMENT THROUGH JAIN POINT

1. Check Veress needle's spring action and its patency with saline.
2. Give 1–2 mm stab incision at Jain point with surgical blade number 15 **(Fig. 4)**.
3. Hold the Veress needle like a dart and place it just perpendicular to the abdominal wall at the stab incision site (without lifting the abdominal wall) **(Fig. 5A)**.

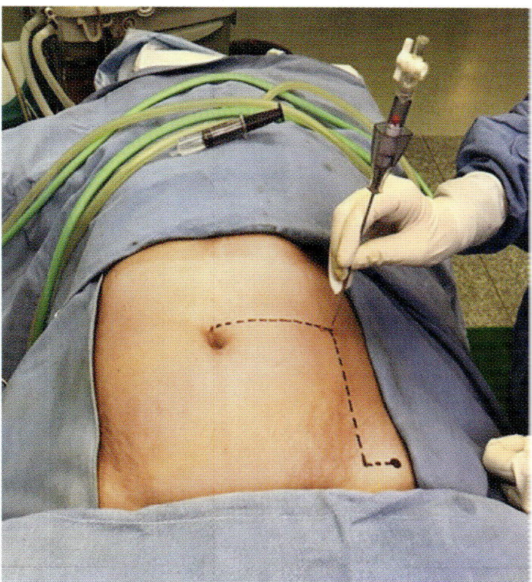

Fig. 5A: Veress needle held as a dart at Jain point.

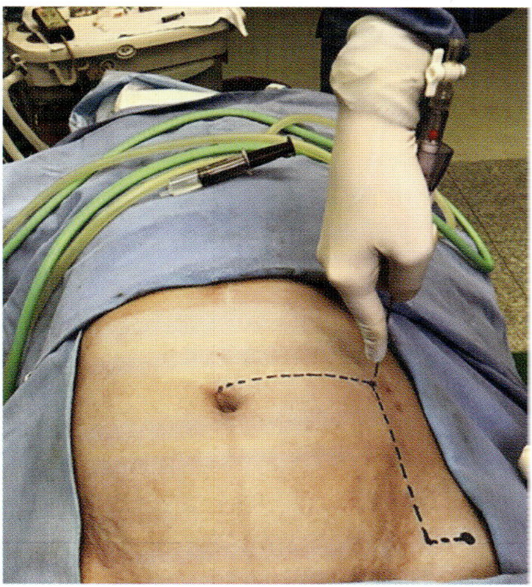

Fig. 5B: Veress needle held with a finger guide at Jain point.

[*Note:* Dr Nutan Jain and other fellows prefers holding it with a finger guide to increase the safety by avoiding over or under shooting of Veress needle **(Fig. 5B)**. However, we have a habit of holding it as a dart, so it is more comfortable for us in that way. Old habits die hard!]

4. Advance the Veress needle through the anterior abdominal wall layers slowly noticing three clicks **(Fig. 6)**:

   i. *1st click:* As the Veress needle passes through the external oblique aponeurosis.

   ii. *2nd click:* When it pierces the fused aponeurosis of internal oblique and transverses abdominis muscle.

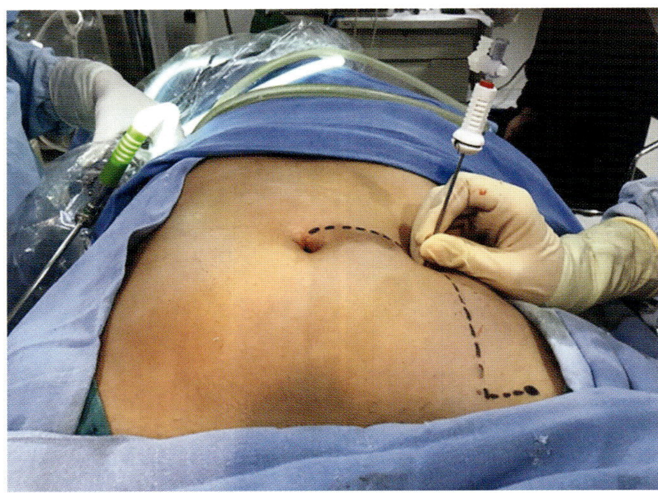

Fig. 6: Veress needle inserted perpendicular to abdominal wall at Jain point.

iii. *3rd click:* As the needle penetrates the parietal peritoneum and enters the peritoneal cavity.

[*Note:* Dr Nutan Jain calls for two clicks followed by lack of resistance. But, what we have noticed, that she being highly experienced with this technique, goes very fast which disables us to appreciate last two clicks distinctly. Thus, as a beginner, it is recommended to insert the needle slowly appreciating all the three clicks, to avoid false entries. Also, the abdominal wall being convex laterally, a slight 1–2 mm of medial shift of the Veress needle from its perpendicular alignment after the 2nd click (particularly in very thin patients), helps avoid track formation inside the lateral abdominal wall and thus prevents preperitoneal insufflation. In multiparous women with very lax abdomen, one may not appreciate all the three clicks distinctly, thus one should always sense for the feeling of give way as the final entry point of Veress needle in the abdomen.]

5. *Ask an assistant to hold the Veress needle in position and attach a 10 mL saline fluid syringe to the Veress needle hub and aspirate.
6. *If no aspirate is seen, irrigate it with 3–4 mL of saline and then again aspirate **(Fig. 7)**.
7. *If again no aspirate comes, it assures that the Veress needle is inside the peritoneal cavity.
8. *Now, attach CO_2 gas insufflation tubing to the Veress needle and check for the intra-abdominal pressure in the insufflator. It should remain ≤8 mm Hg for initial 10 seconds. This further confirms that the needle is intraperitoneal (*see* **Figs. 5A and B)**.

[*Note:* In case your insufflator shows higher pressure, think again. Either your needle is in wrong place or if intraperitoneal, it may be touching the

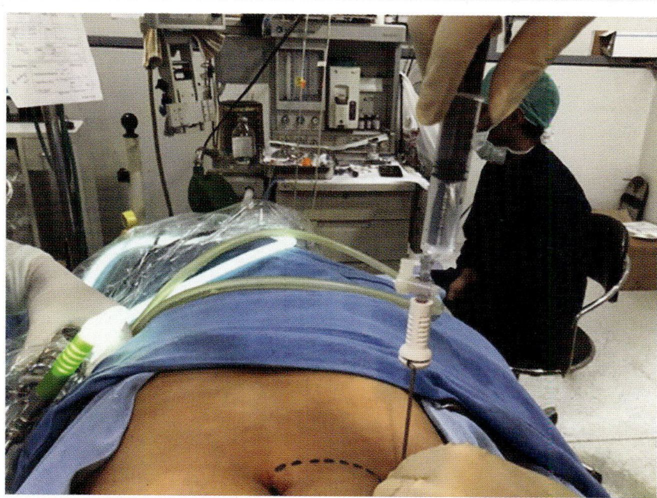

Fig. 7: Saline aspiration and infusion test to determine the correct placement of Veress needle.

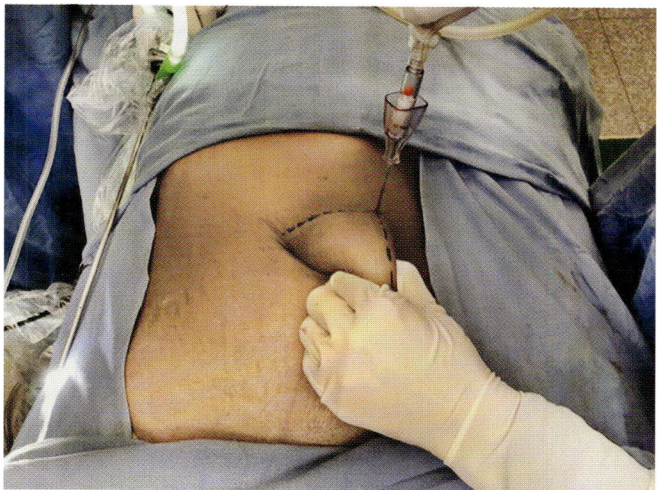

Fig. 8: Abdominal wall lifted up during insufflation in an attempt to raise the Veress needle tip from underlying omental surface to prevent omental insufflation.

omentum or other underneath structures like gut, abdominal mass, etc. In the latter case, one may lift the abdominal wall with left hand **(Fig. 8)**, after securing the Veress needle in its position with right hand, and again look for the pressure readings over the insufflator. If reading shows ≤8 mm Hg pressure, you are in right place, which usually is the case **(Fig. 9)**, otherwise take out the needle and try again by repeating all the above mentioned steps. A maximum of three attempts can be made.]

*Standard safety measures for intraperitoneal insufflation:[2-4]

9. Insufflate the abdomen at the rate of 1 L/min aiming to achieve initial intra-abdominal pressure of 20–25 mm Hg.

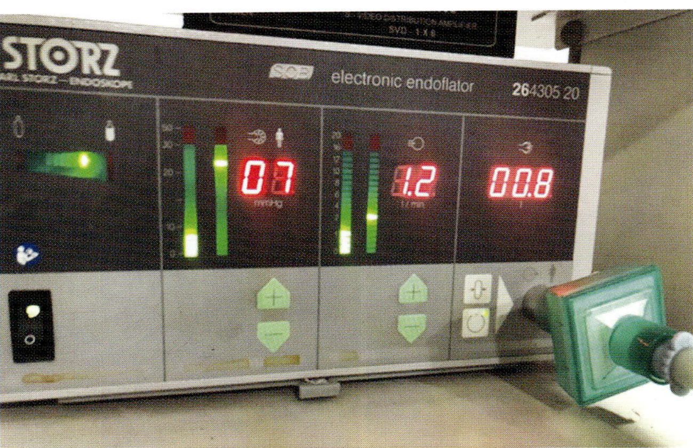

Fig. 9: Insufflator reading showing low initial Veres intraperitoneal pressure (<8 mm Hg).

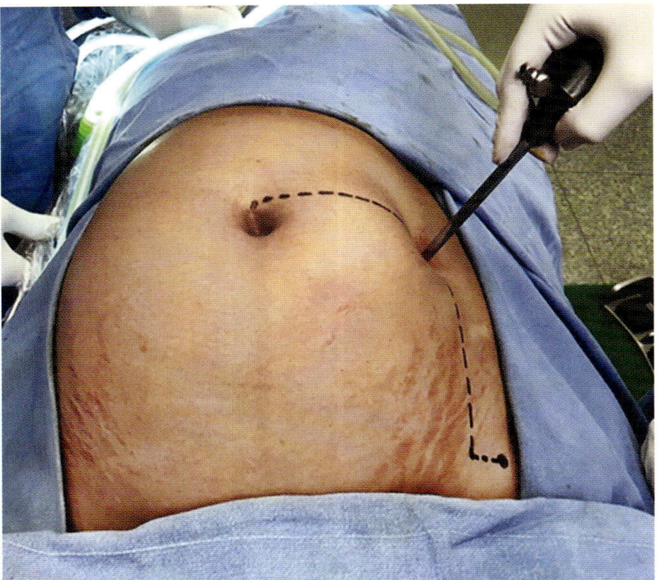

Fig. 10A: Primary trocar entry through Jain point after pneumoperitonization.

10. Once the abdomen is uniformly distended and taut, the Veress needle is removed.
11. The initial stab incision is extended to 5 mm size and a 5 mm trocar with cannula held as a pistol with its vent open is inserted with screwing movements **(Fig. 10A)**.
12. Once the trocar and cannula enters the insufflated peritoneal cavity, a hissing sound is heard. This confirms intraperitoneal entry. Trocar is then removed.
13. A 5 mm telescope is introduced through the cannula and abdominal cavity is checked for any entry related injury and presence of adhesions.

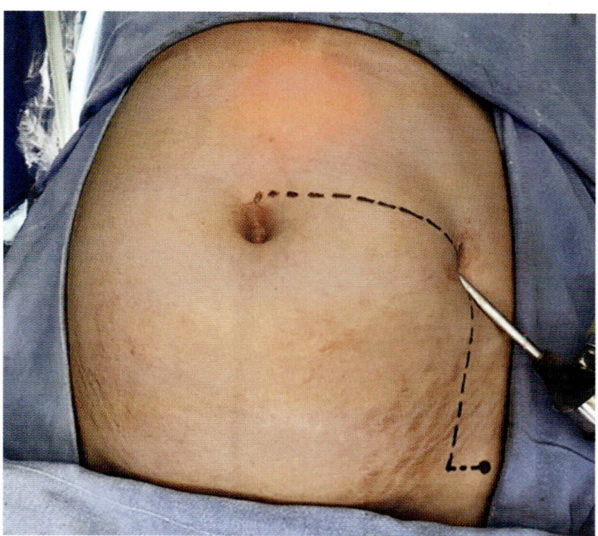

Fig. 10B: Rationalizing the position of 10 mm telescope under direct vision through Jain point.

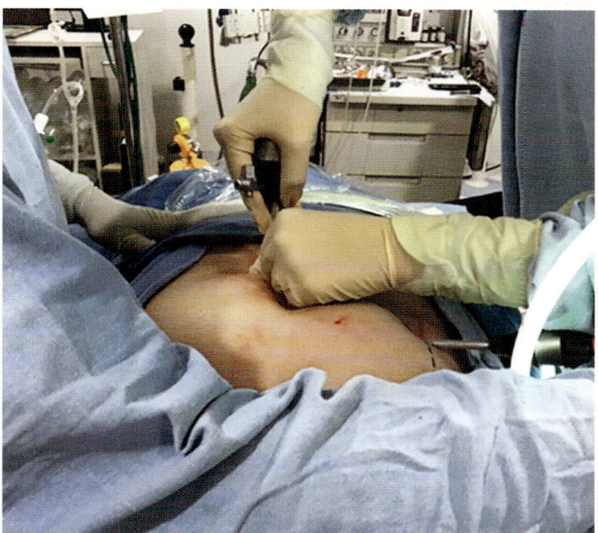

Fig. 10C: Inserting 10 mm trocar cannula under direct vision of 5 mm telescope at Jain point.

14. The pelvic anatomy is inspected and the target area of dissection is looked for, to decide the appropriate placement of 10 mm telescope **(Figs. 10B and C)** and other secondary ports according to the baseball diamond concept[5] **(Figs. 11 and 12)**.

Benefits of Jain Point Entry

- It is one of the best available options for blind entry into the abdomen especially in previous surgery patients, as it is relatively free of adhesions.[6]

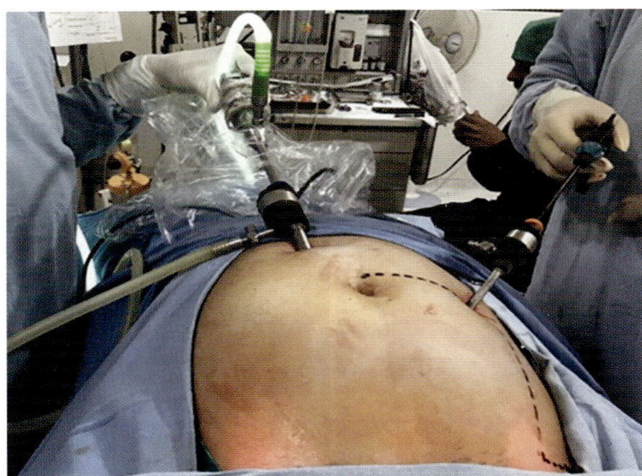

Fig. 11: Inspecting the pelvic anatomy and disease pathology through Jain point working port with 10 mm telescope inserted in upper abdominal wall to decide number of secondary ports needed for appropriate working.

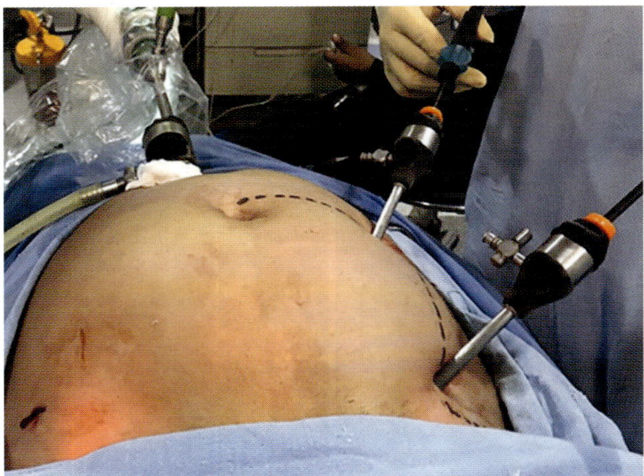

Fig. 12: Ipsilateral working with Jain point port as upper working port.

- The surface marking of Jain point is very easy even in draped patient as compared to Palmer's point where midclavicular line is difficult to appreciate due to layers of drapes over the patient's body.
- There is negligible risk of injury to great vessels as the Jain point is paraumbilical and the tip of usual length of Veress (10–12 cm size) can never reach till the umbilicus, which is 10–13 cm away from Jain point.
- Primary port insertion through the Jain point precludes the need to lift the abdominal wall which allows the surgeon to do the procedure of pneumo-peritonization independently.
- Irrespective of the body makeup of the patient, the Veress needle is inserted perpendicular to the patient's body, which eliminates the technical

challenges faced with umbilical port entry in extremely obese or lean patients.

- It forms excellent main working port for all usual gynecological cases, as it obeys baseball diamond concept and thus avoids extra port insertion as required in Palmer's point entry.
- It is most easily learnt and is replicable by most of the fellows, trainees, and new aspirants of endoscopic surgery with a short learning curve of 5–6 procedures.
- Apart of all the above mentioned benefits, it can also be used in those conditions where umbilical and Palmer point is contraindicated.[7]

Primary optical port entry is the most crucial step of any laparoscopic surgery. Once this hurdle is passed successfully, one can proceed with the actual surgery confidently. We find Jain point entry a very safe and easy way of inserting first blind port. Though honestly, our initial 4–5 entries were not so perfect and were preperitoneal, leading to surgical emphysema involving the left abdominal wall. However, as we understood the abdominal wall anatomy and technique well, we were soon able to enter into the abdominal cavity very precisely and confidently without any failures. We did not experience any vascular or bowel injury so far. Omental insufflation may be encountered few times; however no intervention is required for it, as it resolves on its own.

We would recommend the readers to try the Jain's point for the blind Veress and primary port insertion followed by secondary ports insertion under direct vision. Its application is very easy with short learning curve of 1–2 weeks. This point would not only act as a safety cushion for those who are apprehensive about first blind trocar entry through the umbilicus, but would also serve well in difficult case scenarios where all other entry sites are dangerous.

REFERENCES

1. Drake R, Vogl AW, Mitchell AWM. Gray's Anatomy for Students, 3rd edition. UK: Churchill Livingston Elsevier; 2015. pp. 280-91.
2. Vilos GA. The ABCs of a safer laparoscopic entry. J Minim Invasive Gynecol. 2006;13(3):249-51.
3. Teoh B, Sen R, Abbott J. An evaluation of four tests used to ascertain Veres needle placement at closed laparoscopy. J Min Invas Gynecol. 2005;12(2):153-8.
4. Azevedo OC, Azevedo JL, Sorbello AA, et al. Evaluation of tests performed to confirm the position of the Veress needle for creation of pneumoperitoneum in selected patients: a prospective clinical trial. Acta Cirúrgica Brasileira. 2006;21(6):385-91.
5. Ferzil GS, Fingerhut A. Trocar placement for laparoscopic abdominal procedures: a simple standardized method. J Am Coll Surg. 2004;198(1):163-73.
6. Jain N, Sareen S, Kanawa S, et al. Jain point: a new safe portal for laparoscopic entry in previous surgery cases. J Hum Reprod Sci. 2016;9(1):9-17.
7. Palmer R. Safety in laparoscopy. J Reprod Med. 1974;13(1):1-5.

22

Direct Trocar Entry through Jain Point

Barış Mulayim

INTRODUCTION

Laparoscopy has become a standard way of performing gynecologic surgeries all over the world since laparoscopy has several advantages over laparotomy. However, laparoscopy has unique feature; which needs entering to the abdomen for pneumoperitoneum that also carries a significant risk of bowel and vascular injuries. There are various techniques and different sites for abdominal access.[1]

The traditional way and the most commonly used method of entry to the abdomen for pneumoperitoneum is using Veress needle through the umbilicus among gynecologists.[1] The Veress needle was developed by Veress in 1938.[2]

The other utilized entry techniques are direct trocar insertion without a pre-existing pneumoperitoneum, which was first described by Dingfelder in 1978[3] and classic open Hasson method, which was first described by Hasson in 1971.[4] It remains the preferred entry method for many laparoscopic surgeons, particularly general surgeons.

When there is suspicion of adhesions before entering to the abdomen, especially due to previous surgeries different entry sites rather than umbilicus is recommended. Thus, Palmer's point is the most common known and utilized site of entry among such cases, which was advocated by Palmer in 1974.[5] Besides, in 2001, Lee-Huang technique was published by Lee et al. who used this point for the Veress needle and primary port insertion as an alternative portal for laparoscopic entry.[6] Moreover, in 2016 Jain et al. have recently described a novel technique for laparoscopic entry in previous surgery cases and adds another armamentarium into our arsenal.[7]

Laparoscopic entry has paramount importance because almost 50% of major laparoscopic complications occur before commencement of intended surgery, and this is the reason why there is a great deal of interest on this subject.[8]

DIRECT TROCAR ENTRY THROUGH JAIN POINT: A CRITICAL REVIEW

The direct trocar entry technique, without preinsufflation, requires elevation of the anterior abdominal wall with the nondominant hand while inserting the primary sharp trocar directly and blindly towards the peritoneal cavity. Once the tip of the trocar has been inserted through the skin incision, the trocar is pushed through the fascia and the muscle layer by a continuous twisting motion with constant downward pressure, so that the surgeon can easily realize when the trocar has pierced the peritoneum and entered the peritoneal cavity. The CO_2 gas stopcock must be kept open during the insertion, to relieve the negative intra-abdominal pressure as soon as the vented trocar tip enters the sealed peritoneal space. It is postulated that the viscera falls off its parietal apposition prior to contact with the advancing primary trocar. Once the successful trocar placement is verified by a laparoscope, CO_2 gas is insufflated under direct visualization.[9]

According to Cochrane review written by Ahmad G et al., trial results showed a reduction in failed entry into the abdomen with the use of a direct trocar in comparison with Veress needle. However, evidence was insufficient to show whether there were differences between groups in rates of vascular injury, visceral injury, or solid organ injury.[10]

The potential benefits of this method are reportedly a shorter operating time, immediate recognition of visceral/vascular injuries, and near exclusion of entry failure.[11,12] Direct entry also reduces the number of 'blind steps' from three with Veress needle entry (insertion, insufflation, and trocar introduction) to just one, that of trocar introduction.

Despite those aforementioned advantages, direct trocar entry is probably the least used entry technique because this is a matter of habits and unaware of this technique among gynecologists, we consider.

As mentioned above in the Cochrane review, direct trocar entry has less entry failure; this means that one should possibly have less risk when compared with Veress needle entry because every attempt has lead much more risk for entry complications.[10]

Umbilicus is the rational site for laparoscopic entry because it is the shortest distance to the abdominal cavity through the least vascular area of the abdominal wall. Moreover, the peritoneum is dimpled upward in a cone-shaped configuration at the base of the umbilicus, it is less likely that omentum and intestine will become attached and adheres to its peritoneal surface.[13]

However, guidelines recommended alternative sites in patients with previous laparotomy for laparoscopic entry such as Palmer's and Lee-Huang points.[5,6,14,15]

In patients with previous laparotomy, Palmer advocated insertion of the Veress needle 3 cm below the left subcostal border in the midclavicular line.

This may be considered in the obese as well as in the very thin patient. The stomach should be emptied by nasogastric suction and the needle should be introduced perpendicular to the skin. Patients with previous splenic or gastric surgery, portal hypertension or significant gastropancreatic masses should be excluded.[5] However, there are case reports that Palmer's point is not 100% safe or without adhesions.[16,17]

Lee-Huang point, which used this point for the Veress needle and primary port insertion as an alternative portal for laparoscopic entry in the upper abdomen (in the midline), midway between the xiphoid process and the umbilicus, described by Dr Chyi-Long Lee and Dr Kuan-Gen Huang.[6] The contraindication to using the Lee-Huang point insertion is a patient who has had previous surgery at the supraumbilical region.

Recently, Jain et al. described a novel point for laparoscopic entry in patients with pervious laparotomy. Jain point is placed at the level of umbilicus (paraumbilical) on the left side where usually the operating surgeon stands. It is placed in a straight line drawn vertically upward from a lower point, which is 2.5 cm medial to anterior superior iliac spine (ASIS). Pneumoperitoneum is created through Jain point via Veress needle. They reported that in 624 patients with a history of previous abdominal surgeries intra-abdominal adhesions were found in 487 (78.0%) patients and umbilical adhesions in 404 (64.7%) patients with past abdominal surgeries. They added that, there were no significant entry-related, intraoperative, or postoperative complications with the use of this entry point.[7]

They also claimed that Jain point would be used in patients where Palmer's and Lee-Huang points are contraindicated such as patients with previous splenic or gastric surgery, portal hypertension or significant gastropancreatic masses, and patients who have had previous surgery at the supraumbilical region.[7]

Nowadays in my clinic, we perform Jain point entry with direct trocar insertion in patients who have previous laparotomy; we believe that Jain point entry with direct trocar insertion would be much safer, faster, and successful as aforementioned reasons above.

But are those laparoscopic entry points 100% safe? It is difficult to say 100% yes, of course we need prospective randomized controlled trials with large number of cases. Nevertheless, it is good for us to have alternative sites for laparoscopic entry.

TECHNIQUE

The Jain point is located in the left paraumbilical region at the level of umbilicus, on a straight line drawn vertically upwards from a point 2.5 cm medial to ASIS. The 5 mm trocar is inserted at this point but 10 mm trocar can be used either for direct trocar insertion, depending on your port configuration and you can keep

Jain point trocar through your surgery, as well. Then telescope inserted into the abdomen after then pneumoperitoneum created from Jain point trocar and whole abdomen inspected. Other secondary ports are inserted under vision of this telescope **(Figs. 1 to 5)**. If adhesions are present, adhesiolysis is performed and then according to your port configuration ports are placed. By resorting to this novel entry technique, we may safely overcome all contraindications of Palmer's and Lee-Huang points discussed above.

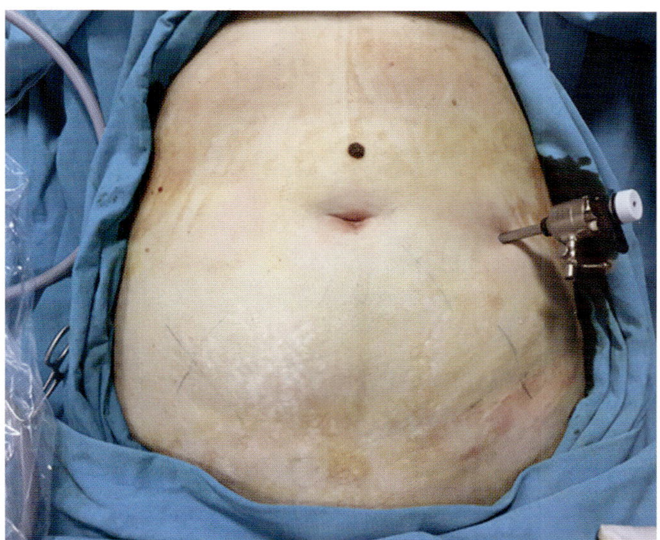

Fig. 1: Direct trocar entry at Jain point.

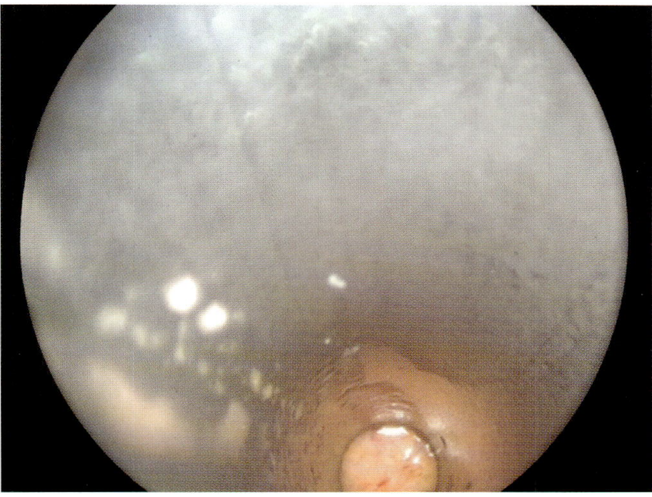

Fig. 2: Omentum is detected when inserting the telescope that is confirmation of correct entry.

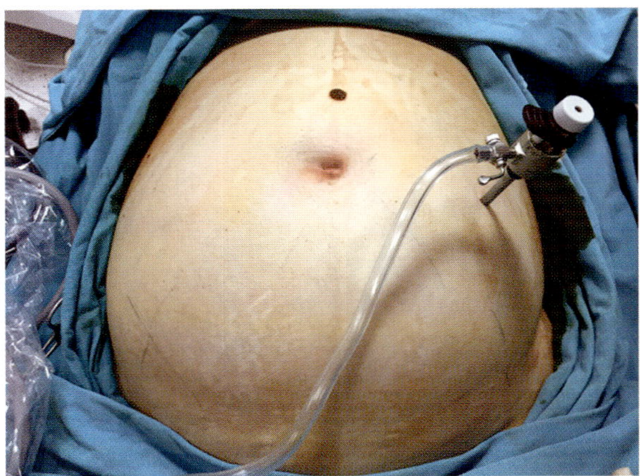

Fig. 3: Pneumoperitoneum is established from Jain point trocar.

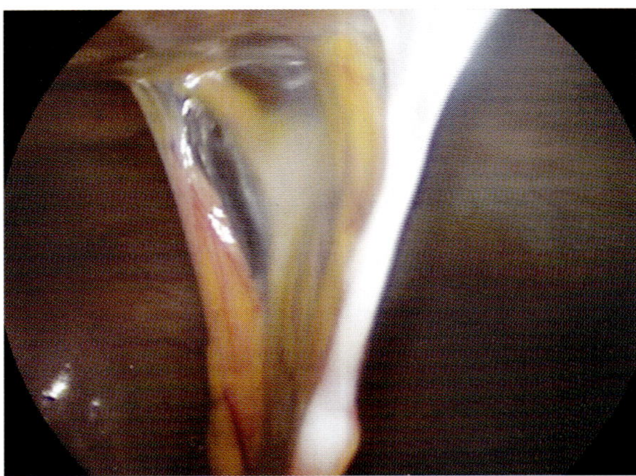

Fig. 4: Omentum and bowel are attached to the anterior abdominal wall detected from Jain point with 5 mm telescope.

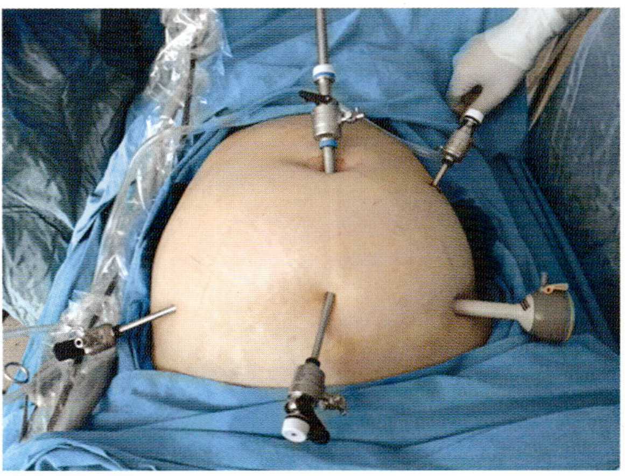

Fig. 5: Suprapubic port configuration.

REFERENCES

1. Molloy D, Kaloo PD, Cooper M, et al. Laparoscopic entry: a literature review and analysis of techniques and complications of primary port entry. Aust NZJ Obstet Gynaecol. 2002;42(3):246-54.
2. Veress J. Neues Instument zur Ausfuhrung von Brust-oder Bauchpunktionen und Pneumothoraxbehandlung. Dtsch Med Wochenshr. 1938;41:1480-1.
3. Dingfelder JR. Direct laparoscope trocar insertion without prior pneumoperitoneum. J Reprod Med. 1978;21:45-7.
4. Hasson HM. A modified instrument and method for laparoscopy. Am J Obstet Gynecol. 1971;110:886-7.
5. Palmer R. Safety in laparoscopy. J Reprod Med. 1974;13:1-5.
6. Lee CL, Huang KG, Jain S, et al. A new portal for gynecologic laparoscopy. J Am Assoc Gynecol Laparosc. 2001;8:147-50.
7. Jain N, Sareen S, Kanawa S, et al. Jain point: a new safe portal for laparoscopic entry in previous surgery cases. J Hum Reprod Sci. 2016;9(1):9-17.
8. Krishnakumar S, Tambe P. Entry complications in laparoscopic surgery. J Gynecol Endosc Surg. 2009;1(1):4-11.
9. Jiang X, Anderson C, Schnatz PF. The safety of direct trocar versus Veress needle for laparoscopic entry: a meta-analysis of randomized clinical trials. J Laparoendosc Adv Surg Tech A. 2012;22(4):362-70.
10. Ahmad G, Baker J, Finnerty J, et al. Laparoscopic entry techniques. Cochrane Database Syst Rev. 2019;1:CD006583.
11. Zakherah MS. Direct trocar versus Veress needle entry for laparoscopy: a randomized clinical trial. Gynecol Obstet Invest. 2010;69(4):260-3.
12. Angioli R, Terranova C, De Cicco Nardone C, et al. A comparison of three different entry techniques in gynecological laparoscopic surgery: a randomized prospective trial. Eur J Obstet Gynecol Reprod Biol. 2013;171(2):339-42.
13. Roy GM, Bazzurini L, Solima E, et al. Safe technique for laparoscopic entry into the abdominal cavity. J Am Assoc Gynecol Laparosc. 2001;8(4):519-28.
14. Vilos GA, Ternamian A, Dempster J, et al. No. 193-Laparoscopic entry: a review of techniques, technologies, and complications. J Obstet Gynaecol Can. 2017;39(7):e69-84.
15. RCOG. (2008). Laparoscopic Injuries (Green-top Guideline No. 49). [online] Available from https://www.rcog.org.uk/en/guidelines-research-services/guidelines/gtg49/ [Last accessed November, 2019].
16. Dar S, Lazer T, Baratz A. Is Palmer's point really safe? J Obstet Gynaecol Can. 2013;35(12):1063.
17. Mulayim B. Laparoscopic entry, but how? Ann Clin Case Rep. 2017;2:1262.

Jain Point in the Practice of General Surgery

Jain Point Port in Ventral Hernia Repair

Siddharth Gupta, Nutan Jain

◼ INTRODUCTION

Repair of incisional hernia and ventral hernia is most commonly performed surgery in day-to-day clinical practice. The commonly seen long-term complications of abdominal surgery is incisional hernia, with the occurrence rate of 11–20%.[1,2] An incisional hernia is defined as a protrusion of intraperitoneal structures through a defect in the anterior abdominal wall fascia.[3]

Predisposing technical factors are related to suture material selection, type of fascial closure, and ratio of suture to incision length.[4] Other factors, such as anemia, hypoproteinemia, malnutrition, diabetes, immunosuppression, male gender, and old age, are related to surgical wound dehiscence and incisional hernias.[5] Conditions that increase abdominal pressure, such as coughing, vomiting, distention, and ascites, also increase the incidence of incisional hernias. Surgeons have to be aware of poor wound healing conditions to prevent incisional hernias. Perioperative efforts to reduce risk factors and to select proper technical methods of wound closure are essential if the incidence of incisional hernias is to be reduced.

It has been seen that approximately 50% of incisional hernias develop in initial 2 years of surgery, and this percentage rises up to 74% after 3 years of duration.[6,7] The use of meshes (prosthetic materials) for repair has reduced the recurrence rate of incisional hernia from 50% (by primary hernia repair) to 10–23% (after mesh repair).[8,9] Infectious complications leading to morbidity in cases of open ventral hernia repair has encouraged the surgeons for laparoscopic repair of ventral hernia. Also, as these days the general surgeon's attention is increasing toward laparoscopic surgery and same time prosthetic materials (mesh) have shown better long-term results. These factors have encouraged the surgeons for laparoscopic repair of ventral hernia. Hence, repair of hernia by laparoscopy is increasing worldwide not only for simple cases but also for complex incisional hernias. Laparoscopic hernia repair followed the same guidelines and principles as the open procedure described by Stoppa.[10] Rives et al.[11] and Wantz[12] Laparoscopic Ventral hernia repair (LVHR) was first described by Leblanc and Booth[13] in 1991. Laparoscopic ventral hernia repair fixes tears or openings in the abdominal wall with the help of small incisions, laparoscopes and a prosthetic mesh to strengthen the abdominal wall. Just like other laparoscopic procedures done by competent surgeons, it offers a quicker return to normal activities with decreased pain. Most of the literatures available on this topic have also supported minimal postoperative complications, a shorter recovery period, and an acceptable recurrence rate.[14-16]

INDICATIONS AND PATIENT SELECTION

The indication to repair a ventral hernia is for symptom relief and/or prevention of future problems related to the hernia such as pain, acute incarceration, enlargement, and skin problems.

Prior hernia repairs, large defect sizes, and incarcerated hernias increase the difficulty and duration of the procedure and should be taken into consideration by surgeons when deciding to take up the case.

Given the variation of technical expertise and institutional infrastructure, along with the gradual acquisition of experience, surgeons must use their judgment when determining whether to perform a laparoscopic or open ventral hernia repair. When considering a laparoscopic approach to a ventral hernia, the surgeon should consider his or her own experience when selecting patients. There is limited evidence on how expertise with laparoscopic ventral hernia repair is developed; however, it appears prudent to recommend that good suturing skills will make the job easier and less experienced surgeons should start with simpler cases and gradually progress to more challenging tasks.[17]

LIMITATIONS AND CONTRAINDICATIONS

- *Loss of domain:* Massive hernia sac (>30% abdominal contents) where reduction would cause major abdominal hypertension leading to abdominal compartment syndrome.
- Abdominal skin grafts overlying the defect makes adhesiolysis difficult. Increased risk of visceral injuries.
- Incarcerated hernia.
- Active enterocutaneous fistula.
- Need to remove previously placed prosthetic mesh.
- Large abdominal wall defects.[17]

TECHNIQUES (FIGS. 1A TO I)

Previous mesh hernia repair cases need special mention in entry technique. In ventral hernia which are going up to umbilicus, obviously the entry technique has to be other than umbilicus. Even if there is no previous surgery and there is a hernia defect over umbilicus, an alternate entry point is needed. The usually used point is the Palmer's point. But if there are scars of previous surgery and/or previously used mesh was of bigger size, the Palmer's point being more medial,

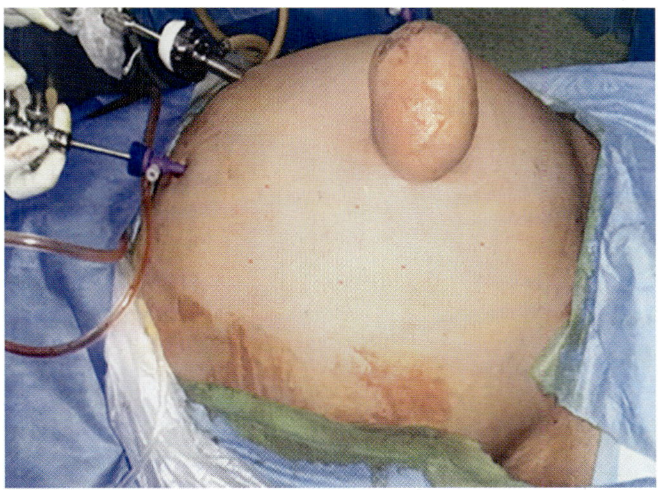

Fig. 1A: External view of port position.
Courtesy: Dr Praveen Bhatia, Sir Ganga Ram Hospital, New Delhi, India.

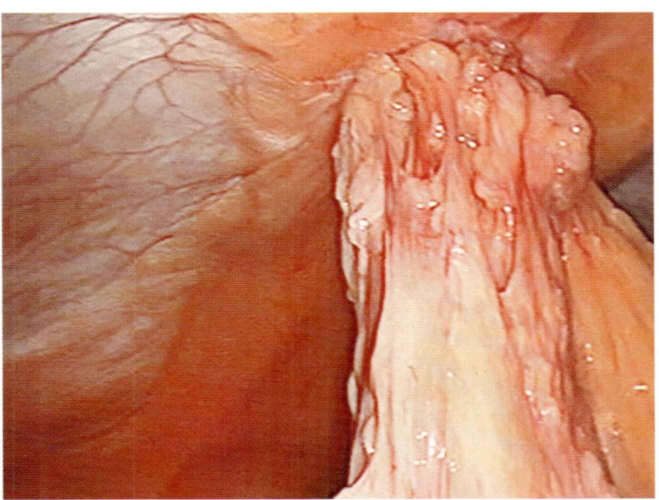

Fig. 1B: Omentum adherent to anterior abdominal wall.
Courtesy: Dr Praveen Bhatia, Sir Ganga Ram Hospital, New Delhi, India.

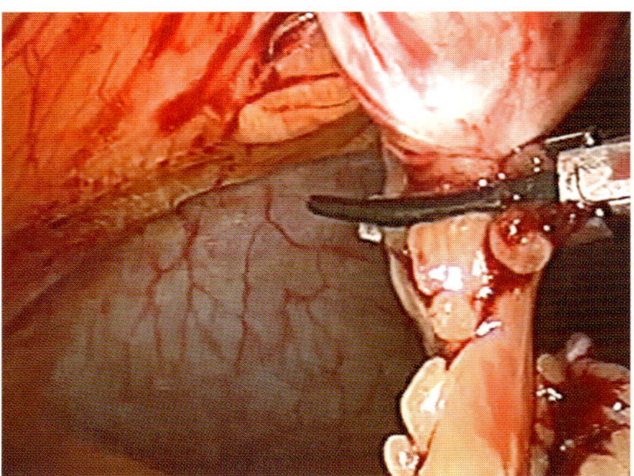

Fig. 1C: Adhesiolysis with Harmonic Ace.
Courtesy: Dr Praveen Bhatia, Sir Ganga Ram Hospital, New Delhi, India.

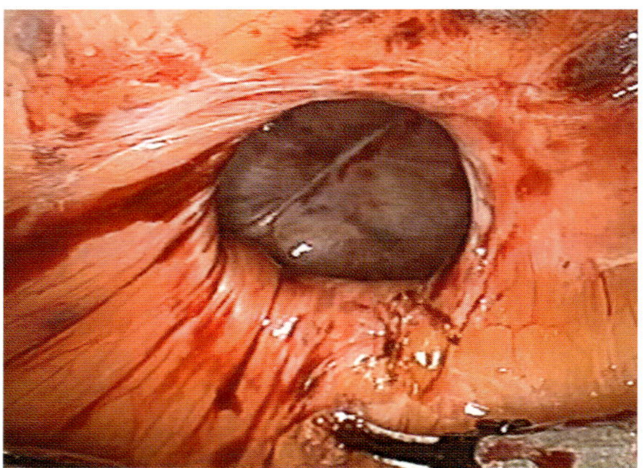

Fig. 1D: Hernial defect seen.
Courtesy: Dr Praveen Bhatia, Sir Ganga Ram Hospital, New Delhi, India.

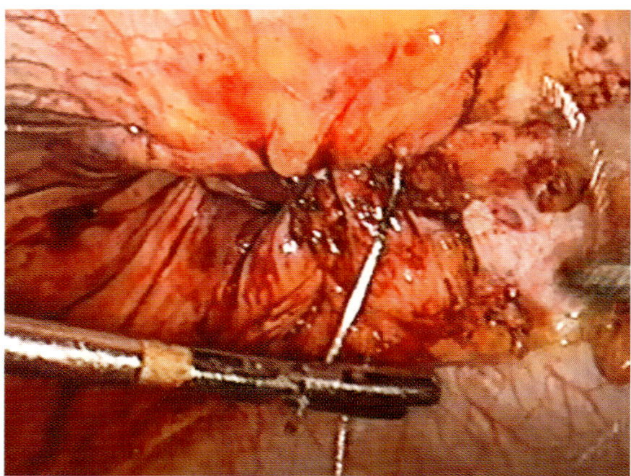

Fig. 1E: Hernial defect being sutured with Stratafix no.1.
Courtesy: Dr Praveen Bhatia, Sir Ganga Ram Hospital, New Delhi, India.

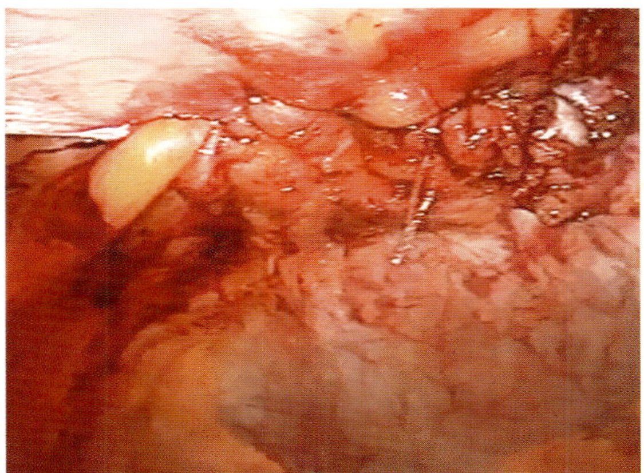

Fig. 1F: Defect completely closed.
Courtesy: Dr Praveen Bhatia, Sir Ganga Ram Hospital, New Delhi, India.

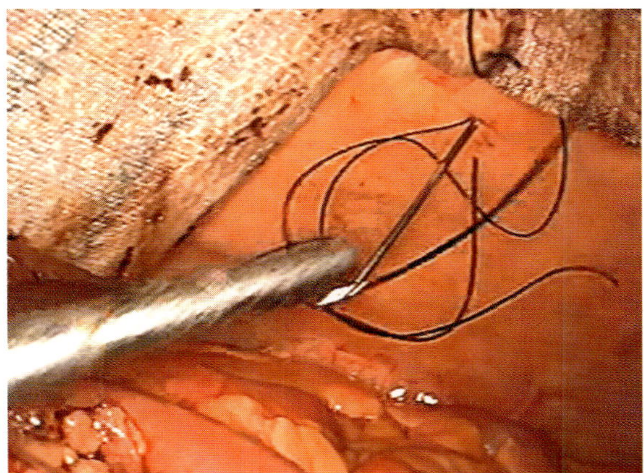

Fig. 1G: Transfascial sutures applied for mesh fixation.
Courtesy: Dr Praveen Bhatia, Sir Ganga Ram Hospital, New Delhi, India.

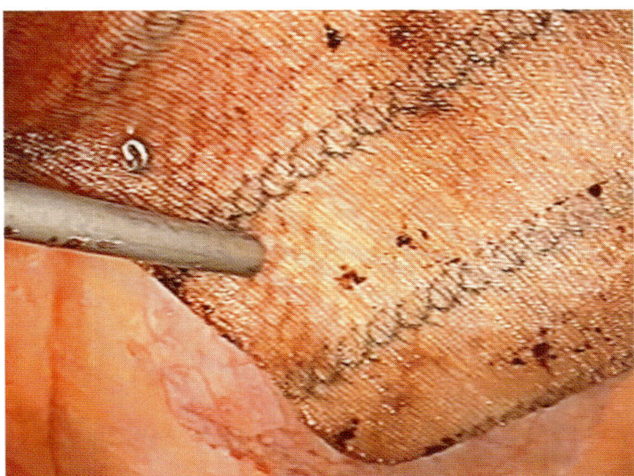

Fig. 1H: Proceed mesh fixed with tacker.
Courtesy: Dr Praveen Bhatia, Sir Ganga Ram Hospital, New Delhi, India.

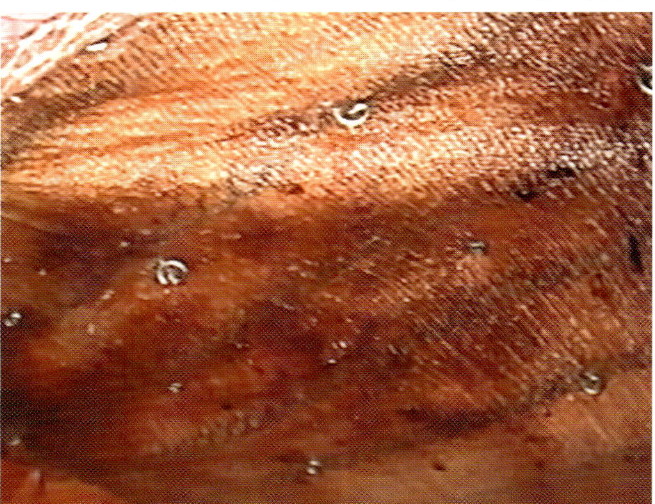

Fig. 1I: Defect completely covered.
Courtesy: Dr Praveen Bhatia, Sir Ganga Ram Hospital, New Delhi, India.

we propose Jain point which is about 10–13 cm from midline and can be more congenial and surer to remain outside the mesh. Jain point is a mid-abdomen outer quadrant port which is safely outside the largest size of hernia or largest size of mesh used for earlier repair. Jain point is a dynamic port which can be made further laterally, as lateral to this point at L4 level there is no concern of vital viscera. Not only for the first blind port entry, Jain port also doubles up as the main working port. As in hernia repair, either for applying tackers or suturing the fascial defects, the left lateral port is used. So, if we use Jain point for first blind port entry, we can also use it all throughout the surgery. Along with the left lower port, Jain point port becomes a good ergonomic ipsilateral working port, enabling the surgeon to accomplish suturing the fascial defect and using the tackers.

Prerequisite of safe entry in hernia is that the primary trocar should be 10 cm[17] from the scars of previous surgeries[18] and also from hernia orifice but should still provide adequate instrument reach. Hence, these two prerequisites are fully met with Jain point first blind port entry. After the initial port placement, rest of the 10 mm port and accessory ports are placed according to mandate of the case. The hernial sac contents are reduced in the peritoneal cavity with atraumatic grasper, and if bowel is also the content, cautery to be avoided and all precautions should be taken to avoid bowel injury. After the contents are reduced, the hernial sac is excised if too large.

Primary Fascial Closure and Mesh Repair (IPOM Plus)

This technique has been developed to reduce postoperative bulging and formation of seroma after laparoscopic ventral hernia repair. According to

LaPlace's law, a central nonfunctional portion of the abdominal wall acts like a "sail in the wind" and is prone to bulging. The advantage of primary fascial closure is in restoring normal anatomy by reapproximating the abdominal wall under physiologic tension, which ultimately may restore abdominal wall function.[19,20] This repair can only be done for hernial defects up to 5 cm.

The different closure techniques used for this are intracorporeal closure, extracorporeal closure, or a mixed technique; out of all these techniques, extracorporeal suturing is most commonly used. Here in this technique, small skin incisions are made and then a suture passer is used to close the defect. By completely removing the dead space, the incidence of seromas and wound complications are reduced. Further, it allows wider lateral mesh overlap which reduces the possibility of recurrence.[20]

Mesh Repair

Peritoneal surface is cleared of adhesions away from the hernia defect. Intra-abdominal pressure is reduced to 5–8 mm Hg, so as to know about the actual size of hernial defect. Craniocaudal and lateral measurements are taken to define the size of mesh. As of basic hernia surgery rule, mesh should overlap 5 cm circumferentially from the edge of defect. Two main types of mesh are used commonly:
1. ePTFE mesh (Dual, Dulex).
2. Composite mesh with coated barrier (Proceed, Parietex, Physiomesh).

Meshes Used Intraperitoneally for the Repair of Ventral and Incisional Hernias (Table 1)

After the selection of mesh, four sutures are placed on the midpoint of each of the four edges of mesh **(Fig. 2)**. The mesh is rolled and inserted in peritoneal cavity through 10 mm trocar. It is unrolled and spread under the defect, four transfascial sutures are used to fix the mesh. It is further secured with titanium tacks applied using fixation devices (Covidien Protack, Securestrap Ethicon). Tacks should be placed circumferentially at 1 cm margin of mesh to prevent bowel from becoming incarcerated between mesh and abdominal wall **(Fig. 3)**.

◼ COMPLICATIONS

- *Hemorrhage*: Initially during insertion of trocars, bleeding may occur, usually from the inferior epigastric artery branches, which could be secured by cautery or by placing the sutures. If vessels are injured during mesh placement, these should be ligated with the help of transfascial suture or a figure of eight transfascial suture.[18] Visualize inferior epigastric artery during mesh fixation to avoid any injury.
- *Iatrogenic enterotomy*: Seen in up to 14% of cases.[21] This may occur because of dense bowel/omental adhesion, recurrent hernias and energy devices

TABLE 1: Meshes used intraperitoneally for the repair of ventral and incisional hernias.		
Group/Mesh	*Material*	*Company*
• *ePTFE*		
– Dulex	ePTFE	Bard Davol, Inc., Warwick, RI
– Dual mesh	ePTFE	WL Gore
• *Composite mesh with absorbable coated barrier*		
– Proceed	PP with ORC layer	Ethicon, Somerville, NJ
– Parietene	PP with collagen coated	Covidien, Mansfield, MA
– Parietex composite	Polyester with collagen coated	Covidien
– Symbotex	Polyester with collagen film	Covidien
– Physiomesh	PP with polyglecaprone 25	Ethicon
• *Composite mesh with permanent coated barrier*		
– Composix	PP/ePTFE	Bard Davol, Inc.
– Ventrio	PP/ePTFE	Bard Davol, Inc.

(ePTFE: expanded polytetrafluoroethylene; PP: polypropylene; ORC: oxidized regenerated cellulose).

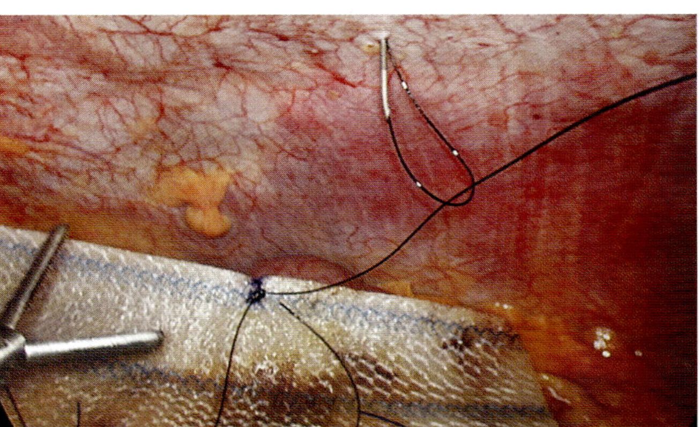

Fig. 2: Suture placed on midpoint of each edge of mesh.
Courtesy: Dr Praveen Bhatia, Sir Ganga Ram Hospital, New Delhi, India.

used for adhesiolysis. In this situation, enterotomy is to be repaired laparoscopically and usual practice is to defer the hernia repair with mesh fixation by 4–6 weeks.

• *Seroma*: Mostly occur at seventh postoperative day, are usually asymptomatic, and are resolved normally by 3 months. Cauterization of

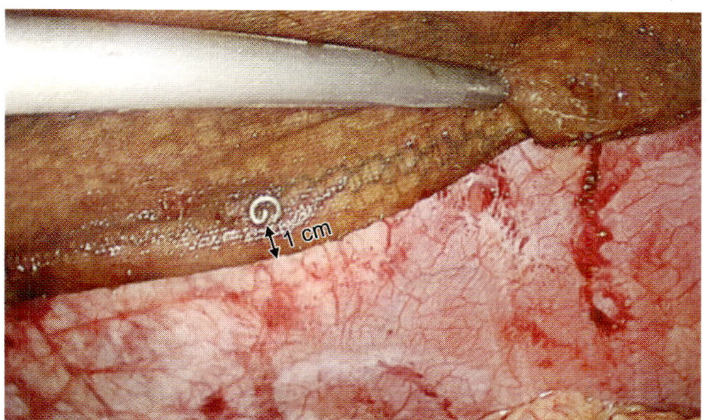

Fig. 3: Tack placed 1 cm from the mesh margin.
Courtesy: Dr Praveen Bhatia, Sir Ganga Ram Hospital, New Delhi, India.

hernia sac and compression dressing for 1 week may reduce the risk of seroma.

- *Abdominal bulging*: With the incidence rate of 1.6–17.4%.[22] To reduce the risk of seroma and postoperative bulging, Orenstein et al. modified their laparoscopic approach to routine shoe lacing technique for hernia defect closure.[23]
- *Chronic pain*: Approximately 20% of patients may experience residual pain. Prolonged pain which may be because of nerve entrapment can be managed by injecting local anesthetic at suture site, or by intercostal nerve block.[24] In some cases pain is relieved by removing suture, tack or even mesh.[25]
- *Mesh infection*: Lower incidence than in open approach.[26] To avoid this complication, we should use preoperative antibiotic, maintain sterility of instruments, change gloves before placing mesh and minimum handling of mesh should be practiced.
- Recurrence is usually reported in 7% of cases.[27]

LEARNING POINTS

- Patience, patience, and patience.
- Role of traction and counter traction for reducing hernia contents.
- Use as little energy as possible for adhesiolysis (cold scissors>harmonic> bipolar>monopolar).
- Do not solve the problem which is not there (avoid extra adhesiolysis).
- There can be a snake (bowel) behind every bush (adhesion and omentum) and even a small snake can be lethal.
- If there is a bleeding, fix it then and there.
- Soar over the clouds like an eagle (remain centrifugal, close to anterior abdominal wall).

- Small bites, small mistakes.
- Preoperative CT scan is must (to diagnose occult hernias, multiple defects, abscess, hematoma, differentiate incarcerated hernia from abdominal wall neoplasms).
- If enterotomy, defer the use of mesh.

ADVANTAGES

Jain point usage as the primary blind entry port may tide over the menace of visceral injury in case of splenomegaly, bloated stomach, and adhesions due to previous surgery in upper quadrant and offers a nonumbilical port in ventral hernia repair where umbilical entry is hazardous.

The adequate closure of hernia defect is achieved with the help of intraperitoneal mesh fixation and minimum soft tissue dissection. Hence, patients experience less postoperative pain, early recovery, less hospital stay in comparison to open repair.[27] This technique also offers complete visibility of interior of abdominal wall, hence fixation of mesh is much accurate. Smaller defects which were not obvious otherwise can also be seen by the magnification offered by the laparoscope.

Patient satisfaction and quality of life are better in laparoscopic repair in comparison to open repair.

ACKNOWLEDGMENT

All surgical snapshots of ventral hernia repair have been provided by Dr Praveen Bhatia, Sir Ganga Ram Hospital, New Delhi, India.

REFERENCES

1. Bloemen A, van Dooren P, Huizinga BF, et al. Randomized clinical trial comparing polypropylene or polydioxanone for midline abdominal wall closure. Br J Surg. 2011;98(5):633-9.
2. Van't Riet M, Steyerberg EW, Nellensteyn J, et al. Meta-analysis of techniques for closure of midline abdominal incisions. Br J Surg. 2002;89:1350-6.
3. Korenkov M, Paul A, Sauerland S, et al. Classification and surgical treatment of incisional hernia. Results of an experts' meeting. Langenbecks Arch Surg. 2001;386(1):65-73.
4. Veljkovic R, Protic M, Gluhovic A, et al. Prospective clinical trial of factors predicting the early development of incisional hernia after midline laparotomy. J Am Coll Surg. 2010;210:210-9.
5. Sorensen LT, Hemmingsen U, Kallehave F, et al. Risk factors for tissue and wound complications in gastrointestinal surgery. Ann Surg. 2005;241(4):654-8.
6. Pollock AV, Evans M. Early prediction of late incisional hernias. Br J Surg. 1989;76:953-4.
7. Anthony T, Bergen PC, Kim LT, et al. Factors affecting recurrence following incisional herniorrhaphy. World J Surg. 2000;24(1):95-100; discussion 101.

8. Shell DH, de la Torre J, Andrades T, et al. Open repair of ventral hernia incisions. Surg Clin North Am. 2008;88(1):61-83.

9. Luijendijk R, Hop W, Van den Tol MP, et al. A comparison of suture repair with mesh repair for incisional hernia. N Eng J Med. 2000;343:392-8.

10. Stoppa RE. The treatment of complicated groin and incisional hernias. World J Surg. 1989;13:545-54.

11. Rives J, Pire JC, Flament JB, et al. Treatment of large eventrations: new therapeutic indications apropos of 322 cases. Chirurgie. 1985;111(3):215-25.

12. Wantz GE. Incisional hernioplasty with Mersilene. Surg Gynecol Obstetr. 1991;172:129-37.

13. Leblanc KA, Booth WV. Laparoscopic repair of incisional abdominal hernias using polytetrafluoroethylene: preliminary findings. Surg Laparosc Endosc. 1993;3:39-41.

14. Franklin ME, Dorman JP, Glass JL, et al. Laparoscopic ventral and incisional hernia repair. Surg Laparosc Endosc. 1998;8:294-9.

15. Heniford BT, Park A, Ramshaw BJ, et al. Laparoscopic ventral and incisional hernia repair in 407 patients. J Am Coll Surg. 2000;190:645-50.

16. LeBlanc KA, Booth WV, Whitaker JM, et al. Laparoscopic incisional and ventral herniorrhaphy: our initial 100 patients. Hernia. 2001;5:41-5.

17. Earle D, Roth S, Saber A, et al. (2016). Sages guideline for laparoscopic vental hernia repair. [online] Available from https://www.sages.org/publications/guidelines/guidelines-for-laparoscopic-ventral-hernia-repair/. [Last accessed January, 2020]

18. Alexander AM, Scott DJ. Laparoscopic ventral hernia repair Surg Clin North Am. 2013;93:1091-110.

19. Kurmann A, Visth E, Candinas D, et al. Long term follow-up of open and laparoscopic repair of large incisional hernias. World J Surg. 2011;35:297-301.

20. Nguyen DH, Ngugen MT, Askenasy EP, et al. Primary fascial closure with laparoscopic ventral hernia repair: systematic review. World J Surg. 2014;38:3097-104.

21. LeBlanc KA, Elieson MJ, Corder JM 3rd. Enterotomy and mortality rates of laparoscopic incisional and ventral hernia repair: a review of the literature. JSLS. 2007;11:408-14.

22. Bittner R, Bingener-Casey J, Dietz U, et al. Guidelines for laparoscopic treatment of ventral and incisional abdominal wall hernias (International Endohernia Society [IEHS]), Part 2. Surg Endosc. 2014;28:353-79.

23. Orenstein SB, Dumeer JL, Monteagudo J, et al. Outcomes of laparoscopic ventral hernia repair with routine defect closure using "shoelacing" technique. Surg Endosc. 2011;25:1452-7.

24. Carbonell AM, Harold KL, Mahmutovic AJ, et al. Local injection for the treatment of suture site pain after laparoscopic ventral hernia repair. Am Surg. 2003;69:688-92; discussion 691-2.

25. Wassenaar EB, Raymakers JT, Rakic S. Removal of transabdominal sutures for chronic pain after laparoscopic ventral and incisional hernia repair. Surg Laparosc Endosc Percutan Tech. 2007;17:514-6.

26. Cuccurullo D, Piccoli M, Agresta F, et al. Laparoscopic ventral incisional hernia repair: evidence-based guidelines of the first Italian Consensus Conference. Hernia. 2013;17:557-66.

27. Poelman M, Apers J, van den Brand H, et al. The INCH-trial: a multicentre randomized controlled trial comparing the efficacy of conventional open surgery and laparoscopic surgery for incisional hernia repair. BMC Surg. 2013;13:18.

Jain Point in the Practice of General Surgery

Siddharth Gupta, Prateek Gupta, Nutan Jain

■ INTRODUCTION

Today laparoscopy has come a long way, evolving day by day in both surgical and gynecological practice and the masters of laparoscopy are able to perform complex surgical procedures such as Whipple's procedure, total colectomy, fundoplication, bariatric surgeries, and Wertheim's hysterectomy. But primary entry into the abdomen still hangs like a naked sword on the neck of surgeons more particularly in cases of previous surgeries, in terms of gastrointestinal and major vascular complications. Statistical data show 50% of such injury occurs at the time of entry.[1]

Routinely, primary trocar is placed at umbilical level, but an alternate entry site is recommended when umbilical placement of a primary trocar is deemed hazardous, like in cases with previous abdominal surgery.

The traditional way of alternative entry site in such cases is by Palmer's point.[2] As general surgeons perform all sorts of laparoscopic procedures in all quadrants of abdomen, other safe options of alternate entry sites are must,[3-5] where Palmer's point is not a feasible option. There are not many acceptable options in literature. One such point is Jain point, which is located in the left paraumbilical region at the level of umbilicus, in a straight line drawn vertically upward from a point 2.5 cm medial to anterior superior iliac spine (ASIS).

Palmer's point is a safe access port, but it is not used much during the later course of surgery due to its anatomically higher location. While Jain point being lower and lateral in position,[6] can be used as the main operating port throughout the surgery. Jain point has been consistently found to be free of adhesions.

At Jain point, adhesions due to infective inflammatory disease are minimum, as these are more in right side of abdomen, e.g. enteritis perforation, intestinal tuberculosis, appendicitis, Crohn's disease. This could be explained by more lymphoid tissue (Peyer's patches)[7] present in the wall of terminal ileum. Along with, there is stagnation of bowel contents in ileocecal region because of more horizontal orientation of this region. These two features together cause infections, inflammation, and adhesions more on the right side of abdomen. This pathological fact along with our observation in laparoscopies for last so many years leads to opine that left side of abdomen is comparatively free from adhesions.

It has been found that despite previous infectious pathologies such as Koch's, septicemia, previous multiple bowel, and pelvic surgery, Jain point has been found to be free of bowel adhesions. There was no major vessel injury. The anatomical location of Jain point is such that there are no superficial or deep vessels underneath and it is far away from major retroperitoneal vessels.

The Jain point derives its safety from the fact that it is more lateral, hence, it avoids intra-abdominal adhesions at previous incision sites. Being lower down at paraumbilical position, it is ergonomic to be used as operating port later on in the surgery. Since it is much lower than the subcostal margin, it can very well be used in cases of hepatosplenomegaly, portal hypertension, and upper abdomen vertical or Kocher's, Chevron incisions.[8,9] It is universally suitable for all body types. Jain point promises to be a safe portal for laparoscopic entry in cases with a history of previous surgery.

Many renal and upper urinary tract surgeries (nephrectomy, pyeloplasty, stone surgeries) are performed in right lateral position (left side up position), where Jain point is a safe point for entry as compared to umbilicus as bowel falls in midline. For surgeries in left lateral position (right side up) also, mirror image of this point can be used on right side, as used by author, which is not possible with Palmer's point. More so in these surgeries, this point can be used as a port site by surgeon or assistant. Another feature which can be of use is that it becomes a working port rather than being redundant after initial entry port is over.

From a general surgeon's perspective, Jain point appears to be a safe, dynamic point which can be of use in various ways:

- As a first blind port and Veress needle insertion in incisional hernia, ventral hernia, and umbilical hernia.
- In gastric surgeries like in sleeve gastrectomy, it can be used as first blind and working port **(Figs. 1A to I)**.
- In diaphragmatic hernia repair, it can be used as first blind and working port **(Figs. 2A to H)**.
- In appendectomy, for Veress insertion, a mirror image of Jain point is used on the right side as working port **(Figs. 3A to F)**.
- For diagnostic laparoscopy in Koch's abdomen, infective pathologies or any second look procedures **(Figs. 4A to C)**.
- Urological procedures like cystectomy **(Figs. 5A to G)**, vesicovaginal fistula repair, and ureteric reimplantation **(Figs. 6A to M)**.

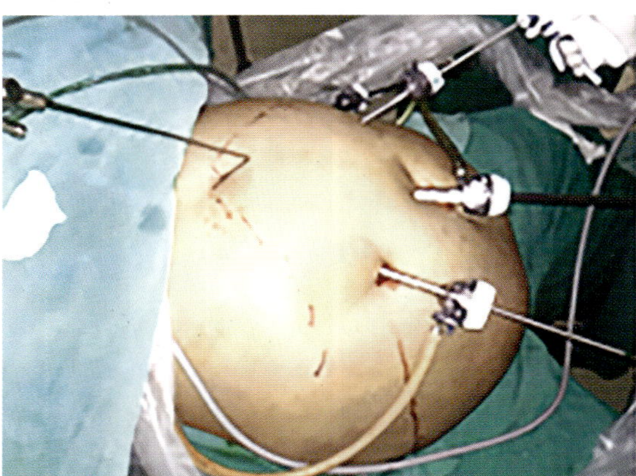

Fig. 1A: External view with port position.
Courtesy: Dr Praveen Bhatia, Sir Ganga Ram Hospital, New Delhi, India.

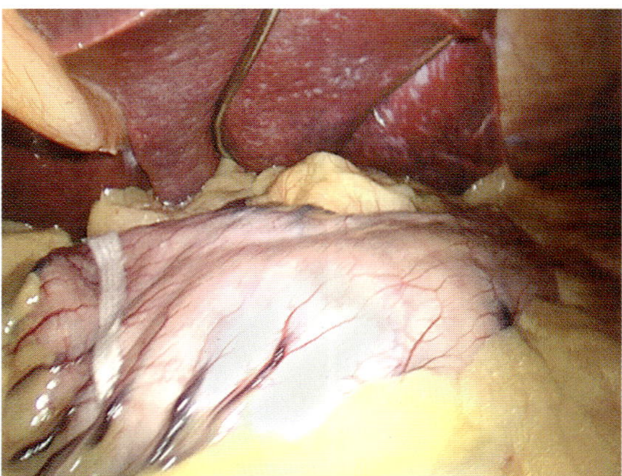

Fig. 1B: Gastrolysis started 5 cm proximal to pylorus.
Courtesy: Dr Praveen Bhatia, Sir Ganga Ram Hospital, New Delhi, India.

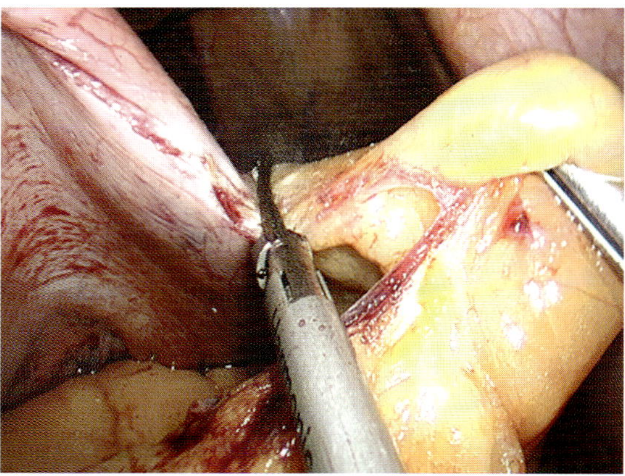

Fig. 1C: Gastrolysis done using Harmonic ACE.
Courtesy: Dr Praveen Bhatia, Sir Ganga Ram Hospital, New Delhi, India.

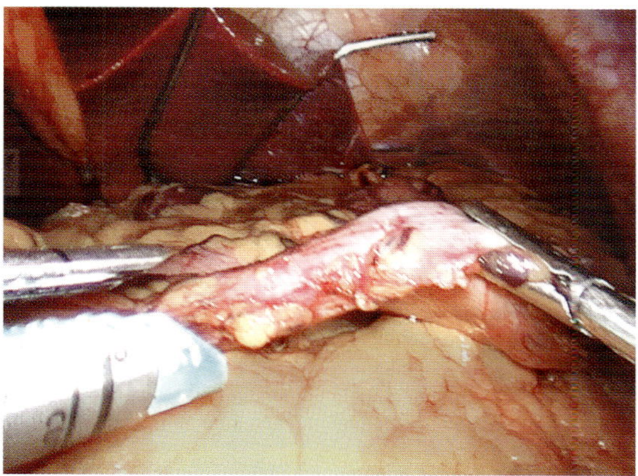

Fig. 1D: 1st stapling done with GST 60 (green).
Courtesy: Dr Praveen Bhatia, Sir Ganga Ram Hospital, New Delhi, India.

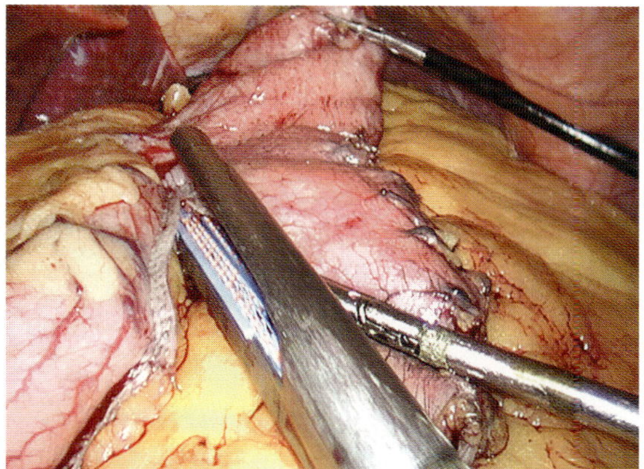

Fig. 1E: Stapling done with GST 60 (blue).
Courtesy: Dr Praveen Bhatia, Sir Ganga Ram Hospital, New Delhi, India.

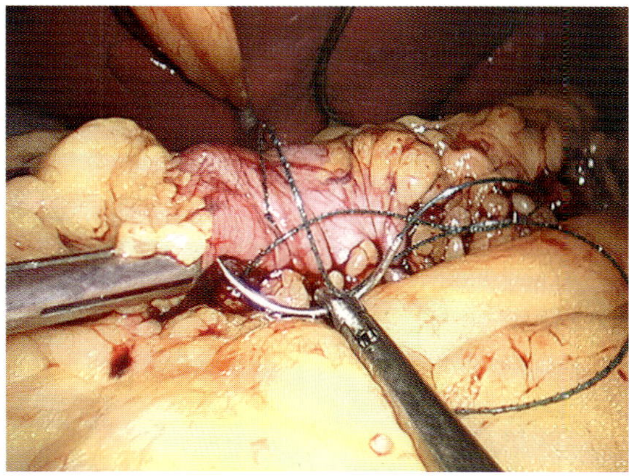

Fig. 1F: Staple line imbricated with V-loc suture.
Courtesy: Dr Praveen Bhatia, Sir Ganga Ram Hospital, New Delhi, India.

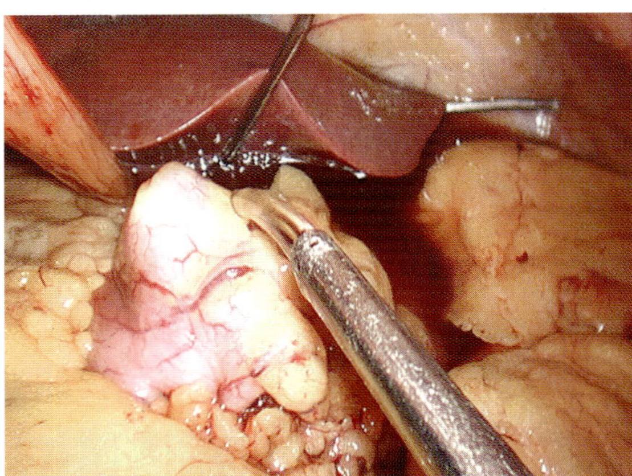

Fig. 1G: Confirmatory endoscopic leak test done.
Courtesy: Dr Praveen Bhatia, Sir Ganga Ram Hospital, New Delhi, India.

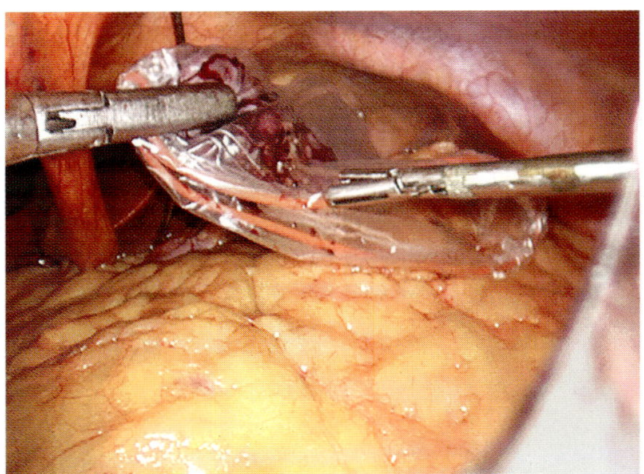

Fig. 1H: Specimen removed in endobag.
Courtesy: Dr Praveen Bhatia, Sir Ganga Ram Hospital, New Delhi, India.

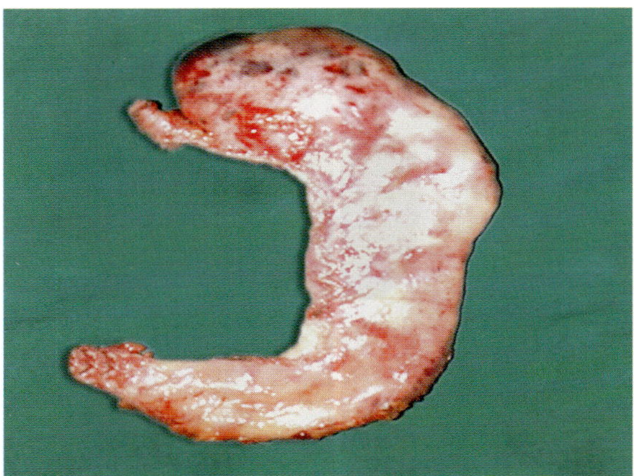

Fig. 1I: Resected specimen.
Courtesy: Dr Praveen Bhatia, Sir Ganga Ram Hospital, New Delhi, India.

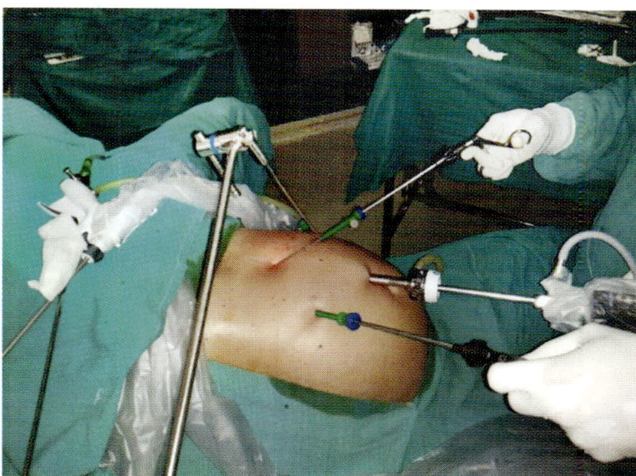

Fig. 2A: External view of port placement.
Courtesy: Dr Praveen Bhatia, Sir Ganga Ram Hospital, New Delhi, India.

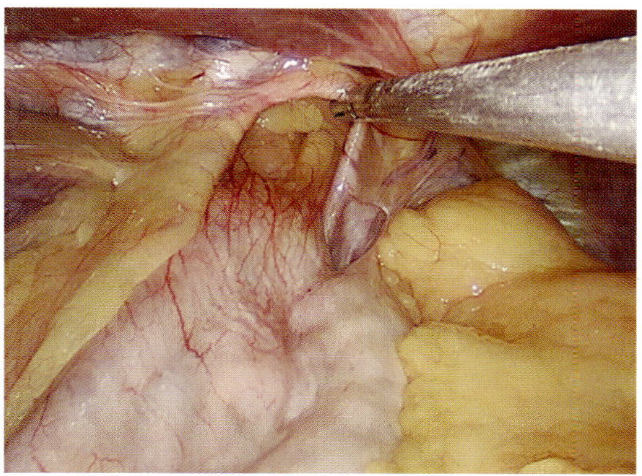

Fig. 2B: Hernial defect visualized.
Courtesy: Dr Praveen Bhatia, Sir Ganga Ram Hospital, New Delhi, India.

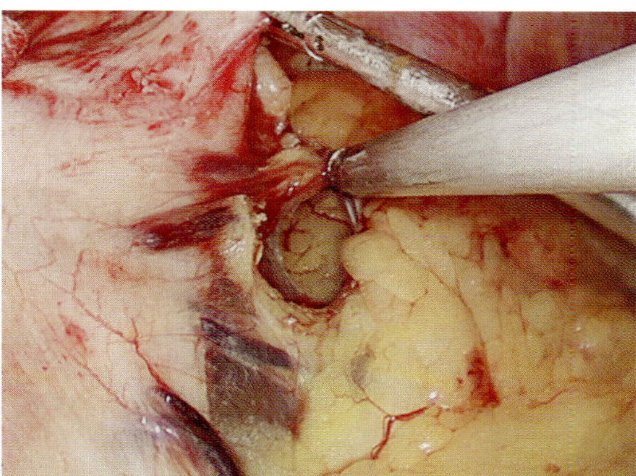

Fig. 2C: Short gastric vessels desiccated with Harmonic Ace.
Courtesy: Dr Praveen Bhatia, Sir Ganga Ram Hospital, New Delhi, India.

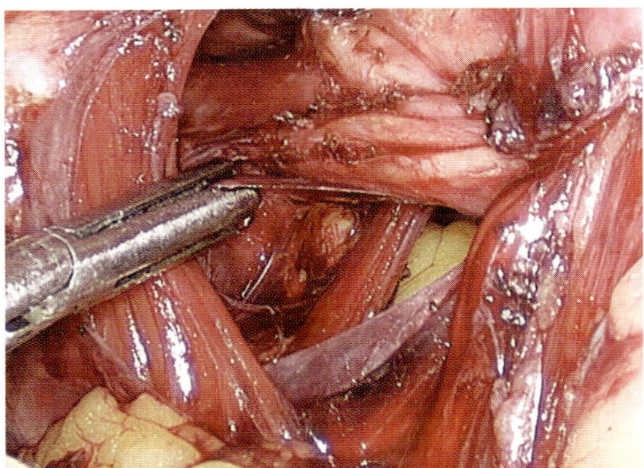

Fig. 2D: Right and left crus being exposed.
Courtesy: Dr Praveen Bhatia, Sir Ganga Ram Hospital, New Delhi, India.

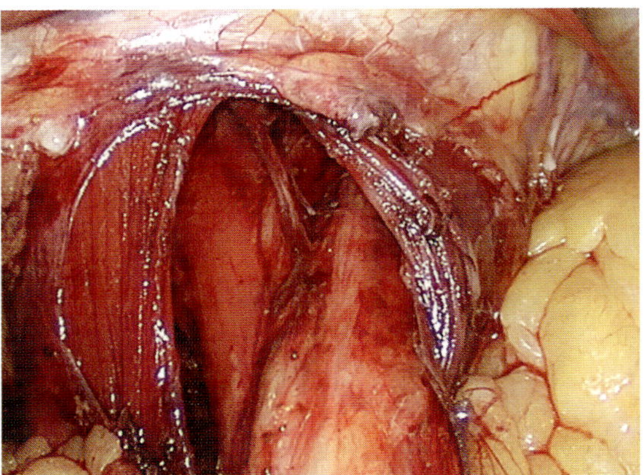

Fig. 2E: Dissection completed.
Courtesy: Dr Praveen Bhatia, Sir Ganga Ram Hospital, New Delhi, India.

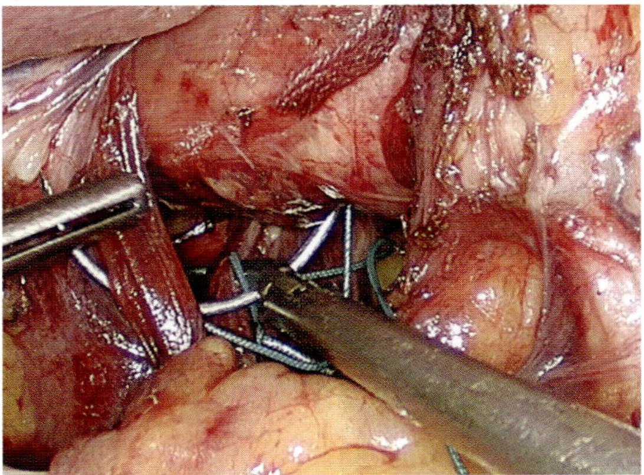

Fig. 2F: Cruroraphy being done with no. 2 Ethibond suture.
Courtesy: Dr Praveen Bhatia, Sir Ganga Ram Hospital, New Delhi, India.

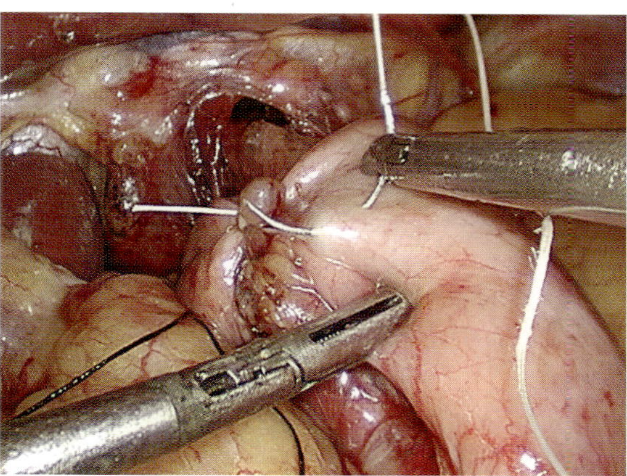

Fig. 2G: Suturing of fundal wrap with Ethibond no. 2/0.
Courtesy: Dr Praveen Bhatia, Sir Ganga Ram Hospital, New Delhi, India.

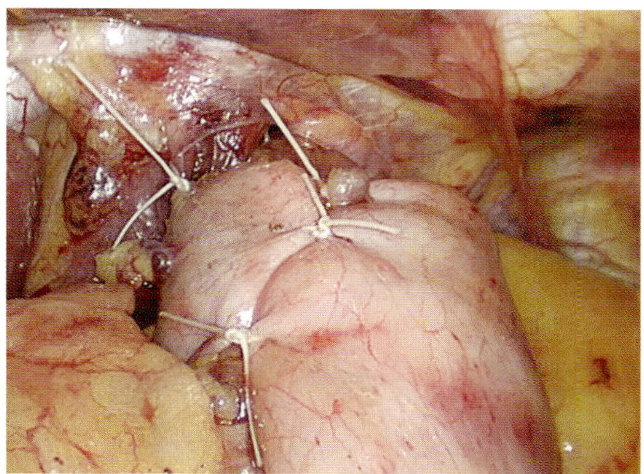

Fig. 2H: Complete 360° wrap.
Courtesy: Dr Praveen Bhatia, Sir Ganga Ram Hospital, New Delhi, India.

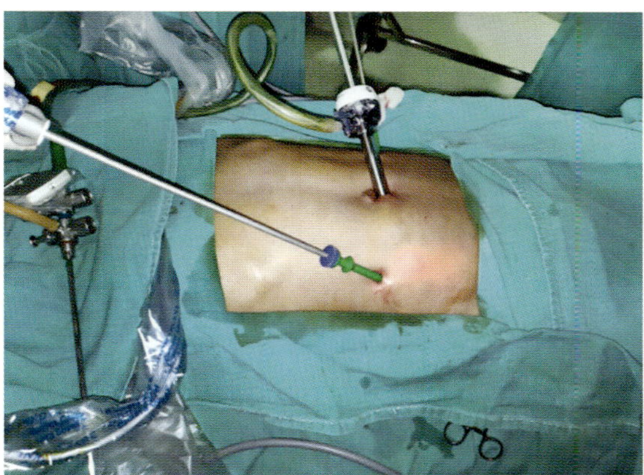

Fig. 3A: External view of port position.
Courtesy: Dr Praveen Bhatia, Sir Ganga Ram Hospital, New Delhi, India.

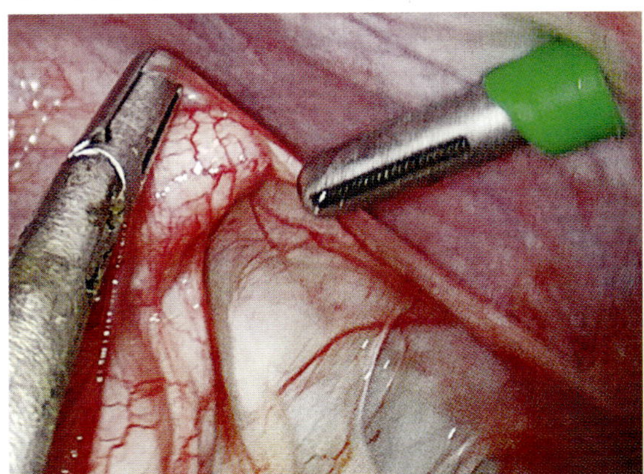

Fig. 3B: Appendix visualized.
Courtesy: Dr Praveen Bhatia, Sir Ganga Ram Hospital, New Delhi, India.

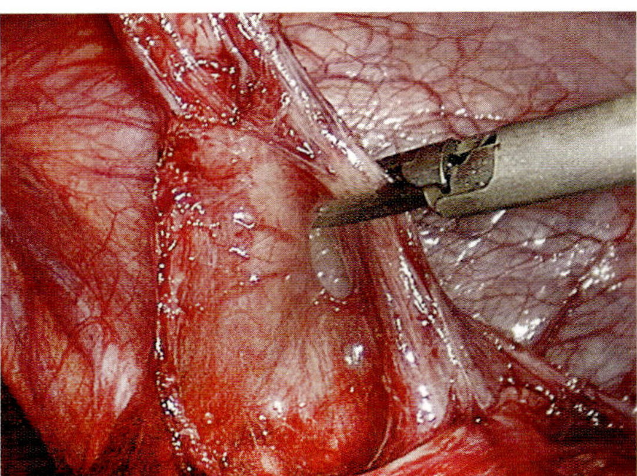

Fig. 3C: Appendicular artery dissected.
Courtesy: Dr Praveen Bhatia, Sir Ganga Ram Hospital, New Delhi, India.

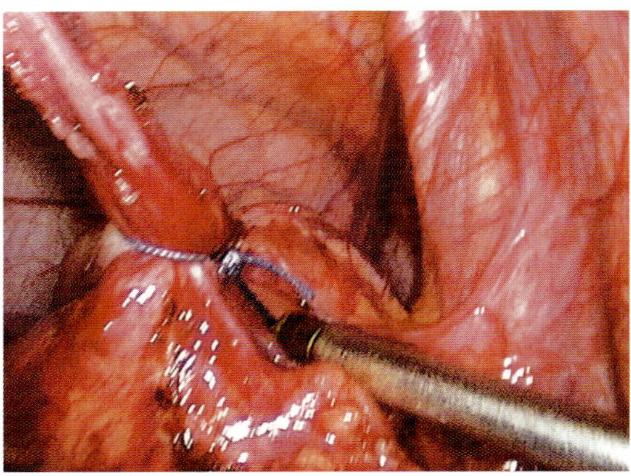

Fig. 3D: Endoloop tightened at base of appendix.
Courtesy: Dr Praveen Bhatia, Sir Ganga Ram Hospital, New Delhi, India.

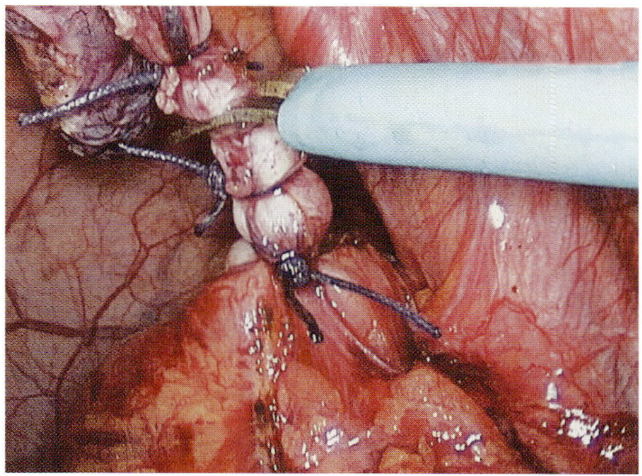

Fig. 3E: Appendix being cut.
Courtesy: Dr Praveen Bhatia, Sir Ganga Ram Hospital, New Delhi, India.

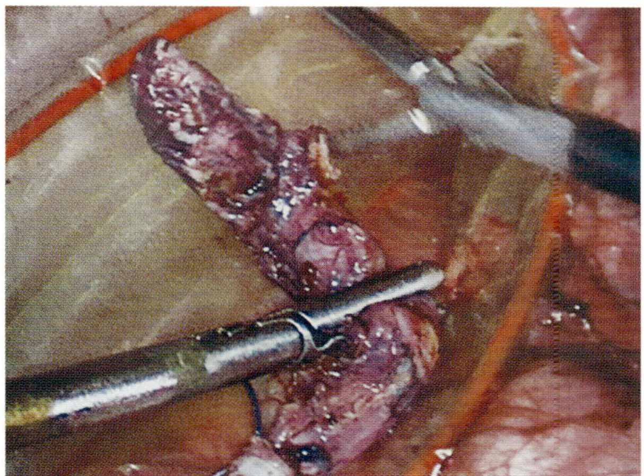

Fig. 3F: Appendix extracted in an endobag.
Courtesy: Dr Praveen Bhatia, Sir Ganga Ram Hospital, New Delhi, India.

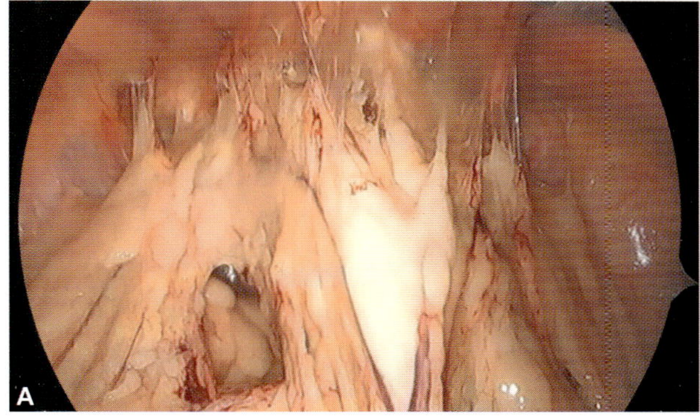

Fig. 4A

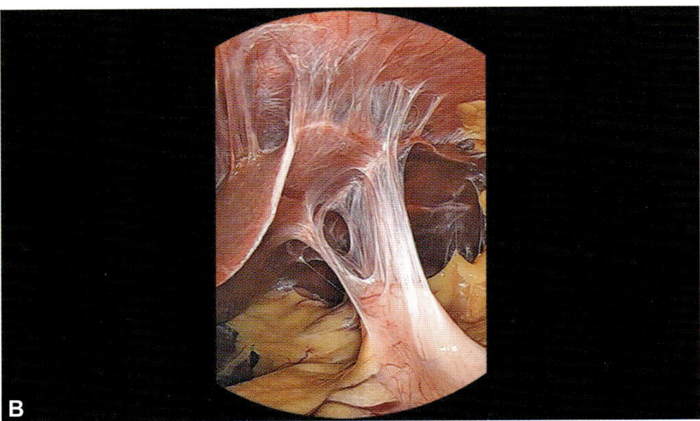

Figs. 4A and B: Koch's abdomen showing intraperitoneal dense adhesions.

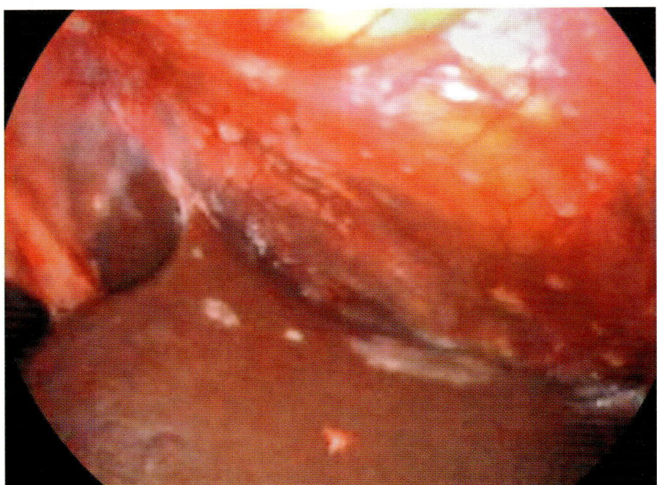

Fig. 4C: Tubercle nodules.

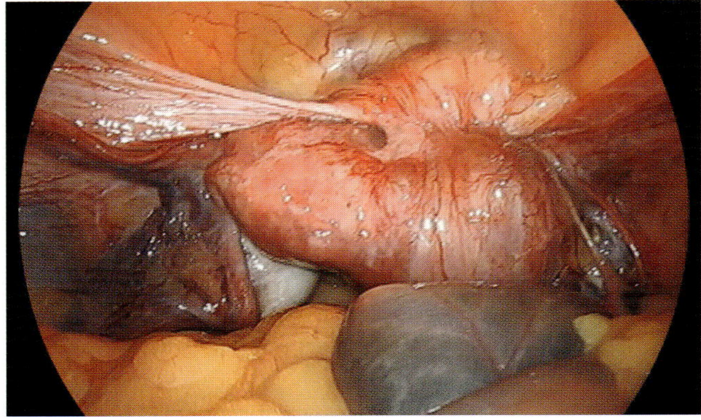

Fig. 5A: Puckering and scarring in UV fold.

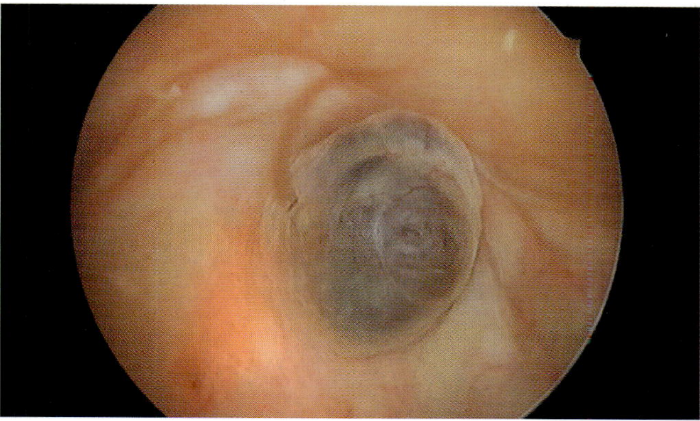

Fig. 5B: Big endometriotic nodule seen in cystoscopy.

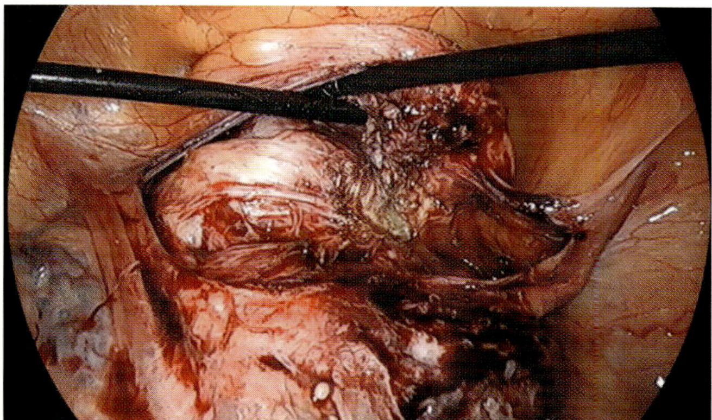

Fig. 5C: Dissection done in the prevesical space to push the bladder down and exposed the nodule.

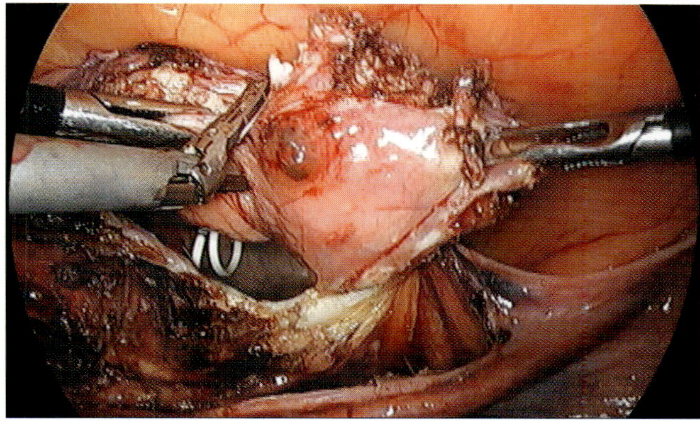

Fig. 5D: Excision of the big endometriotic nodule, ureteric stent seen in place.

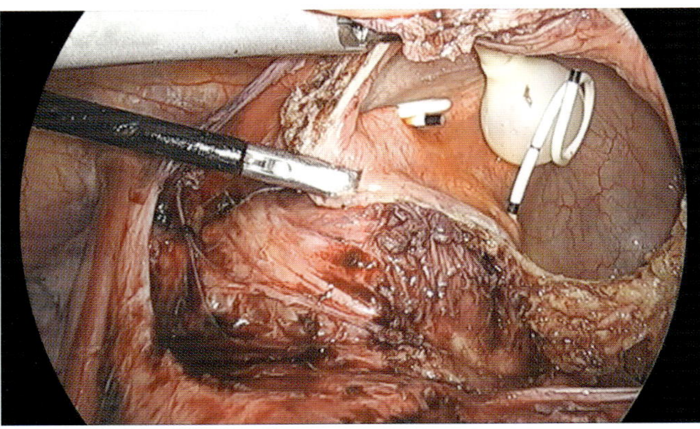

Fig. 5E: Both D.J. stent seen which are placed in situ before starting the nodule excision.

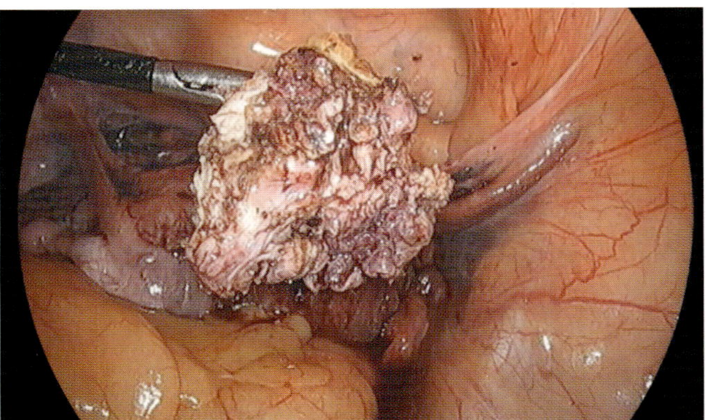

Fig. 5F: Fully excised nodule.

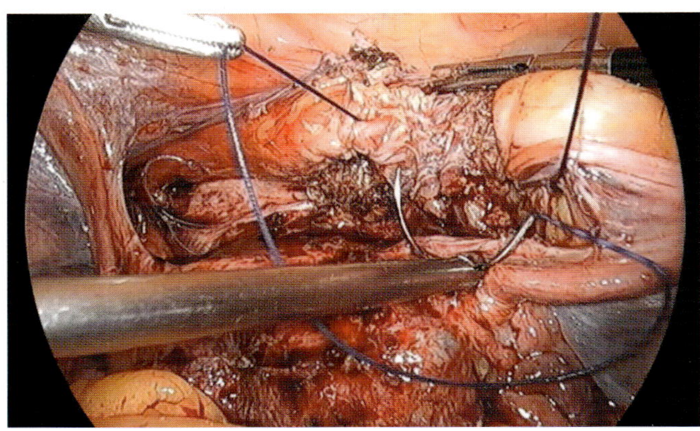

Fig. 5G: Suturing back the bladder in three layers.

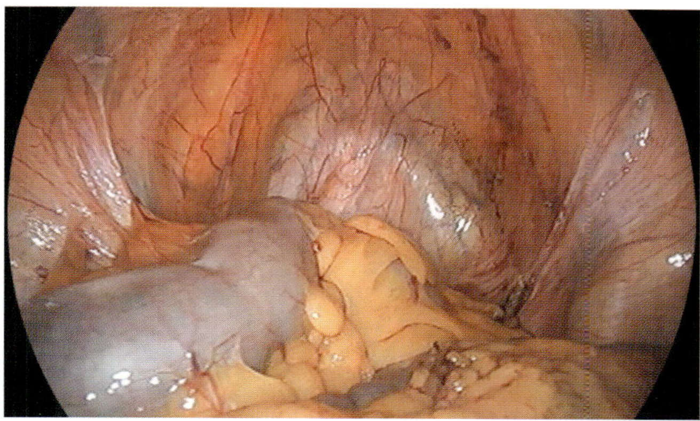

Fig. 6A: Dense adhesions in a case of recurrent endometriosis.

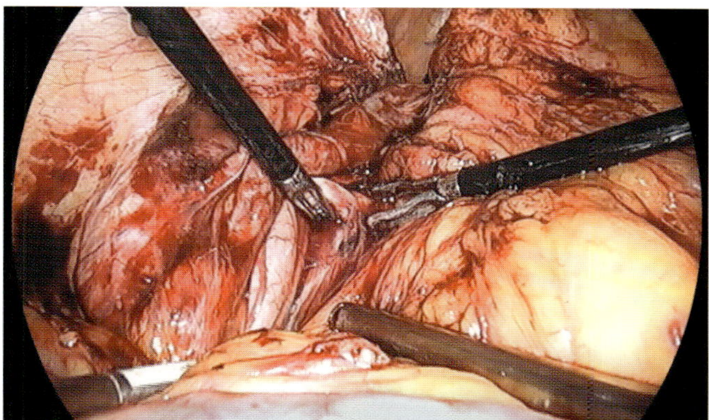

Fig. 6B: Dilated ureter proximal to stricture side.

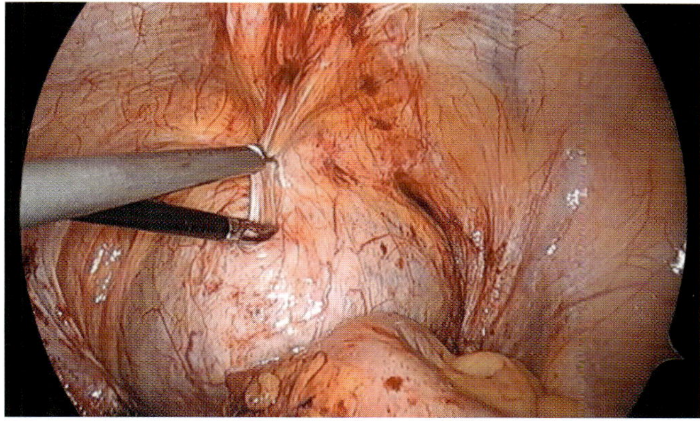

Fig. 6C: Opening the space of Retzius to push the bladder down and bring it close to the ureter for tension free implantation.

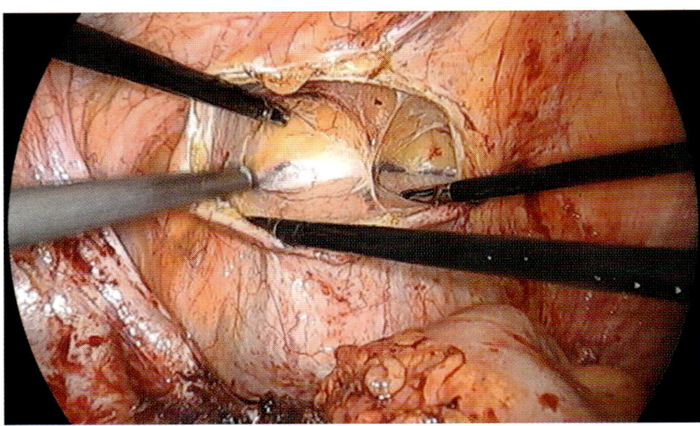

Fig. 6D: Entry into the space of Retzius.

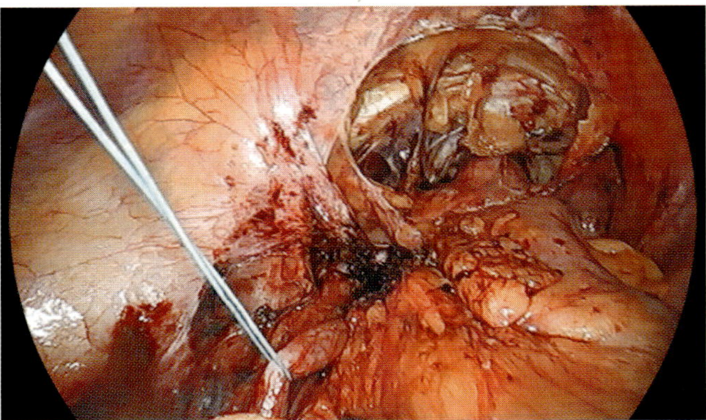

Fig. 6E: Ureter is lifted up by no. 2 Ethibond suture, in the lower frame completed dissection of bladder is seen.

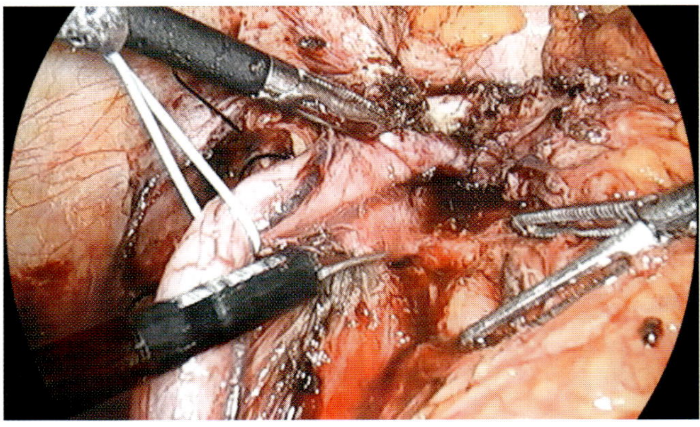

Fig. 6F: Ureteral exposure done proximal to the stricture side.

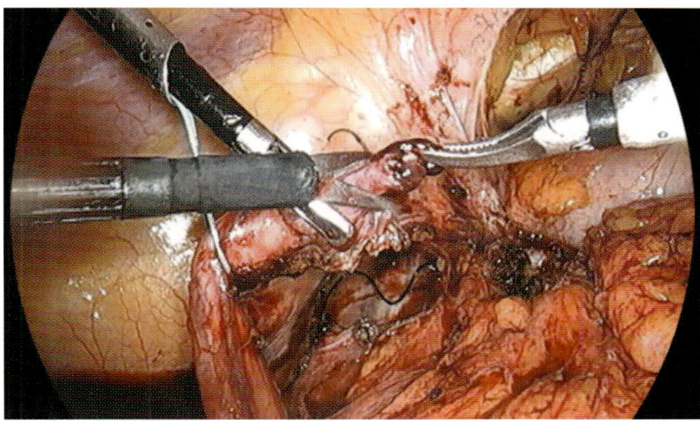

Fig. 6G: Cutting the stricture end of the ureter.

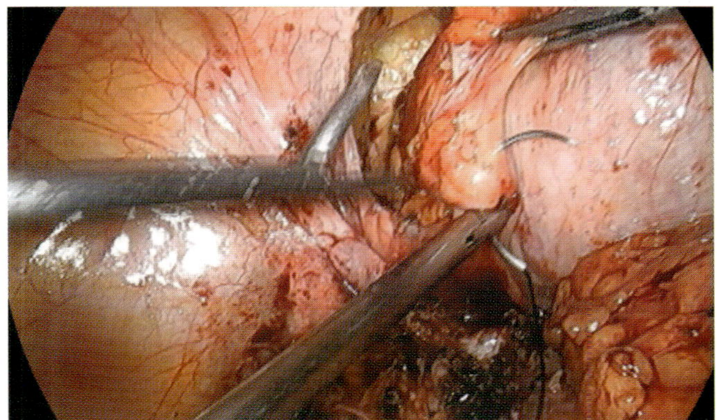

Fig. 6H: Passing the psoas hitch suture with no. 2 silk.

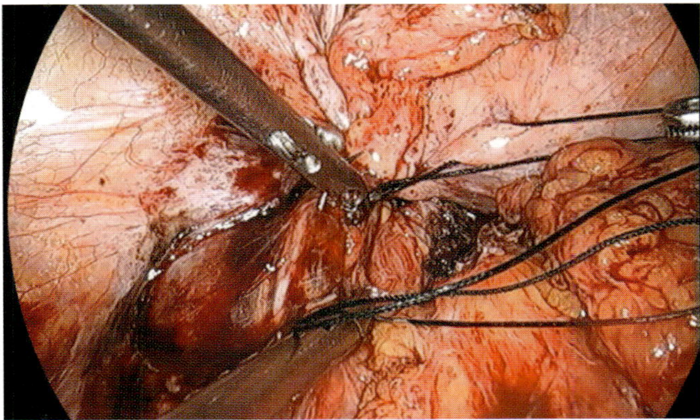

Fig. 6I: Suture over the psoas muscle, avoiding the genitofemoral nerve.

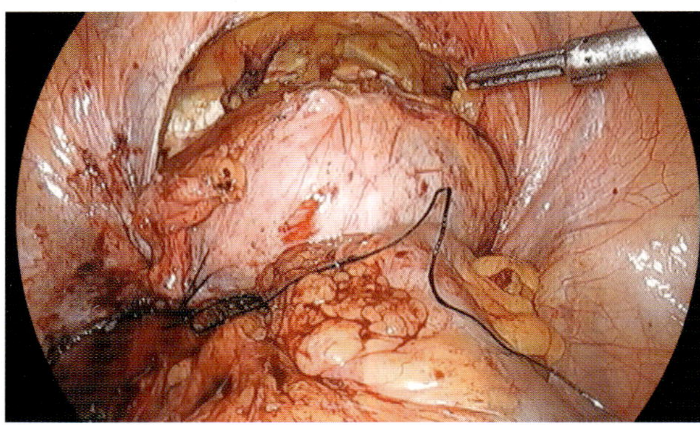

Fig. 6J: Two psoas hitch sutures passed to approximate the bladder to the ureter.

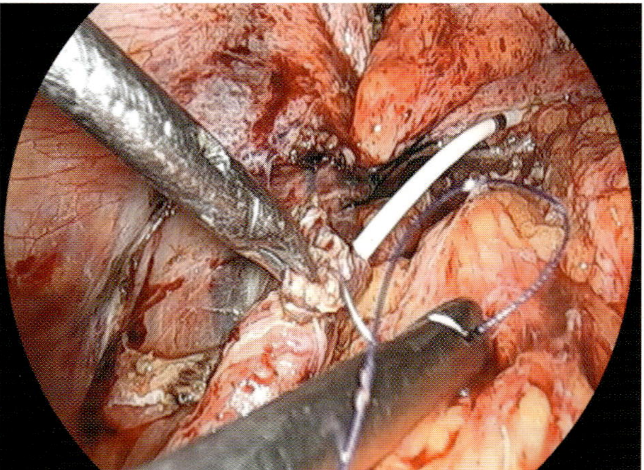

Fig. 6K: Cut end of ureter fish mouthed and suture passed with 4-0 vicryl.

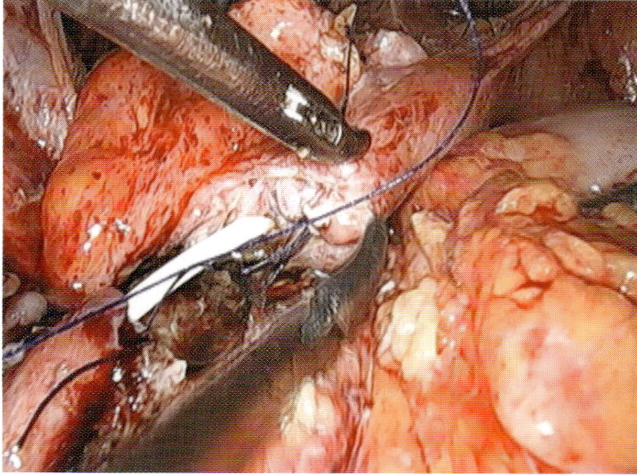

Fig. 6L: Suture passed through the bladder.

- Urinary incontinence procedures like Burch colposuspension procedure and paravaginal defect repair.
- In surgeries with previous upper abdomen scars such as Kocher's incision, Chevron incision, and exploratory laparotomy midline scars **(Figs. 7A to C)**.
- Hemicolectomy, for cancer of colon.
- Segmental resection of bowel as in endometriosis of right sigmoid junction.
- Jain point can be used as direct trocar entry as has been tried by and published from other centers. The author has no first-hand experience of direct trocar entry technique but surgeons who are well-conversant with

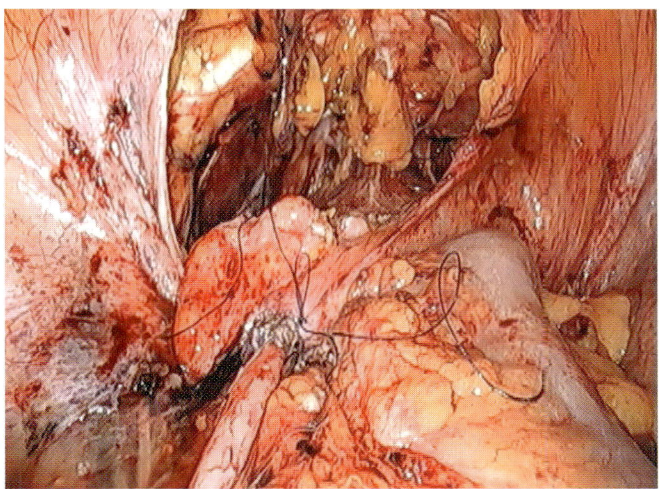

Fig. 6M: Final view, ureteric reimplantation.

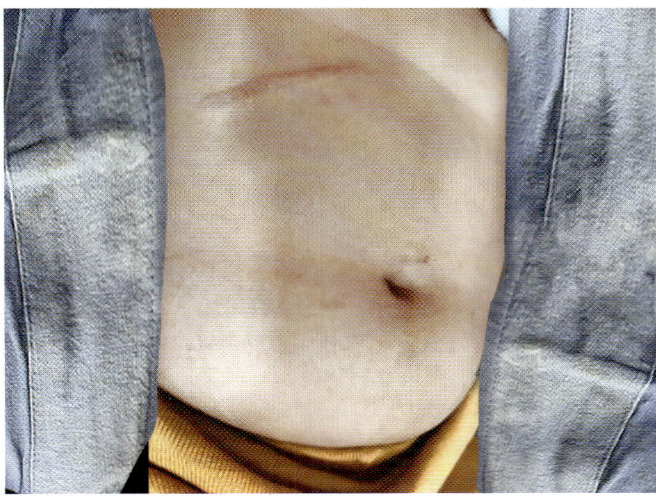

Fig. 7A: Previous Kocher's incision for open gallbladder surgery.

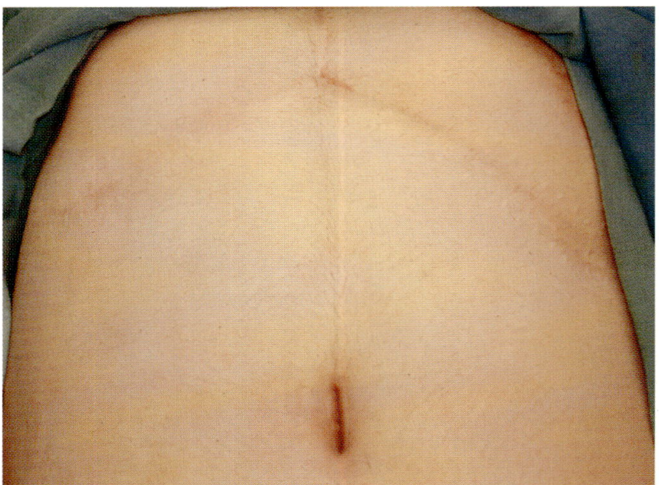

Fig. 7B: Chevron incision given for hydatid cyst removal.

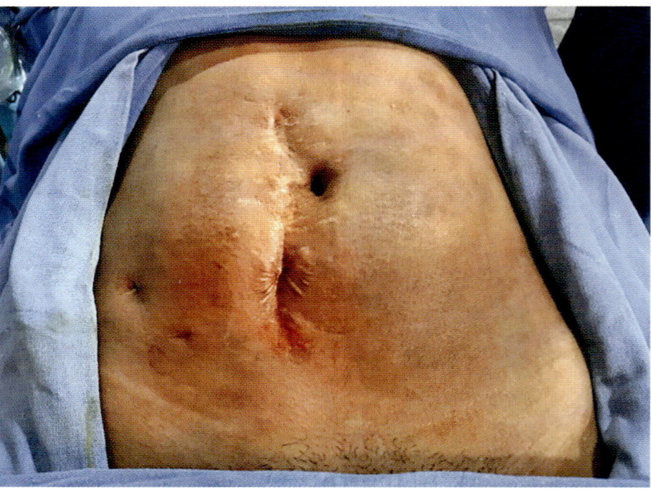

Fig. 7C: Previous laparotomy for intestinal obstruction with drain site on right side of abdomen.

direct trocar entry find it convenient to switch over to Jain point whenever needed.[10]

In today's era, fast learning from interdepartmental expertise can be a catalyst to fast propagation of safe practices. What has been good and safe in gynecology practice can be taken as a base to build on its usage in the practice of endoscopy in general surgery and urology. Safe primary laparoscopic access can be done by Jain point by both experienced and budding endoscopists in wide variety of clinical applications. Thus this point, being safe and ergonomically better alternative in wide spectrum of laparoscopic surgeries, can be used by general surgeons as well.

REFERENCES

1. Jansen FW, Kapiteyn K, Trimbos-Kemper T, et al. Complications of laparoscopy: a prospective multicentre observational study. Br J Obstet Gynaecol. 1997;104(5):595-600.
2. Palmer R. Safety in laparoscopy. J Reprod Med. 1974;13(1):1-5.
3. Hasson HM. Open laparoscopy as a method of access in laparoscopic surgery. Gynaecol Endosc. 1999;8(6):353-62.
4. Lee CL, Huang KG, Jain S, et al. A new portal for gynecologic laparoscopy. J Am Assoc Gynecol Laparosc. 2001;8(1):147-50.
5. Agarwala N, Liu CY. Safe entry techniques during laparoscopy: left upper quadrant entry using the ninth intercostal space: a review of 918 procedures. J Minim Invasive Gynecol. 2005;12(1):55-61.
6. Sharp HT. (2019). Overview of gynecologic laparoscopic surgery and non-umbilical entry sites. [online] Available from https://www.uptodate.com/contents/overview-of-gynecologic-laparoscopic-surgery-and-non-umbilical-entry-sites [Last accessed January, 2020].
7. Jung C, Hugot J-P, Barreau F. Peyer's patches: the immune sensors of the intestine. Int J Inflam. 2010;2010:823710.
8. Jain N, Sareen S, Kanawa S, et al. Jain point: a new safe portal for laparoscopic entry in previous surgery cases. J Hum Reprod Sci. 2016;9(1):9-17.
9. Jain N, Jain V, Aggarwal C. Left lateral port: safe laparoscopic port entry in previous large upper abdomen laparotomy scar. J Minim Invasive Gynecol. 2019;26(5):973-6.
10. Mulayim B, Aksoy O. Direct trocar entry from left lateral port (Jain point) in a case with previous surgeries. J Gynecol Surg. 2019.

25   Entry-related Complications and their Management

Kiran Kumari Mandal, Nutan Jain

INTRODUCTION

Laparoscopy has gradually become popular in gynecology practices because of its many benefits. Laparoscopy is frequently used for the diagnosis and treatment of various gynecologic conditions. Overall, there is a low incidence of serious complications associated with laparoscopic surgeries. The advancement in laparoscopic instruments and optic transmission contribute to lower complication rate. Although most complications occur at the time of entry for camera or port placement, they can also arise from abdominal insufflation, tissue dissection, and during the process of hemostasis. The overall incidence of major injuries at the time of entry is 1.1/1,000. Bowel injuries have occurred in 0.7/1,000 laparoscopies and major vascular injuries in 0.4/1,000 laparoscopies.[1] The incidence of bowel and major vessel injuries are low, but both of these types of injuries are potentially life-threatening, especially during the initial access.

The incidence of complications for individual laparoscopic procedures is discussed below in more detail. According to a survey which assessed the complications related to laparoscopy from 1980 to 1999, the incidence of injury related to abdominal access was 5–30 per 10,000 procedures. About 76% of all the injuries comprised of bowel and retroperitoneal injuries; and almost half of the small and large bowel injuries remained unrecognized for at least 24 hours.[2] The proportion and type of organ injury during abdominal access are stated below:

- Small bowel (25%)
- Iliac artery (19%)
- Colon (12%)
- Iliac or other retroperitoneal vein (9%)
- Secondary branches of a mesenteric vessel (7%)
- Aorta (6%)

- Inferior vena cava (4%)
- Abdominal wall vessels (4%)
- Bladder (3%)
- Liver (2%)
- Other (<2%).

COMPLICATIONS RELATED TO ABDOMINAL ENTRY

Abdominal access and the creation of a pneumoperitoneum carry a limited risk of visceral injury. Pneumoperitoneum is created most commonly for the accomplishment of transabdominal laparoscopic surgery. Visceral injury during abdominal access and creation of pneumoperitoneum is divided into broad groups, i.e. injuries of blood vessels, gastrointestinal organs, and the genitourinary system. Although these fatal injuries are rare, they represent a major reason for mortality from laparoscopic procedures, for conversion to open procedures, and a significant source of the morbidity associated with any laparoscopic procedure. In one large review of gynecologic laparoscopy, over 50% of these complications occurred during abdominal access.[3] Knowledge of proper access techniques is pivotal to avoid these complications. However, no significant differences in overall complication rates have been found for closed compared with open techniques for primary abdominal insufflation, when performed by experienced surgeons. Most severe injuries are due to blind insertion of access device.

Vascular Injury

The comprehensive reported rate of vascular injury (arterial or venous injury) is ranging from 0.1 to 6.4 per 1,000 laparoscopies.[1] Vascular injuries related to abdominal access are grouped in major and minor vascular injuries. Minor vascular injuries affect vessels of the abdominal wall, mesentery, or other organs. Most injuries involve minor vessels, which is common but it is underreported. These minor vascular injuries are often the reason for reoperation, conversion to open, and transfusion. Most common minor vascular injury is laceration of the inferior epigastric vessels during lateral port placement **(Fig. 1)**. Injury to these vessels is reported to occur in up to 2.5% of laparoscopic hernia repairs.[4] Injuries are more likely with cutting trocar with sharp blades in contrast with smooth and conical-tip trocars that push the vessel out of the way.[5] Partial lacerations of the inferior epigastric artery vessels may not spontaneously stop bleeding because the vessel is tethered and cannot retract and contract. Similar to the inferior epigastric vessels, other abdominal wall vessels can be injured, particularly if the trocar is not placed under direct vision, and if secondary trocars are placed without transilluminating the abdominal wall to identify the vessels. Epigastric vascular injuries can

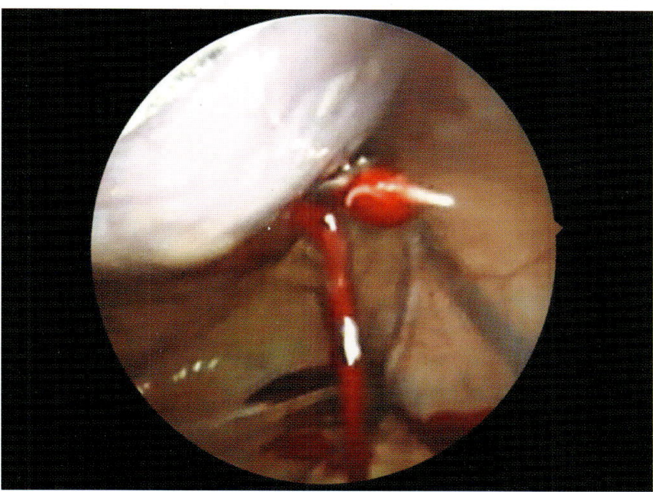

Fig. 1: Acute inferior epigastric artery bleed.
Courtesy: Dr Aruna Tantia, ILS Hospital, Kolkata, West Bengal, India.

be treated with various techniques, including application of direct pressure with the operating port, open or laparoscopic suture ligation, or tamponade with a Foley catheter inserted into the peritoneal cavity.[6] For suture ligation, cut down over the area to pinpoint and ligate the vessels, or by blind suture ligation of the bleeding site.

Patients with an abdominal wall hematoma from laparoscopic access who are hemodynamically stable and with no signs of hematoma expansion can be managed conservatively. The hematoma may drain spontaneously through one or more port sites. If the hematoma expands, the patient becomes hemodynamically unstable, or the hematoma becomes infected, prompt intervention is needed.

Major vascular injuries include major vessels such as the aorta, inferior vena cava, and iliac vessels. Major vascular injury during the initiation of pneumoperitoneum is a well-recognized and much-feared complication of laparoscopic procedures, because of the significant mortality associated with it. Vascular injury is a major cause of death from laparoscopy, second only to anesthesia, with a reported mortality rate of 15%.[7] These injuries occur due to the close proximity of anterior abdominal wall to the retroperitoneal vascular structures. Major vascular injuries may be recognized either by direct visualization of pool of blood in the abdominal cavity or more commonly by a retroperitoneal hematoma. Since these injuries most often occur with a Veress needle, the hole is not large and the only visual indication of injury may be a hematoma **(Fig. 2)**. The laparoscopy view may be reduced or poor initially because of the red pigment in blood absorbs light. This can be used as a clue to an occult injury.

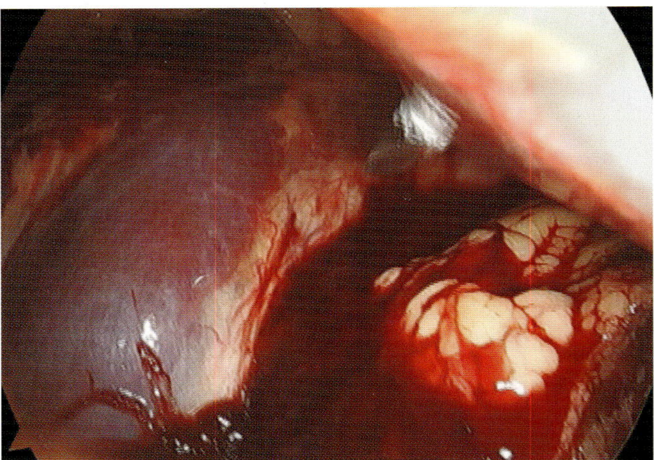

Fig. 2: Retroperitoneal hematoma.

Other factors that may indicate injury are hypotension, tachycardia or a fall in end tidal CO_2 from embolization of CO_2 gas.

Factors responsible for large vessel injury are as follows:

- Inexperienced or unskilled surgeon
- Failure to sharpen the trocar
- Entering of trocar in Trendelenburg position
- Failure to elevate or stabilize the abdominal wall
- Lateral deviation of the needle or trocar
- Inadequate pneumoperitoneum
- Forceful thrust
- Failure to note anatomic landmarks
- Inadequate incision size.

The distal aorta, which lies directly underneath the umbilicus, and right common iliac artery, which crosses the midline, are each particularly susceptible to major injury. If a major vascular injury occurs, the first thing is not to panic and to stay calm. Let the anesthesiologist know the situation so that he/she can ensure there is adequate intravenous (IV) access and fluid or blood resuscitation or both can be initiated. If the injury cannot be repaired with speed and efficiency by laparoscopically due to lack of visualization or inexperience, then open quickly and of course carefully. The abdomen should be rapidly opened with a midline incision, pressure should be applied directly to the bleeding site for initial control, and the abdominal cavity can be packed, if needed. These maneuvers allow for fluid resuscitation. Meanwhile vascular surgeon need to be informed for further management. Control should be gained directly, or if this is not possible, by gaining proximal and distal control then the injury should be repaired.

Visceral Injury

Visceral injury includes injury to greater omentum, stomach, bowel, liver or spleen. After major vascular injury and anesthesia-related deaths, bowel injury is the third most common cause of death from a laparoscopic procedure.[7] Unlike major vascular injuries where the risk and presentation are immediate, many bowel injuries go unnoticeable and remain concealed at the time of the procedure. Accordingly, patients present postoperatively, often after discharge, with the specific and nonspecific features of peritonitis. The small bowel is the most commonly injured gastrointestinal structure during abdominal access for laparoscopic surgery, but stomach, liver, and colon injuries **(Figs. 3 to 5)**

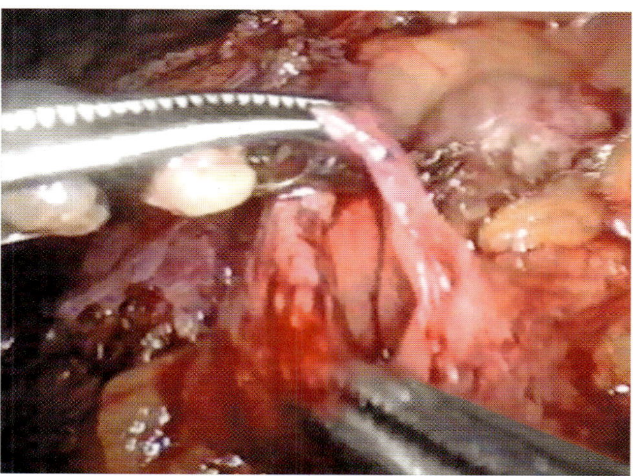

Fig. 3: Bowel injury.
Courtesy: Dr Aruna Tantia, ILS Hospital, Kolkata, West Bengal, India.

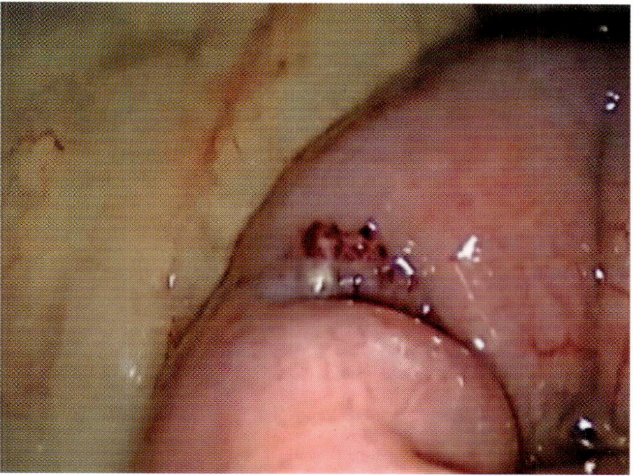

Fig. 4: Bowel laceration.
Courtesy: Dr Aruna Tantia, ILS Hospital, Kolkata, West Bengal, India.

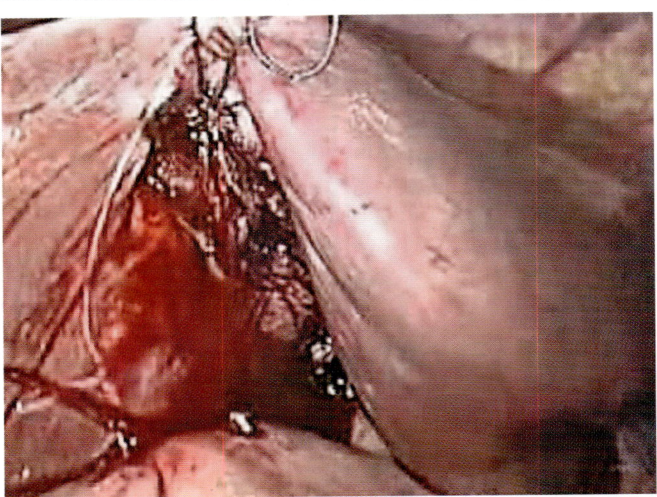

Fig. 5: Liver bed suture.
Courtesy: Dr Aruna Tantia, ILS Hospital, Kolkata, West Bengal, India.

have been reported when subcostal access techniques (Palmer's technique) are used.[8-10] Decompressing the stomach with an orogastric or nasogastric tube prior to Veress insertion may minimize the potential risk for accidental stomach injury. The absence of peritoneal signs does not rule out the probability of bowel perforation and spillage of gastrointestinal contents within the peritoneal cavity. Delayed diagnosis of an access-related gastrointestinal injury is a significant cause for morbidity and mortality. Gastrointestinal injury should be managed as early when it recognized. Iatrogenic small and large bowel injuries are managed as with other traumatic intestinal injuries, based upon the grade of injury. Injuries due to the pneumoperitoneum needle (e.g. Veress) may be able to be managed conservatively. Most other trocar punctures require simple primary closure, reappose the bowel wall with simple sutures in one or two layers. Colostomy is rarely required for discrete large bowel injuries. If the operating surgeon is inexperienced or uncomfortable performing such a repair, we advise consultation with a surgeon.

Bladder Injury

Bladder injury is a rare but reported injury during abdominal access for laparoscopy. A history of prior pelvic surgery increases the risk of bladder injury.[11] Injury to the bladder is more commonly associated with dissection during the course of the operation, rather than primary or secondary trocar insertion. In general, puncture of the bladder results when a midline, suprapubic trocar is placed in a patient with an over distended bladder. Previous pelvic surgery places the patient at additional risk. The diagnosis of injury to the bladder is often made by distention of the urinary drainage bag during the procedure.[12] In addition, instillation of indigo carmine into the bladder may abet in identifying an injury. The major step in preventing this complication is ensuring satisfactory drainage of the bladder before the procedure. Though it is common to advice patients to void immediately before the procedure, besides it is safer to drain the bladder with a catheter after the induction of anesthesia. This confirms that dystonic bladders will be completely emptied. Furthermore, it allows for easy recognition of the complication when it occurs if the catheter is left in place for the duration of the operative procedure. A small 3 mm or 5 mm puncture injury in the dome of the bladder resolve spontaneously with keeping the indwelling bladder catheter for 7–10 days.[11] Large or irregular defects will require a two-layer suture closure with absorbable sutures (vicryl 3-0) either through an open or laparoscopic approach.[13] A bladder catheter should be left in place for 4–10 days depending on the location and size of the puncture or tear.

Nerve Injury

Location of port site should be chosen accordingly to avoid abdominal wall nerve injury. Site specific and procedure-related dissection should be carried out to spare nerve injury as it leads to severe constipation postsurgery.

COMPLICATIONS RELATED TO PNEUMOPERITONEUM

Complications related to creation of pneumoperitoneum include subcutaneous emphysema, extraperitoneal insufflation **(Fig. 6)**, mediastinal emphysema, pneumothorax, cardiac arrhythmia, carbon dioxide retention, postoperative pain related to retained intra-abdominal gas, and air embolism due to venous injury. The complications such as subcutaneous emphysema and extraperitoneal insufflation are mainly due to improper placement of Veress needle during creation of pneumoperitoneum. And other complications are due to poor cardiopulmonary reserve and prolonged surgery. Extraperitoneal insufflation can be decompressed with needle insertion and aspiration **(Figs. 7 and 8)**. Patients complain about postoperative pain radiating to shoulder, it is due to irritation of diaphragm related to retained CO_2. Tips for coping include applying a heating pad to affected shoulder, lying flat or on your side, judicious use of postoperative analgesia, and ambulating.

COMPLICATIONS RELATED TO TISSUE DISSECTION AND HEMOSTASIS

Electrosurgical complications are an inescapable reality of laparoscopy, it is important to have a consciousness of the types of complications and how to respond appropriately and deal with complications. Bipolar electrosurgical injury, compared with monopolar injury, is easily identified by viewing the area of blanch on the surface of the colon. The spread of electrothermal injuries is

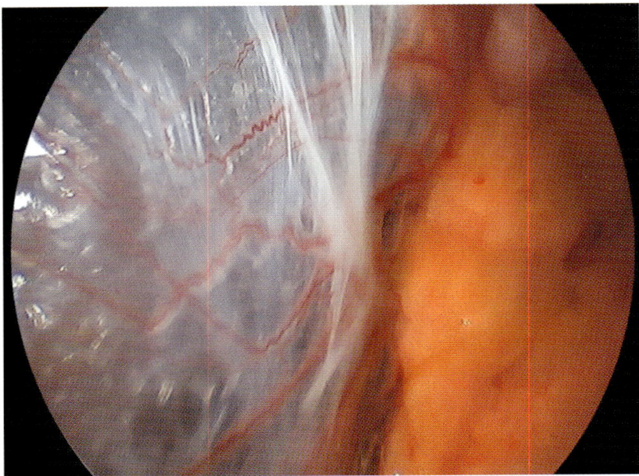

Fig. 6: Extraperitoneal insufflation.

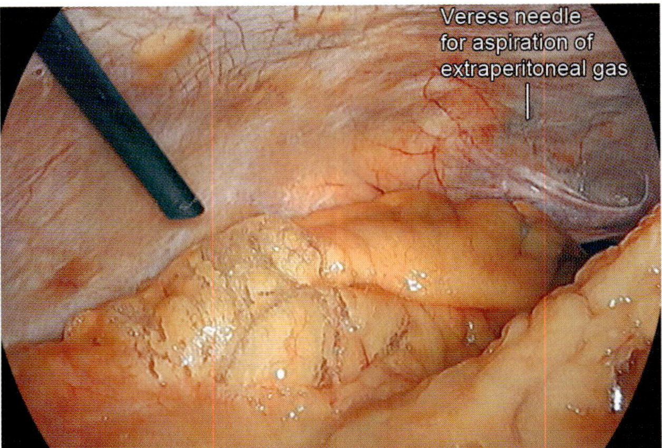

Fig. 7: Needle aspiration of extraperitoneal gas.

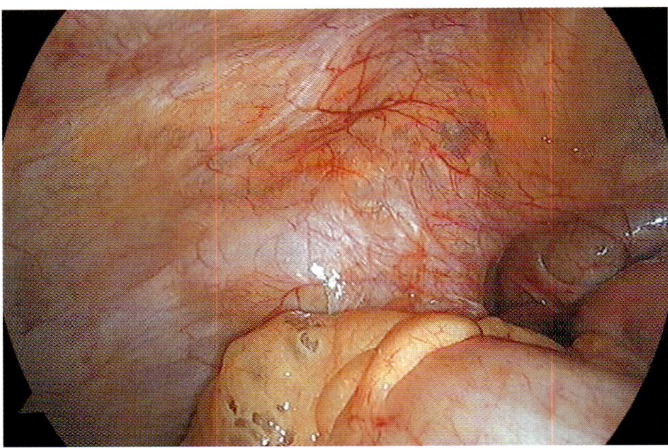

Fig. 8: Normal anatomy restored.

greater than the initial area of blanching, creating a large area of necrosis. Thus, the depth of injury is difficult to assess even if it is noticed intraoperatively. It should be turned and oversewn to healthy tissue at the margins, or resected with a 1–2 cm margin around the injury site. It is important to remember that the visible thermal injury is always less than the actual injury. Resection and anastomosis is a reasonable approach if the electrosurgical injury is a significant size and there is any risk of not getting a healthy tissue margin.

When bladder injury is recognized intraoperatively, it can be repaired vaginally, laparoscopically, or by laparotomy. Bladder injury is more encountered during dissection in cases of previous surgery. Early recognition with immediate salvage procedure, along with extended use of an indwelling catheter, may help overcome further sequelae. Large or irregular defects will require a two layer suture closure with absorbable sutures (vicryl 3-0) **(Figs. 9A and B)**.

Ureteral injury occurs in less than 2% of pelvic procedures and can result from pelvic dissection during the course of distal colon/rectal, gynecologic, or urologic surgery,[14] or as a result of thermal injury by excessive use of an energy source adjacent the ureter.

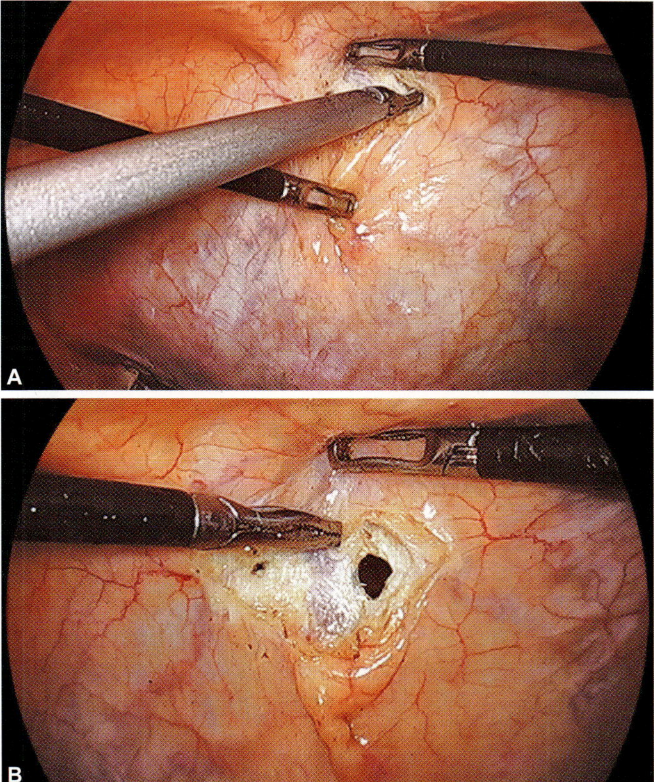

Figs. 9A and B: A case of bladder injury while performing Burch colposuspension.

The most relevant factors related to ureteral damage are: (1) inadequate knowledge of pelvic anatomy; (2) failure to open the peritoneum and dissect retroperitoneally; (3) the use of energy devices with marginal knowledge of their physics and tissue interaction; (4) imprecise application of stapling devices; and (5) pelvic adhesions, particularly dense adhesions located in and around the ovarian fossa.

If pelvic dissection is anticipated to be in an inflamed operative field or reoperative field, ureteral stents can be used to help identify the ureters to minimize ureteral injury; however, injury can still occur with a prophylactic stent in place. The best means of preventing inadvertent ureteral injury is identification of the ureter during the procedure using anatomic landmarks and observation of peristalsis.[15] With complex surgeries or where anatomy is unclear, dissection and mobilization of the ureter may be needed. At the conclusion of any laparoscopic procedure in which the operative field is in the vicinity of the ureter(s), the surgeon should confirm and document the integrity of the ureters before closing. **Figures 10A to C** is showing the ureter transections and its repair during intraoperative period by absorbable suture (vicryl 5-0) after cystoscopy guided stenting. As here in our setup we routinely perform cystoscopy after each case of total laparoscopic hysterectomy to rule out ureteric injury. In preoperative period patients are given oral Pyridium 200 mg two tablets a night before surgery so that reddish orange tinge of urine can be easily appreciated during the cystoscopy **(Figs. 11A and B)**. This effect is harmless and will go away on stopping the medicine.

■ COMPLICATIONS RELATED TO EXIT

Port-site Hernia (Richter's Hernia)

When there is a strangulated hernia which involves part of the circumference of the bowel wall, it is known as Richter's hernia. As the passage of bowel contents through the bowel lumen remains unaffected, there is absence of intestinal obstruction despite strangulation. These comprise about 10% of strangulated hernia.[16,17]

Trocar site hernias are classified in three categories.[18] The *early-onset type* hernia represents dehiscence of the anterior and posterior fascial plane as well as the parietal peritoneum. It usually develops in the early postoperative period, often presenting as small bowel obstruction. The *late-onset type* trocar hernia occurs when there is dehiscence of the anterior and posterior fascial plane. It is the most frequent type of trocar-site hernia and generally develops several months after the original surgery.

A *special type* of trocar-site hernia usually arises because of dehiscence of the whole abdominal wall. There is absence of hernial sac but the bowel or omentum may protrude, sometimes as early as when the trocar sheath is

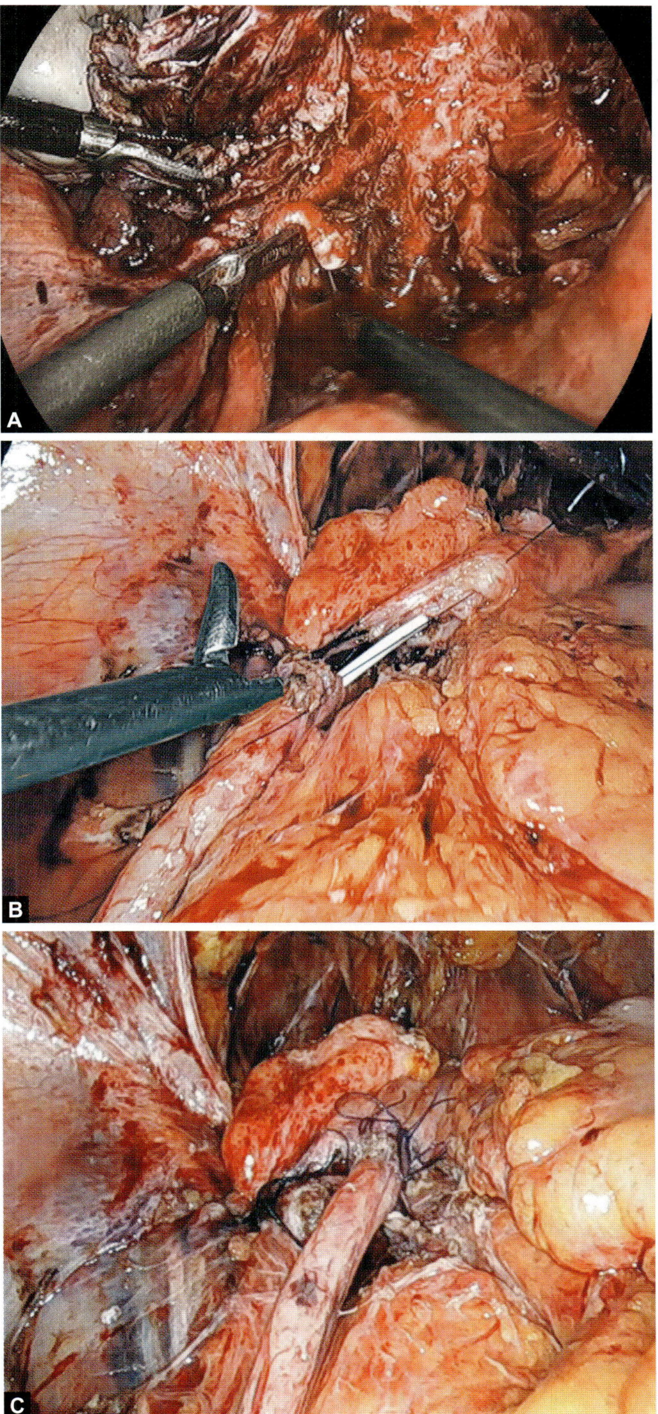

Figs. 10A to C: Ureter transection during total laparoscopy hysterectomy in case of previous multiple surgery.

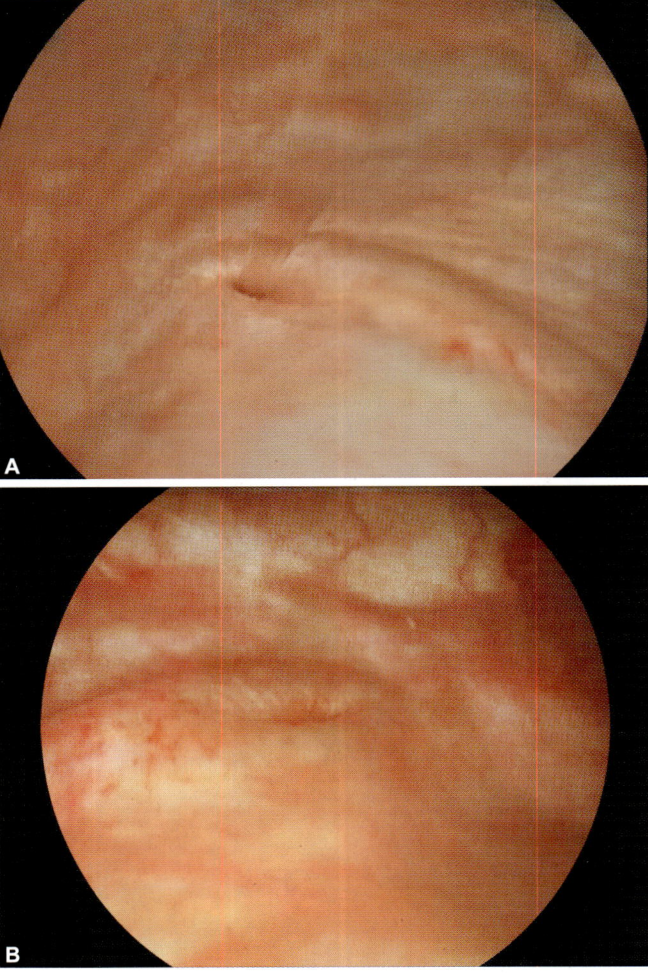

Figs. 11A and B: Cystoscopy view of ureteric peristalsis showing orange tinge urine after oral pyridium.

withdrawn during surgery. Some surgeons have reported an *unclassified type* of trocar-site hernia called Richter's hernia.

Various risk factors are the cause for the pathogenesis of hernias like large trocar size, incomplete closure of fascia at port site, midline ports, stretching the port site for organ retrieval, effect of partial vacuum while port withdrawal, obesity, parity, poor nutrition, and operation site infection.[19-23]

Richter's hernia is a highly ambiguous entity. Patients present with nontoxic symptoms and very few clinical finding like nausea, vomiting, abdominal pain, and swelling and tenderness over hernia orifice. Bowel function remains normal without any abdominal distension. It has a high mortality rate of 17–21% and prognosis is poor if complicated with peritonitis.[24] Radiological investigations like ultrasonography and/or computed tomography are excellent tools for clear visualization and diagnosis. Abdominal X-ray is helpful in showing ileus like dilated bowel loops and air fluids level.

Once the diagnosis is made, immediate surgery must be done as if delayed in intervention increases the risk of bowel perforation. Most of these hernias are accessed by extending the trocar site, laparoscopy or an explorative laparotomy followed by reduction of hernia. Manual removal avoided as it may ended in fatal complication such as perforation due to unintentional reduction of gangrenous bowel. On the operating table, findings are reconfirmed followed by resection and anastomosis of gangrenous gut. Postprocedure patient kept for nil per oral with supplements of IV fluids and IV antibiotics. On seeing patient improvement accordingly patients are allowed orally.

It is estimated that 16–56% of patients remain asymptomatic with umbilical fascial defect, hence, thorough abdominal examination must be performed pre- and intraoperatively before any laparoscopic surgery.[25] Incidence of hernia decreases when surgeons perform fascial closure when trocar of size 10 mm or more is used. Others preventive measures include deflation of pneumoperitoneum prior to removal of ports, fascial closure techniques using fascial closure device, suture carrier, Deschamps needle and port plugs. Some authors have also reported a lower incidence of hernias with the use of a paramedian incision and nonbladed trocars, but these are not foolproof.[26]

Measures to prevent postoperative Richter's hernia **(Figs. 12A and B)** are as follows:

- Do not remove trocar with their valves open
- Use the smallest diameter trocar and conical tip trocar possible
- Visualize removal of the trocar with closed tip instrument kept flush with the tip of cannula
- Close the fascia at all port sites greater than 5 mm in diameter
- Shake the abdominal wall after the trocars are removed
- Close the peritoneum tightly.

Surgical Site Infection

Wound infection is less common following laparoscopic compared with open procedures and if occur, it can produce significant morbidity. The presence of fever, wound drainage, and significant erythema around incision may point towards development of a necrotizing fascial infection. Although the umbilicus is more commonly associated with surgical site infection than other trocar sites, this finding correlates with the use of the umbilicus as a specimen extraction site and also poor hygiene at umbilicus makes it more liable to surgical site infection. The incidence of wound infections can be minimized by appropriate administration of prophylactic antibiotics, sterile technique, and use of bags during specimen extraction. Once established, surgical site infection is treated with drainage, packing, and appropriate antibiotics.

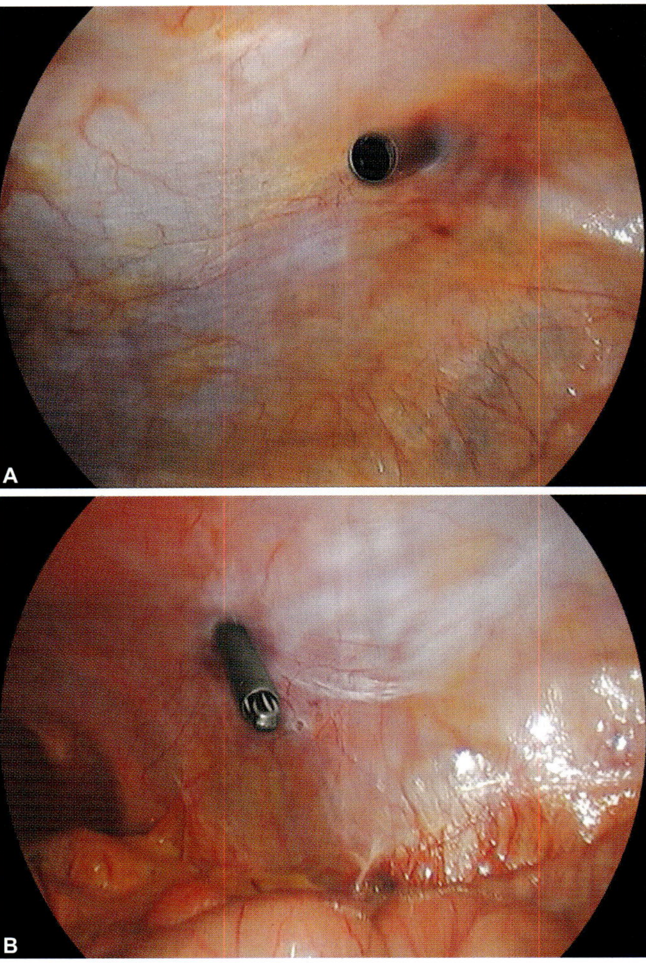

Figs. 12A and B: Visualize removal of the trocar with closed tip instrument kept flush with the tip of cannula.

OTHER COMPLICATIONS

Port-site Metastasis

It refers to growth of cancer at a port-site incision after laparoscopic tumor removal. Port-site metastasis occurs after 1–2% of laparoscopic procedures performed in the presence of intraperitoneal malignancy, which is equivalent to the rate of wound metastasis after laparotomy performed under similar conditions.[27] Proposed mechanisms include hematogenous spread or direct contamination by tumor cells, secondary effects from pneumoperitoneum (e.g. immune suppression), and surgical technique.[27,28] Port-site metastasis may observed in as little as 10 days following laparoscopy. Although it is not clear whether port-site metastases can be prevented, suggested measures to minimize the risk of port-site metastases include the use of wound protectors and specimen extraction bags, instillation of agents to prevent tumor growth, and port-site excision.

Vulvar Edema

Few case reports have been published describing unilateral vulvar edema **(Fig. 13)** after operative laparoscopy. It is self-limited event whose exact mechanism is unclear till now. Conservative management such as pressure 'T' bandage ice packs, bladder catheterization, and analgesia can be used in some cases.[29-31] However, swelling in this setting can also be related to vascular bleeding which should be ruled out and may require intervention.[31]

COMPLICATIONS COMMONLY ENCOUNTERED IN JAIN POINT ENTRY TECHNIQUE

In our decades of experience, minimal complications were seen. Entry related major complication was seen in one case and it involved the small bowel injury, was immediately detected after trocar insertion. Laparoscopic primary reparative surgery performed successfully. Preperitoneal insufflation and omental insufflation were seen in few cases. There was no case of intra-abdominal hemorrhage/hemotoma. No case was converted into open surgery and no mortality was reported. Lesser complications rate with respect to viscera, vessel, adhesion and bowel (VVAB) makes this port side an ideal condidate for first blind entry in the abdomen.

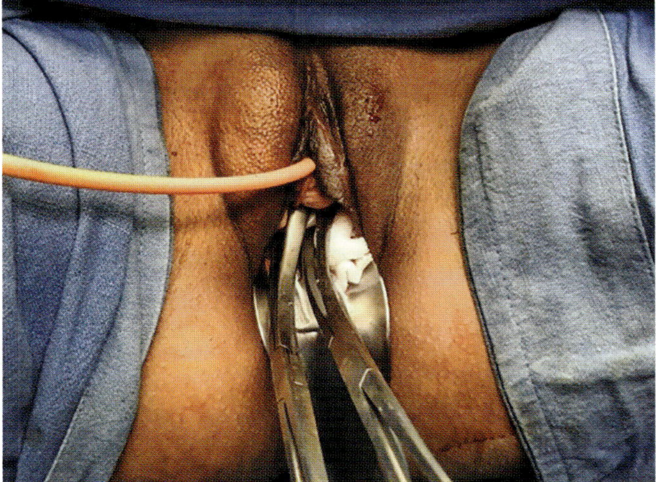

Fig.13: Right sided labial swelling just after pneumoperitoneum.

CONCLUSION

Laparoscopic techniques are uprising ladder in the field of surgery. Before performing any laparoscopic surgery risk evaluation (obesity, previous surgery, hernia, large masses, and inflammatory masses) need to be done, simultaneously abdominal wall and cavity need to be assessed before entry and placing the ports because major complications take place during abdominal access. As well as alertness required at the end of surgery during the removal of trocars to avoid late complications. The overall rate of these complications is low with safe entry techniques which are done through Jain point at our hospital setup.

ACKNOWLEDGMENT

Figures of complications (acute inferior epigastric injury, bowel injury, liver bed injury) are contributed by Dr Aruna Tantia.

REFERENCES

1. Krishnakumar S, Tambe P. Entry complications in laparoscopic surgery. J Gynec Endosc Surg. 2009;1:4-11.
2. Chandler JG, Corson SL, Way LW. Three spectra of laparoscopic entry access injuries. J Am Coll Surg. 2001;192:478-90.
3. Magrina JF. Complications of laparoscopic surgery. Clin Obstet Gynecol. 2002;45:469-80.
4. Quilici PJ, Greanery EM, Quilici J, et al. Transabdominal preperitoneal laparoscopic herniorrhaphy: results of 509 repairs. Am Surg. 1996;62:849-52.
5. Tews G, Arzt W, Bohaumilitzky T, et al. Significant reduction of operational risk in laparoscopy through the use of a new blunt trocar. Surg Gynecol Obstet. 1991;173:67-8.
6. Bailey RW, Flowers JL. Complications of Laparoscopic Surgery. St. Louis, MO: Quality Medical Publishing, Inc.; 1995. pp. 26-57.
7. Nordestgaard AG, Bodily KC, Osborne RW, et al. Major vascular injuries during laparoscopic procedures. Am J Surg. 1995;169:543-5.
8. Ahmad G, Duffy JM, Phillips K, et al. Laparoscopic entry techniques. Cochrane Database Syst Rev. 2008;(2):CD006583.
9. Kaali SG, Bartfai G. Direct insertion of the laparoscopic trocar after an earlier laparotomy. J Reprod Med. 1988;33:739-40.
10. Philosophe R. Avoiding complications of laparoscopic surgery. Fertil Steril. 2003;80 (Suppl 4):30-9.
11. Georgy FM, Fetterman HH, Chefetz MD. Complication of laparoscopy: two cases of perforated urinary bladder. Am J Obstet Gynecol. 1974;120:1121-4.
12. Sia-Kho E, Kelly RE. Urinary drainage by distention: an indication of bladder injury during laparoscopy. J Clin Anesth. 1992;4:346-7.
13. Poffenberger RJ. Laparoscopic repair of intraperitoneal bladder injury. Urology. 1996;47:248-9.
14. Grainger DA, Soderstrom RM, Schiff SF, et al. Ureteral injuries at laparoscopy: insights into diagnosis, management, and prevention. Obstet Gynecol. 1990;75:839-43.

15. Shirk GJ, Johns A, Redwine DB. Complications of laparoscopic surgery: How to avoid them and how to repair them? J Minim Invasive Gynecol. 2006;13:352-9.
16. Skandalakis PN, Zoras O, Skandalakis JE, et al. Richter hernia: surgical anatomy and technique of repair. Am Surg. 2006,72(2):180-4.
17. Le HD, Odom SR, Hsu A, et al. A combined Richter's and de Garengeot's hernia. Int J Surg Case Rep. 2001:5(10):662-4.
18. Tonouchi H, Ohmori Y, Kobayashi M, et al. Trocar site hernia. Arch Surg. 2004;139:1248-56.
19. Montz FJ, Holschneider CH, Munro MG. Incisional hernias following laparoscopy: a survey of the American Association of Gynecologic Laparoscopists. Obstet Gynecol. 1994;84:881-4.
20. Sanz-Lopez R, Martinez-Ramos C, Nunez-Pena JR, et al. Incisional hernias after laparoscopic vs open cholecystectomy. Surg Endosc. 1999;13:922-41.
21. Lee JH, Kim W. Strangulated small bowel hernia through the port site: a case report. World J Gastroenterol. 2008;14(44):6881-3.
22. Trehan AK. Richter's hernia following operative laparoscopy. Gynaecol Endosc. 1996;5:353-4.
23. Mayol J, Garcia-Aguilar J, Ortiz-Oshiro E, et al. Risks of the minimal access approach for laparoscopic surgery: multivariate analysis of morbidity related to umbilical trocar insertion. World J Surg. 1997;21:529-33.
24. Medical Joyworks. (2016). Richter's Hernia. [online] Available from https://www.medicaljoyworks.com/prognosis-your-diagnosis/catalog/Surgery/Richters-Hernia# [Last accessed November, 2019].
25. Ramchandran CS. Umbilical hernial defects encountered before and after abdominal laparoscopic procedures. Int Surg. 1998;83:171-3.
26. Coda A, Bossoti M, Ferri F, et al. Incisional hernia and fascial defects following laparoscopic surgery. Surg Laparoscopic Endosc Percutan Tech. 2000;10:34-8.
27. Ramirez PT, Wolf JK, Levenback C. Laparoscopic port-site metastases: etiology and prevention. Gynecol Oncol. 2003;91:179-89.
28. Ost MC, Tan BJ, Lee BR. Urological laparoscopy: basic physiological considerations and immunological consequences. J Urol. 2005;174:1183-8.
29. Pados G, Vavilis D, Pantazis K, et al. Unilateral vulvar edema after operative laparoscopy: a case report and literature review. Fertil Steril. 2005;83:471-3.
30. Guven S, Guven ES, Ayhan A. Vulvar edema as a rare complication of laparoscopy. J Am Assoc Gynecol Laparosc. 2004;11:429-32.
31. Marcovici I, Shadigian E. Operative laparoscopy and vulvar hematoma: an unusual association. JSLS. 2001;5:87-8.

Extrocation

Nutan Jain, Vandana Jain

INTRODUCTION

In laparoscopy as much the importance of entire techniques, so is the value of good port removals. At our center, as much importance is given to this step that gradually the term extrocation come into being. It simply means removal of the trocars after finishing laparoscopic surgery in a gradual, scientific set pattern to avoid exit-related complications. The most common and dreaded complication related to trocar removal is "Richter's hernia"[1,2] or the sliding hernia.[3,4] It is the entrapment of large bowel in the trocar as it is being removed from the abdominal cavity. Two factors are contributory to this complication. First, the hollow trocar which allow *space* for the *bowel* or omentum to be pulled in. Secondly, the high pressure and pneumoperitoneum which is congenial to the phenomena of bowel or omentum getting sucked in to hollow channel of the trocar. To prevent this occurrence, two steps in extrocation are important. Firstly the abdominal pressure should be released gradually and trocars removal only after the *high* pressure due to CO_2 *pneumoperitoneum* has been released. Secondly the hollow channel of the trocar to be kept occupied with an atraumatic grasper inside the trocar. This instrument to be kept flushed with the inner abdominal end of trocar, this prevents the *sucking* in of the bowel or omentum as the trocar is being pulled out. CO_2 pneumoperitoneum creates a high pressure environment inside the peritoneal cavity, so while extrocation the CO_2 should be released gradually.

TECHNIQUE

After finishing the laparoscopic procedure, a thorough check is made for any left suture or tissue which is to be removed. A thorough check for hemostasis is done. If any saline or ringers *lactate* fluid is to be instilled in the cavity, that is done and then, finally the process of extrocation is begun. First step is to close the CO_2 supply and then the surgeon's main working port is focused

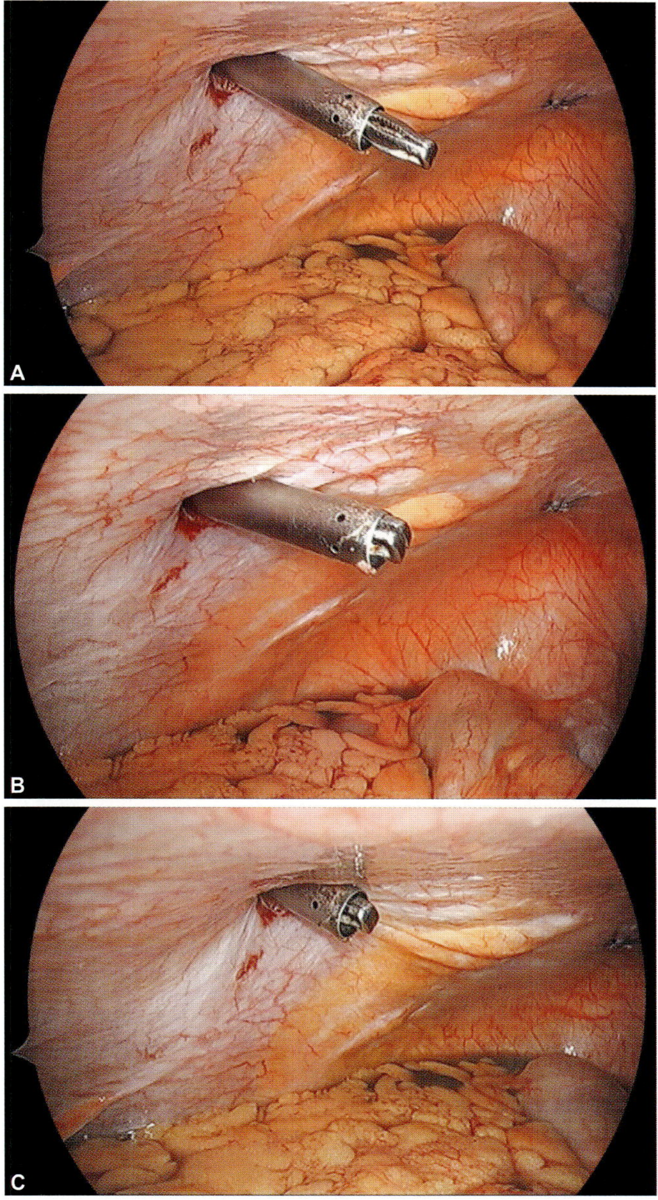

Figs. 1A to C: Pulling out the 5 mm trocar along with the instrument under direct visualization.

by the telescope. The vent of this trocar is opened to release the CO_2 gas and before this is done an instrument is placed in the trocar and it is *brought* flush with the tip of the abdominal end of the trocar. After releasing sufficient pneumoperitoneum, the trocar and *atraumatic* grasper in a closed jaw position is brought out **(Figs. 1A to C)**. Similarly all accessory trocars brought out one by one under direct vision with the *atraumatic* grasper in their cannula. This

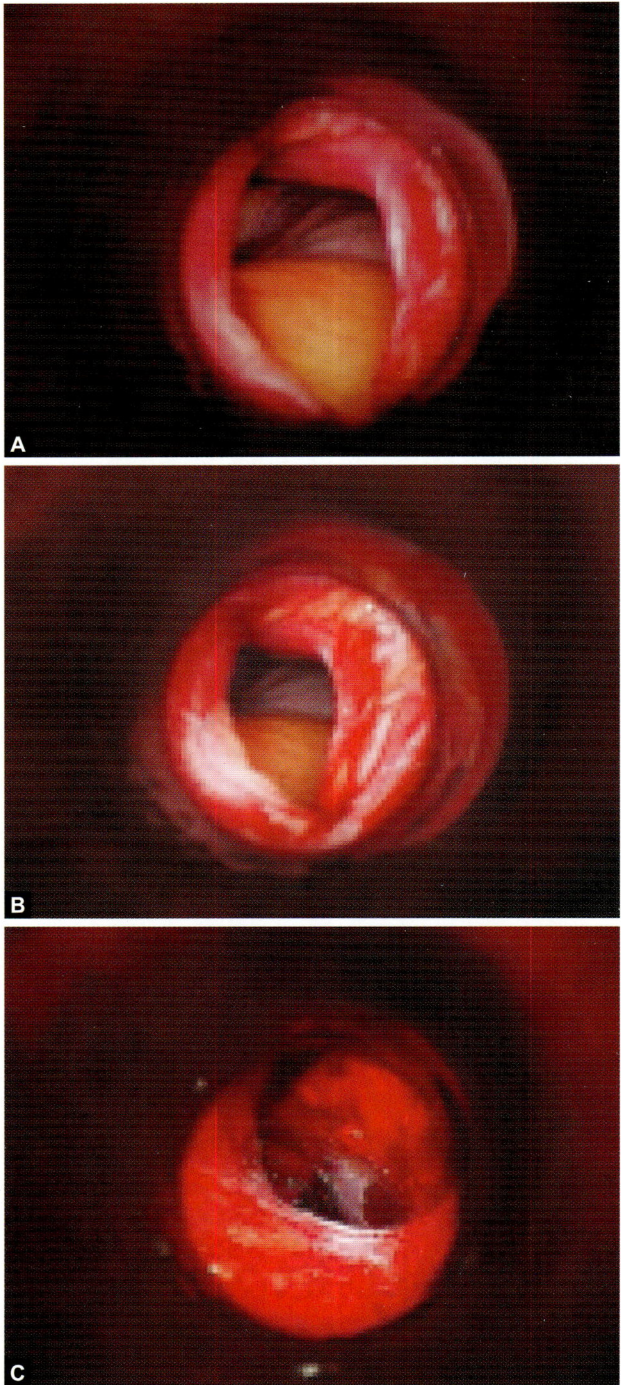

Figs. 2A to C: To remove 10 mm trocar under direct visual control, the telescope is pulled 1 cm inside the trocar sleeve and the cannula is rotated gradually taking out the trocar and telescope assembly visualizing each layer as it comes out.

precludes any bowel or omentum getting sucked in. Then, lastly it is very important to clear the abdominal cavity of all CO_2 gas, which if left inside, is *an important* cause of patient's postoperative discomfort by *causing* shoulder pain. It is acute, almost unbearable and at *most* totally avoidable. So, a good clinician will almost always try to take preventive measures to avoid *shoulder pain.* Then after emptying the abdominal cavity of all gas the last ritual/step of extrocation is the removal of 10 mm telescope trocar. This is to be brought out layer by layer visualizing the peritoneum, then, the muscle, the rectus health and then finally brought over the abdominal wall **(Figs. 2A to C)**. This step is most important in cases of previous surgery and abdominal adhesions where the first blind trocar has been the 10 mm trocar.[5,6] In a very rare occurrence, the blind trocar may have passed both the anterior and posterior walls of bowel loop adherent or plastered over the anterior abdominal wall. This is a disastrous situation, very rare, but with traditional laparoscopy with the first blind step of 10 mm trocar insertion, can pose this complication. It can be confidently excluded by removing the 10 mm trocar with the telescope *still inside it*, and visualized the abdominal wall parietes layer by layer. So with all these precaution extrocation becomes safe, hassle free, and prevents the occurrence of postoperative shoulder pain. Hence the need of coining this new term learning point, *extrocation.*

LEARNING POINTS

- Remove all accessory ports under direct vision of 10 mm telescope.
- Keep a laparoscopic grasper flush with the trocar tip during removal.
- Remove optic trocar at last visualizing all layer of abdominal wall layer by layer.
- Release CO_2 gradually and completely.

REFERENCES

1. Boughey JC, Nottingham JM, Walls AC. Richter's hernia in the laparoscopic era: four case reports and review of the literature. Surg Laparosc Endosc Percutan Tech. 2003;13:55-8.
2. Uslu HY, Erkek AB, Cakmak A. Trocar site hernia after laparoscopic cholecystectomy. J Laparoendosc Adv Surg Tech A. 2007;17:600-3.
3. Martis JJ, Rajeshwara KV, Shridhar MK, et al. Strangulated Richter's Umbilical Hernia—A Case Report. Indian J Surg. 2011;73(6):455-7.
4. Ime A, Cardi F. Incisional hernia at the trocar site in laparoscopic surgery. Chir Ital. 2006;58:605-9.
5. Ternamian A. Laparoscopic access. In: Jain N (Ed). State of the Art Atlas of Endoscopic Surgery in Infertility and Gynecology. New York, United States: McGraw-Hill Education; 2004. pp. 22-35.
6. Vilos GA, Ternamian A, Dempster J, et al. Laparoscopic entry: a review of techniques, technologies, and complications. J Obstet Gynaecol Can. 2007;29: 433-65.

Index

Page numbers followed by *f* refer to figure and *t* refer to table.